# LUNG CANCER IN WOMEN

# Lung Cancer in Women

Varetta N. Torres
Editor

Nova Biomedical Books
*New York*

For permission to use material from this book please contact us:
Telephone 631-231-7269; Fax 631-231-8175
Web Site: http://www.novapublishers.com



**LIBRARY OF CONGRESS CATALOGING-IN-PUBLICATION DATA**

Lung cancer in women / Varetta N. Torres (editor).
p. ; cm.
Includes bibliographical references and index.
ISBN-13: 978-1-60021-659-6 (hardcover)
ISBN-10: 1-60021-659-5 (hardcover)
1. Lungs--Cancer. 2. Cancer in women. 3. Lungs--Cancer--Sex factors. I. Torres, Varetta N.
[DNLM: 1. Lung Diseases. 2. Sex Factors. 3. Women's Health. WF 600 L9628 2007]
RC280.L8L778 2007
616.99'4240082--dc22

2007012454

*Published by Nova Science Publishers, Inc. ✦ New York*

# CONTENTS

# PREFACE

Lung disease is fatal for 86 percent of its victims within five years of a diagnosis, and is the leading cause of cancer death among women, exceeding even breast cancer. Researchers continue to study the causes of lung cancer and to search for ways to prevent it. But, about 90% of all lung cancer deaths among women are from smoking. Even though it is well known that the effects of smoking are harmful, an alarming number of women continue to smoke. The effects of tobacco seem to be far more damaging to women than to men. Scientists have discovered that a gene that accelerates lung cancer growth is more active in females. This new book presents the latest research in this dynamic field.

Chapter 1 – Lung cancer is now the most common cause of cancer death in both men and women in the United States and is the leading cause of cancer death overall in the world, with over 1,000,000 deaths occurring yearly. Postsurgical mortality has declined from the early days of the 1950s but 5-year cure rates have only barely improved. The addition of chemotherapy to radical radiotherapy, together with novel radiotherapy techniques, is gradually improving the outcome for locally advanced, inoperable non–small cell lung cancer. The most important and cost-effective management for lung cancer is smoking cessation, but for those with the disease, novel treatment approaches are urgently needed. Combining conventional cancer treatments with gene therapy offers exciting prospects for improved lung cancer control. Novel strategies that specifically target damage to tumor cells, while sparing normal tissue, will be particularly effective. The authors outline two new approaches for targeting anti-tumor therapy. The first uses clinically relevant radiation doses to activate gene therapy vectors, via radiation-responsive gene promoters, following delivery to the tumor volume. This system could be applied to lung cancer patients, especially those that are highly resistant to current cancer treatments. The second approach exploits the physiological condition of hypoxia, which occurs commonly in lung cancer but is rarely seen in normal tissues. Hypoxia-regulated gene promoters can be used to drive expression of therapeutic genes in intratumoral areas of low oxygen. Furthermore, gene therapy vectors that respond both to radiation and hypoxia stimulation have recently been developed, allowing more tumor cell populations to be targeted. Such tailoring of gene therapy vectors to lung cancer treatment and environment, in combination with an efficient delivery system, is likely to produce significantly more efficacious clinical treatments in the near future.

Chapter 2 - Accelerated glycolysis is one of the biochemical characteristics of cancer. Tumor cells require a steady source of metabolic energy in the form of adenosine triphosphate (ATP) in order to continue their uncontrolled growth and proliferation. Glucose transport and metabolism are important determinants of post-treatment survival in tumor cells, leading to poor prognosis. Glycolytic breakdown of glucose is preceded by the transport of glucose across the cell membrane, a rate-limiting process mediated by facilitative glucose transporter proteins (GLUTs). Tumors frequently exhibit over-expression of GLUTs, especially the hypoxia-responsive GLUT1 and GLUT3 proteins. Significant associations between GLUT expression and proliferative indices have been reported suggesting that GLUT expression may be of prognostic significance. Here the authors review the recent clinical and basic research on glucose metabolism in cancer. They explore the involvement of GLUT proteins as potential coordinators of metabolic processes in the tumour microenvironment. With the discovery of the oxygen-sensitive transcription factor hypoxia-inducible factor (HIF) has come a new understanding of the molecular link between hypoxia and deregulated glucose metabolism. HIF induces a number of genes integral to angiogenesis, e.g. vascular endothelial growth factor (VEGF), a process intimately involved with metastatic spread. The authors discuss the links between HIF, glucose transporters, angiogenic factors and tumour development. This knowledge may enhance existing chemotherapeutic strategies so that treatment can be more rationally applied and personalized for cancer patients.

Chapter 3 - Although breast cancer is the most common malignant disease diagnosed in women, lung cancer has become the most common cancer-related death in women. Noteworthy, lung cancer mortality in women is superior to mortality rate seen from breast, ovarian, and uterine cancers combined. Cigarette smoking is one of the causes directly responsible for this malignancy; however, the disease appears to be different in women, as can be demonstrated by variations in histologic types in men and women. There are also differences in terms of survival where women have shown to have better survival rates after surgical resection in earlier stage or even in the metastatic setting. Recently, genetic variation among men and women and its possible role in oncogenesis has become evident, including those of CYP1A1 gene or gastrin-releasing peptide receptor. Furthermore, studies have shown that estrogens may be involved in lung tumorigenesis at many different levels, as they may act as estrogen-receptor ligands, activating cellular proliferation or may be activated into reactive intermediates that can cause oxidative damage. The possible role of estrogen in lung tumorigenesis has been shown in case control studies where factors such as early menopause, association between tobacco use and estrogen, and hormonal replacement therapy have been associated with an increased risk of lung cancer. Nevertheless, the role and impact of genetic and hormonal variations in lung carcinogenesis in women is still under study.

Interestingly, younger women with lung cancer seem to have better responses with tyrosine kinase inhibitors like gefinitib and erlotinib. In fact, the identification of mutations in the ATP-binding domain of the epidermal growth factor receptor has been shown to predict dramatic responses and introduced the possibility of more individualized therapy. It is already known that factors such as Asian descendant, never-smoker, and female gender confer a better response to epidermal growth factor receptor inhibitors mainly because mutations on that domain appear to be more prevalent in these patients. Thus, it is expected that a better understanding of tumor biology and genetic profile differences among both gender may lead to a more precisely targeted therapy in lung cancer, and consequently, better outcomes.

Chapter 4 - Lung cancer had been considered a disease of men. However, incidence and morality rates of lung cancer among women have risen rapidly in the past few decades. The increase in lung cancer among women parallels their cigarette consumption as had been earlier demonstrated in men. Currently, lung cancer is the leading cause of cancer mortality in women, exceeding the second and third causes (breast and colon cancers) combined. 73,020 deaths from lung cancer in women are estimated in 2006 in the US, slightly fewer than the estimated men's lung cancer mortality. There is controversy whether women have a higher relative risk of developing lung cancer than men. Previous studies reported that women do not have a greater susceptibility to lung cancer than men, given equal smoking exposure. However, this hypothesis has not received universal support. The purpose of this chapter is to review the literature addressing: 1) whether women have a higher susceptibility to tobacco carcinogens than men, 2) whether women have better survival after the diagnosis of lung cancer, and 3) the potential biological mechanisms for a gender difference in lung cancer risk and survival. This information may change strategies for cancer prevention, such as smoking cessation efforts toward women, and has implications for targeted lung cancer therapy.

Chapter 5 - Lung cancer was a rare condition in the early twentieth century. It was only after World War I that this disease assumed epidemic proportions. Unfortunately, a century later, it is estimated that lung cancer will cause 72,130 deaths in women and a much higher estimated 90,330, in men. This is despite the publication of the U.S. Surgeon General's report, in 1964, that cigarette smoking was injurious to health and that the tobacco habit needed to be curbed. Statistics related to smoking and lung cancer mortality have reflected male dominion, since reporting began a few decades ago. However, in the post World War II era, women increasingly picked up the tobacco habit and their lung cancer incidence has risen since then. Lung cancer is now the foremost killer of women amongst all cancers, and kills more women than breast and colon cancer combined. Lung cancer incidence in women has increased fourfold over the last three decades, and is expected to increase further. There are several differences between lung cancer in men and women of growing import. Women may be at increased risk of developing lung cancer as compared to men for any given rate of smoking. Women who have never smoked have a 30% increased risk of lung cancer if they lived with spouses who smoked than if they lived with non-smokers. It is possible that genetic mutations leading to lung cancer may be more frequently found in women. The inability of women to repair DNA damage related to smoking vis-à-vis their male counterparts may lead to increased susceptibility to cancer. Moreover, disease manifestations in pre-menopausal women may be different from post-menopausal women. However, intriguingly, survival in women with lung cancer seems to be better than men with the same disease. Lung cancer in women apparently tends to be detected at an earlier stage, is of different histology and appears to be less aggressive. It is now known that there are important differences in the biology of the tumors in the two sexes. These differences are the focus of the following discussion.

Chapter 6 - With 4.9 million people being killed each year due to smoking worldwide, tobacco is the only product that kills half its consumers. Across the E.U. countries, it is estimated that around 106,000 women die prematurely each year as a result of smoking.

Women are affected by the main smoking-related diseases in the same way as men, but are also at risk of developing a number of gender-specific problems including cancer of cervix and problems related to reproductive health and osteoporosis.

An important question regarding quitting smoking is whether men and women should receive different cessation treatments. Although smoking cessation clinical trials reveal that the same pharmacotherapy treatments (Bupropion SR, Nicotine Replacement Therapies) benefit both men and women, there is strong evidence that the approach should be different towards female smokers. In fact, women may face different stressing parameters and barriers to quitting that may be useful to address in treatment decisions. These include greater likelihood of depression, greater weight control concerns, and hormonal cycle abnormalities. This suggests that women may benefit from tobacco dependence treatments that address these topics, although only few studies have examined programs targeted to one gender.

With regard to motivation in a smoking cessation program for females, one should underline benefits such as physical appearance and lower incidence of osteoporosis. In particular, women, who are candidates to become pregnant, may be more receptive to stop smoking because of the serious risks imposed on the fetus.

In conclusion, different smoking cessation treatment strategies with augmented psychosocial interventions and more intensive counseling about weight gain, osteoporosis, physical appearance, depression, and pregnancy may be needed for female smokers in order to achieve better abstinence rates.

Chapter 7 - Lung cancer is the leading cause of cancer deaths in women. There is increasing evidence to suggest that lung cancer develops and behaves differently between men and women based on the genetic profile of the tumor, as well as the outcome and responses to treatment. It is highly plausible that female hormones play a part in lung cancer development as the two sexes are inherently exposed to different hormonal environment. The female sex hormones, in particular estrogen, have been shown to affect the metabolism of substances, including nicotine and possibly other tobacco carcinogens. In addition, studies in rodents have demonstrated that estrogen or their catechol metabolites can be carcinogenic in various tissues. Estrogen receptors (ER) mediate the cellular response to estrogen and two ERs have been identified, ERα and ERβ. Recent studies suggest that the ERα protein present in the lung are mainly splice variants that may or may not be functional while ERβ may be a more important receptor in lung cancer development. Estrogen receptors, when activated, are known to cause transcriptional activation of several growth factor genes. Laboratory studies have found that estrogen can induce lung tumor growth and the effect of which can be blocked by anti-estrogen therapy. Clinical studies further support the role of female hormones in lung cancer development as early age at menopause has been shown to be associated with a reduced risk while the use of estrogen replacement therapy is associated with a higher risk of adenocarcinoma of the lung. It is possible that the estrogen metabolites and ER-mediated genomic and nongenomic signaling could affect cellular proliferation, which can then contribute to the development of lung cancer in women.

Chapter 8 - We are now living in an exciting new era that the understanding of tumor biology and oncogenesis has begun to evolve. Molecular techniques have allowed insight into specific biological pathways involved in tumorigenesis and these same techniques have developed a cascade of novel therapies directed towards molecular factors critical to the pathogenesis of cancer growth and survival. With lung cancer being the leading cause of world-wide cancer mortality, and with a fourfold increase of incidence in women, the need for new treatment strategies is obvious. In fact, the epidermal growth factor receptor (EGFR) autocrine pathway has a major contribution to a number of processes which are essential for tumor progression and that somatic mutations of the EGFR gene, which are associated with clinical response to the EGFR oral tyrosine kinase inhibitors gefitinib and erlotinib, are more frequently detected in women. At the same time women are three times more likely to have K-ras mutation than men and often express HER-2/neu (one of the four members of EGF receptors). HER-2/neu is also most commonly expressed in the adenocarcinoma histology, the most common subtype in women. All these data raise an issue about the different pathobiology of lung cancer in women and the emerging role of targeted therapies designed specifically for female lung cancer patients.

Chapter 9 - In the past decade the incidence of lung cancer among women has risen, whereas among men it has slightly declined. The link between smoking and lung cancer has been well established in both men and women. However, gender-based difference in susceptibility to smoking-related lung cancer have been found, with women showing a higher risk than men of developing lung cancer for a given level of tobacco consumption. An increasing number of lung cancer cases have also been documented in non-smokers and a disproportionate number of these are adenocarcinomas and occur in women. Several case-control studies showed that long-term, regular exposure to either residential or occupational environmental tobacco smoke is associated with increased lung cancer risk in never-smoking women. Exposure to coal fumes, as well as hormonal effects, have been suggested as potential risk factors for lung cancer in non smoking women. Individual susceptibility factors may also be important in the development of lung cancer. These factors may include family history of lung cancer, personal history of lung disease (asthma, chronic bronchitis, pneumonia, or tuberculosis), diet and specific xenobiotic metabolic profiles.

In never-smoking women several lung cancer susceptibility genes have been proposed, and enzymes activating or detoxifying chemical carcinogens have been investigated. Some studies analyzed germline polymorphisms in genes that have been associated with cancer susceptibility and whose products activate (cytochrome P450 1A1=CYP1A1) and detoxify (glutatione S-transferases M1=GSTM1 and T1=GSTT1) chemical carcinogens found in tobacco smoke.

The authors extensively reviewed the published scientific literature on this topic in order to investigate the clinical and genetic profiling underlying lung cancer in women and to use this information as a tool for medical therapy.

This review is divided in two parts, in the first one the authors illustrated the clinical and pathological carachteristics of lung cancer in women and the differences between women and men in terms of results and toxicity to therapies. In the second part they analysed the molecular targets focusing on women and the future perspectives in particular based on target therapies.

Chapter 10 - The yearly number of new lung cancer cases in women is increasingly contrary to that of men. Women present an increased susceptibility in getting lung cancer, respond better to chemotherapy and biological therapies and live longer regardless of histology and stage. These statistical observations may be explained through molecular differences between the sexes.

K-ras gene mutations are three times more frequent in women, are associated mainly with adenocarcinoma and pose conflicting prognostic significance. CYP1A1 (P4501A1) overexpression alone or in combination with loss of expression of GSTM1 gene (glutathione S-transferase M1) is also correlated with the development of lung cancer in women. Decreased DNA repair capacity and increased levels of DNA adducts due to p53-pathway alterations or different bioavailability of phase I and phase II detoxifying enzymes correlate with the formation and progression of lung cancer in women. It is worthwhile noting that HER-2/neu is overexpressed in adenocarcinoma without overall survival improvement after the addition of monoclonal antibodies to standard chemotherapy. These basic molecular pathways in carcinogenesis as seen in women will be studied and analyzed with the hope of a better management.

Chapter 11 – Background: Lung cancer is the leading cause of cancer-related mortality in both men and women. Emerging data demonstrate sex-specific differences in lung cancer incidence and trends.

Aim: To estimate lung cancer incidence and trends in women and to find whether there are significant differences in treatment modalities and survival between men and women.

Subjects and Methods: This retrospective analysis included all cases with bronchopulmonary cancer registered in the Thoracic Oncology Department database in Albert Calmette University Hospital in Lille, France, between 1990 and 2005. Lung cancer histologic pattern and staging, main treatment modalities and survival data were analyzed by gender and by two different time periods, 1990-1999 and 2000-2005.

Results: The proportion of new lung cancer cases in women significantly increased over the last five-year period compared to the last decade (18.8% vs 9.6%, $p=0.001$). Adenocarcinoma was the histologic type of cancer which predominated in women (51%). A change in the histologic pattern in men, from squamous cell towards lung adenocarcinoma, was observed. Women presented less often complications to chemotherapy than men, especially in the period between 1990 and 1999 ($p=0.001$). The overall median survival time was better in women than men ($p=0.01$) although there were no significant gender differences in median survival time when each treatment modality was considered separately.

Conclusion: In view of the increased number of new lung cancer cases in women, tobacco control and early detection screening programs for lung cancer with reference to gender should be high priorities for health care services.

Chapter 12 - Lung cancer accounts for more than 1 million deaths worldwide per year. Even if most of them are caused by tobacco smoking, the role of environmental causes, including outdoor air pollution, is now generally recognized.

Early evidence for a higher risk of developing lung cancer for populations residing in highly polluted areas came from ecological studies published in the '60s. Such evidence was repeatedly confirmed by many other ecological and semi-ecological investigations, including migrant studies and point source analyses. However, the more compelling evidence came from analytical investigations (case-control and cohort studies), which allow a more strict control for potential confounding. In particular, population-based cohort studies made in the

USA and, more recently, in Northern Europe, have definitively demonstrated the role of air pollution as a risk factor for lung cancer.

In many recent investigations, expecially case-control studies, females have been found to have a higher susceptibility than males to tobacco smoking, which contains many known or alleged carcinogens also present in urban and industrial air pollution (*e.g.*, benzene, polycyclic aromatic hydrocarbons, thin particulate matter and formaldehyde). Moreover, such a finding was confirmed by a recent large screening survey and supported by results from many genetic and biochemical investigations, even if some recent cohorts studies have reported similar rates between female and male smokers. The difficulty of assessing the individual past exposure both to air pollution and to possible confounding factors has hampered the production of reliable estimates of the excess risk due to the exposure to air pollutants. As a consequence, comparisons between risks in males and in females are often lacking, while studies reporting estimates of the impact of air pollution separately in the two sexes have provided conflicting results. However, some recent investigations, especially ecological comparisons and point source analyses, have occasionally shown a higher risk for the female gender. Uncontrolled smoking habits, including passive smoking, indoor exposures to other pollutants, occupational exposures, chronic pulmonary diseases, dietary habits and socio-economic status are all factors that may account for most of differences in the risks observed by gender, but the hypothesis of a higher susceptibility of women cannot be completely ruled out. This chapter reviews the evidence both in favour of and against this hypothesis, using the more relevant epidemiological literature from the last 20 years.

Chapter 13 - Despite the remarkable reduction in the incidence of lung cancer among men in many developed countries, there has been a fourfold increase in lung cancer in women over the past 30 years associated with a rising trend in female lung cancer related mortality. Early diagnosis and appropriate treatment of lung cancer are two important determinants of prognosis and overall disease outcome. Functional imaging has recently gained a prominent role in the management of numerous pulmonary malignancies. The successful introduction of $^{18}$F-fluorodeoxyglucose ($^{18}$F-FDG) along with PET/CT image fusion has revolutionized diagnostic imaging in lung cancer. Currently, $^{18}$F-FDG PET/CT is considered the most precise diagnostic test for a wide range of pulmonary malignancies. This is primarily attributed to its unique ability to assess the global metabolic state of each individual tumor. In fact, the high sensitivity and the whole body mode of data acquisition are two critical advantages that favor $^{18}$F-FDG PET/CT over other cross sectional imaging modalities like CT and MRI. Noteworthy, however, is the complementary role of dynamic contrast enhanced CT in characterizing indeterminate pulmonary nodules and adrenal lesions. Besides its distinguished diagnostic potentials, especially in unmasking occult tumor foci, $^{18}$F-FDG PET/CT can precisely delineate the locoregional tumor burden for an accurate radiotherapy treatment planning. Furthermore, PET can offer reliable prognostic information since the avidity of both de novo and previously treated cancerous lesions to $^{18}$F-FDG has been shown to correlate with the overall disease outcome and patient survival. In the near future, further brilliant horizons are expected since the development trials of other radiotracers that target tumor proliferation, apoptosis, and hypoxia are emerging.

Chapter 14 - Lung cancer is not only the most common cancer in the world, a wide variety of secondaries affect this organ too. Although females are affected much less compared to males, the lung cancer prevalence has been reported to increase among females during the recent years in parallel to the increment in cigarette consumption. Various tissue diagnostic techniques used for lung cancer are conventional cytologic and histopathologic methods as well as fine needle aspiration (FNA) cytology. Of all the diagnostic tools, FNA cytology is simple, safe, accurate and cost effective, which can be practiced on an out patient basis. In a review of literature, the adequacy rate of material obtained by FNA in thoracic lesions, ranged from 68.9% to 95.5% with an average of 82.4% and the diagnostic yield ranged from 67.4% to 91.7% with an average of 81.7%. Examination of routinely stained smears (by Papanicolaou and May-Grünwald-Giemsa/ Diff-Quik methods) showed that nearly two thirds of the intrathoracic FNAs are malignant (36.3% to 88.5% with an average of 65.6%). Where as adenocarcinoma and epidermoid (squamous cell) carcinoma are common primary cancers, small-cell carcinoma (SCC) is relatively less frequent and large cell carcinoma is rare. In the material, the male to female ratio was 2.6:1 for malignancies of the lung. It was 7:1 for squamous cell carcinoma, 2.25:1 for adenocarcinoma, and 4:0 for small cell carcinoma.

In a review of 15 studies, the sensitivity of FNA for intrathoracic lesions ranged from 76.0% to 99.0% (average, 87.7%), the specificity from 68.0% to 100.0% (average, 96.8%), and diagnostic accuracy from 65.0% to 99.0% (average, 88.9%). The clinical utility of FNA, especially in patients with mediastinal compression syndrome and those with poor surgical risk, can be realized from the fact that the rate of more invasive diagnostic methods such as diagnostic mediastinoscopy and futile thoracotomies are greatly reduced by FNA cytology, which provides a tissue diagnosis in minutes with high degree of success.

The major limitation of FNA includes complication like pneumothorax. Sampling and interpretation errors in the hands of inexperienced cytopathologists also contribute to limitations of this diagnostic tool. Diagnostic dilemma may be due to inflammatory pseudo-tumors and cytologic atypia in benign tumors. Diagnostic difficulty may also be encountered in small round cell tumors and poorly differentiated carcinomas/malignancies. In such situations, adoption of ancillary studies like cytochemistry, immuno cytochemistry, florescent insituhybridization (FISH), and electron microscopy can improve the diagnosis of lung cancer.

Chapter 15 – Purpose: The aim of this study was to analyze the effect of cancer diagnosis on employment status, social interactions at work, commitment to the organization, and motives for work among women who have been diagnosed with breast cancer or Hodgkin's or Non-Hodgkin's lymphoma.

Methods: Survivors, aged 25-57 at the time of diagnosis, were selected from female breast and lymphoma cancer survivors in four Nordic countries listed at registers of hospitals or in cancer registers. The reference group was a random sample, with the same age distribution as the cancer survivors, taken from the national population registers. A questionnaire was sent to 2247 cancer survivors and 4710 referents. Ordinary least squares multiple regression was used for continuous dependent variables. Binary logistic regression was used for dichotomous dependent variables.

Results: In all 1580 cancer survivors (70.3%), 1490 diagnosed with breast cancer, 90 diagnosed with Hodgkin's or Non-Hodgkin's lymphoma, and 2516 (53.4%) of the referents answered the questionnaire. The employment participation of breast cancer survivors in this study was not less than that of the referents whereas the lymphoma survivors were less likely to be working. Breast cancer survivors were on average less committed to the organization, perceived less social support at work and scored lower on work motives, but experienced less discrimination than the referents. The lymphoma survivors were less content with the working climate in their unit/department than the referents and like the breast cancer survivors, perceived less social support at work.

Conclusions: This study provides information on differences between cancer survivors and a non-cancer reference group regarding factors that are important for return to and well-being at work. It also shows that the cancer type plays a role, therefore all cancer survivors can not be grouped together.

In: Lung Cancer in Women
Editor: Varetta N. Torres, pp. 1-43
ISBN: 978-1-60021-659-6


*Chapter I*

# Hypoxia-Targeted and Radiation Induced Gene Therapy for Lung Cancer

***Wei-Dong Wang[1], Zheng-tang Chen[1] and Rong Li[2]***

[1] Department of Radiation Oncology, Xinqiao Hospital, Chongqing 400037, China;
[2] Institute of Combined Injury, School of Preventive Medicine at Third Military Medical University, Chongqing 400038, China

## Abstract

Lung cancer is now the most common cause of cancer death in both men and women in the United States and is the leading cause of cancer death overall in the world, with over 1,000,000 deaths occurring yearly. Postsurgical mortality has declined from the early days of the 1950s but 5-year cure rates have only barely improved. The addition of chemotherapy to radical radiotherapy, together with novel radiotherapy techniques, is gradually improving the outcome for locally advanced, inoperable non–small cell lung cancer. The most important and cost-effective management for lung cancer is smoking cessation, but for those with the disease, novel treatment approaches are urgently needed. Combining conventional cancer treatments with gene therapy offers exciting prospects for improved lung cancer control. Novel strategies that specifically target damage to tumor cells, while sparing normal tissue, will be particularly effective. We outline two new approaches for targeting anti-tumor therapy. The first uses clinically relevant radiation doses to activate gene therapy vectors, via radiation-responsive gene promoters, following delivery to the tumor volume. This system could be applied to lung cancer patients, especially those that are highly resistant to current cancer treatments. The second approach exploits the physiological condition of hypoxia, which occurs commonly in lung cancer but is rarely seen in normal tissues. Hypoxia-regulated gene promoters can be used to drive expression of therapeutic genes in intratumoral areas of low oxygen. Furthermore, gene therapy vectors that respond both to radiation and hypoxia stimulation have recently been developed, allowing more tumor cell populations to be targeted. Such tailoring of gene therapy vectors to lung cancer treatment and environment, in combination with an efficient delivery system, is likely to produce significantly more efficacious clinical treatments in the near future.

## INTRODUCTION

Lung cancer is the most common cause of cancer-related death in the United States with an estimated 171,900 new cases and 157,200 deaths in 2002[1]. Deaths from lung cancer in women surpassed those due to breast cancer in 1987 and are expected to account for about 25% of all female cancer deaths in 2002. Thirty-one percent of cancer deaths in men are attributable to lung cancer. Lung cancer causes more deaths than the next three most common cancers combined (colon cancer, 48,100 deaths; breast cancer, 40,000 deaths; and prostate, 30,200 deaths).

The status of the treatment of lung cancer is no more encouraging. The expected 5-year survival rate for all patients in whom lung cancer is diagnosed is 15%, compared with 61% for colon cancer, 86% for breast cancer, and 96% for prostate cancer [1]. The median survival time of patients with untreated metastatic non-small cell lung cancer is 4 to 5 months, with a survival rate at 1 year of 10% [2]. In 2002, state-of-the-art treatment for this population provides a median survival time of approximately 8 months (an extension of a mere 3 to 4 months) and a 1-year survival rate of 33% [2]. For localized lung cancer, the expectations of treatment are better but not good. The 5-year survival rate for patients with potentially resectable lung cancer is significantly < 100% (stage IA, 67%; stage IB, 57%; stage IIA, 55%; stage IIB, 39%; and stage IIIA, 23%) [3]. Furthermore, progress in treatment has been slow. The current overall 5-year survival rate of 15% is only slightly better than the 8% survival rate of the early 1960s. Given these data, many physicians have assumed a nihilistic approach to the patient with lung cancer.

Although a 15% 5-year survival rate is meager and still dismal, the near doubling of the 5-year survival rate has provided some room for optimism and has begun to shift the nihilism associated with lung cancer treatment into a guarded optimism. One might take solace from the fact that 7% of newly diagnosed patients (or nearly 12,000 patients) will survive in 2002 but would not have been successfully treated in 1960. In addition, a number of promising new drugs have been incorporated into clinical trials, and many more are in the pipeline. Specifically targeted biological therapies are particularly promising. New diagnostic modalities, such as positron emission tomography, are finding widespread tumor and may alter our diagnostic and therapeutic algorithms. New surgical procedures and techniques have been developed and perfected. Safer and more effective methods of delivering radiation and some novel strategies such as radiogenetic therapy, are coming into clinical use. Radiogenetic therapy is a novel strategy for cancer treatment, in which an ionizing radiation-inducible regulatory sequence is linked with an adjuvant tumor-therapeutic cytokine sequence, and transfected into tumor cells. The expression of therapeutic gene, therefore, will be induced by radiation in cancer radiotherapy. The transfected cancer cells will be destroyed by both radiation and the radiation-inducible gene. Hypoxia-targeted gene therapy is a newly developed approache for cancer treatment based on the low oxygen microenviroment in solid tumor. Recently, we have constructed the gene therapy vector that responds to both radiation and hypoxia stimulation allowing more tumor cell populations to be targeted. The progressions in these newly developed approaches will be described in the following sections.

# Radiation Induced Gene Therapy

## Radio-Responsive Genes

Ionizing radiation (IR)-induced alterations in cellular RNA and protein levels, described more than 30 years ago [4], could be seen to occur in distinct temporal phases. The earliest nuclear targets, which are induced in the absence of de novo protein synthesis, are referred to as the immediate-early genes. A subclass of these genes encodes transcription factors that constitute the first step in a cascade of protein–DNA interactions. Thus, genes encoding immediate-early transcription factors serve as nuclear couplers of cytoplasmic events to the longer-term cellular response. The human genome contains more than 2000 hypothetical genes encoding putative transcriptional regulators. The factors c-FOS, c-JUN, AP-1, NFκB and EGR-1 are among the best-characterized. In the following paragraphs, we shall examine how the genes encoding these important modulators of the transcriptome respond to IR [5].

## The Fos Family

The viral *Fos* gene (*v-Fos*) was isolated in 1982 as the oncogene of the Finkel–Biskis–Jinkins (FBJ) murine osteogenic sarcoma virus, and its cellular counterpart, *c-Fos*, was described shortly afterwards. In 1984, Greenberg and Ziff [6] discovered that addition of serum to quiescent cells in culture rapidly stimulated *c-Fos* gene transcription. This finding led to a series of important discoveries in the area of transcriptional regulation, as it could be demonstrated that both c-Fos and v-Fos were nuclear DNA-binding proteins with gene activator properties. Since that time, several other members of the *Fos* family, such as *FosB*, *Fra1* and *Fra2*, have been identified.

*c-Fos* belongs to a category of genes known as protooncogenes, because overexpression of *c-Fos* results in cellular transformation and leads to development of osteosarcomas. *c-Fos* was found to be inducible at the level of transcription by a large number of agents including growth factors, lipopolysaccharides (LPS), cytokines and ultraviolet (UV) light. Treatment with IR could also be shown to induce *c-Fos* in different cell lines [5, 7–9]. The common effect observed upon induction of *c-Fos* by all the above-listed stimuli was the extremely rapid accumulation of *c-Fos* mRNA, followed by its fast degradation. Inevitably, research then focused on the signaling events leading to the activation of the *c-Fos* gene, in particular on how extracellular stimuli could activate transcription. Mutational analysis identified several regions in the human *c-Fos* promoter that responded to extracellular signals in transient transfection systems or in *in vitro* studies [10]. The key sequences are located within a 400 base pair (bp) segment directly upstream from the transcription initiation site. In this region, a combination of four regulatory elements, the sis-inducible element (SIE), the serum response element (SRE), the AP-1 site (FAP) and the cAMP response element (CRE), could be shown to be necessary for the correct transcriptional response of the promoter to any of the inducers investigated. A short sequence located ~300 bp upstream from the transcription start site, called SRE, cArG box or dyad symmetry element (DSE) was shown to be necessary and sufficient to render a heterologous promoter responsive to serum [11]. It is a 22 bp segment that contains the inner core sequence CCATATTAGG. This element has been described to be also responsible for radio-inducibility of *c-FOS* [12]. About 30 genes, e.g. *c-Fos*, *FosB*, *JunB*, *Egr-1* and *Egr-2*, have to date been found to contain the SRE (consensus sequence CC (A/T) 6GG) in their promoter region [13]. The SRE could be shown to act as a binding site for Elk-1, a member of the ETS family, which acts as a ternary complex factor (TCF) in concert with other transcription factors, such as the serum response factor p68/SRF [10]. Elk-1 is recruited to the SRE by a combination of protein–DNA and protein–protein interactions [13]. The interaction of Elk-1 with the dimer of SRF is a pre-requisite for Elk-1 binding to the SRE of *c-Fos*. In addition, the complex assembly requires SRF to be phosphorylated by GTPases of the Rho family. Phosphorylation of Elk-1 by mitogen activated protein kinases (MAPKs) is also necessary. MAPKs constitute the main regulatory cascades that control gene expression in response to various extracellular stimuli. This superfamily consists of numerous protein kinases organized into five known cascades. The principal ones are the extracellular-regulated kinase (ERK) cascade, the c-Jun NH2-terminal kinase/stress activated protein kinase (JNK/SAPK) cascade and the p38 MAPK cascade [14]. These differentially-regulated, but partly-overlapping MAPK cascades converge to phosphorylate Elk-1. The MAPK phosphorylation sites are located in the transcriptional activation domain of Elk-1, where the modification of two serine residues (Ser383 and Ser389) leads to enhanced DNA binding of Elk-1 and thus to a more effective transactivation of the target genes. Thus, the response to extracellular signals appears to be mediated at the level of Elk-1 [15]. The actual model proposes that protein kinase C (PKC) [16], activated by IR, activates the MAPKs through the small Raf/Ras G-protein kinases leading to the phosphorylation of Elk-1 and ultimately *c-FOS* transcription [17].

The cyclic AMP response element (CRE) consensus sequence is located at position-63 from the transcription start site of the *c-FOS* gene and controls the basal level of transcription as well as the response of the promoter to cAMP and calcium. CRE binding protein (CREB), the cognate transcription factor, contains a leucine zipper motif and binds as a dimer to the CRE sequence TGACGTCA of the c-*FOS* promoter. Phosphorylation of CREB on Ser133 by protein kinase A (PKA) promotes recruitment of the co-activator CREB binding protein (CBP), which in turn activates the transcription of the *c-FOS* gene. The recent experiments of Amorino et al. [18] highlighted a potential role of CREB also in radiation response. They showed that upon irradiation with a therapeutical dose of 2 Gy, CREB was phosphorylated on Ser133, which correlated with the phosphorylation of ERK/MAPK and its downstream effector p90 ribosomal S6 kinase. They suggested that CREB could play an important role in the regulation of its target genes upon IR.

## The Jun Family

The members of the *Jun* gene family are *c-Jun*, *JunB* and *JunD*. Like *c-Fos*, *c-Jun*, has an oncogenic viral counterpart *v-Jun*, which is found in the avian sarcoma virus 17. *c-Jun* is a proto-oncogene, because its ectopic over-expression can lead to cellular transformation and fibrosarcoma development.

*c-Jun* is transcriptionally inducible by serum, 12-*O*-tetradecanoyl- phorbol-13-acetate (TPA), and various growth factors and cytokines, with kinetics similar to *c-Fos*. The *c-Jun* promoter was also found to be responsive to several stress factors, such as $H_2O_2$, UV light and IR [5, 8, and 9]. Transcriptional activation of *c-JUN* upon IR exposure in the human HL-60 promyelocytic leukemia cells was described by Sherman et al. [9]. The increase in *c-JUN* transcripts upon IR treatment was time- and dose-dependent. Moreover, the half-life of *c-JUN* mRNA was extended in the absence of protein synthesis, indicating that its levels were regulated by both transcriptional and post-transcriptional mechanisms. In an extension of these studies, Datta et al. [19] and Hallahan et al. [20] studied the induction by X-rays of *c-JUN*, *c-FOS*, and a third, early growth response (*EGR-1*) gene. They showed that while all three genes are similarly induced by serum and TPA, the response of *c-FOS* to X-rays was distinct from that of the other two genes. This suggested that the response of the immediate early genes to IR is variable and that it is cell type-dependent. Recent experiments performed by Kool et al. [21] confirmed these results by demonstrating an increase in c-JUN, but not c-FOS expression after exposure to IR of normal human diploid VH 10 fibroblast.

Activation of the human *c-JUN* gene by IR was later found to be mediated by two AP-1/ATF (activating transcription factor)-like binding elements, *Jun1* and *Jun2*. In vitro binding studies, using extracts of various primary and transformed cell lines, have shown that these elements can bind the c-JUN/ATF2 and c-JUN/ATF3 heterodimers, where ATF2 and ATF3 are members of the ATF/CREB family. Activation of the *c-JUN* promoter through the *Jun1* and *Jun2* elements by DNA-damaging agents appears to be mediated by post-translational modification of the pre-existing JUN/ATF complexes. Oxidative damage triggers an intracellular signal that stimulates JNK/SAPK activity, which enhances the transactivation function of c-JUN and ATF2 by phosphorylating Ser63 and Ser73 of c-JUN and Thr69 and Thr71 of ATF2 [14]. However, in response to the same stimulus, ATF2 was also found to be a substrate of the p38 MAPK cascade in HeLa cells [22] and the substrate of both p38 and JNK/MAPK cascades in VH 10 fibroblasts [21]. This finding highlights the fact that the regulation of transcription factors that control the expression of immediate early genes results from a convergence of multiple MAP kinase cascades. Another regulatory element in the *c-JUN* promoter was found to be important in the induction of *c-JUN* mRNA upon IR. This element, adjacent to the *Jun1* site and referred to as the CCAAT box domain, is also found in the promoters of *JUNB* and *JUND*. The studies of Hallahan et al. [23] showed that the AP-1/ATF-like binding elements and the CCAAT box combine to control the activity of the *c-JUN* promoter in response to IR.

# ACTIVATING PROTEIN-1 TRANSCRIPTION FACTOR (AP-1)

FOS and JUN family proteins function as dimeric nuclear transcription factors that bind to AP-1 regulatory elements in the promoter and enhancer regions of numerous genes. JUN proteins form both homodimers and heterodimers with FOS proteins, whereas FOS does not form homodimers and requires heterodimerization to bind DNA. The JUN dimerization partners JDP1 and JDP2, and the closely-related activating transcription factors ATF2, ATF3 and B-ATF subfamilies can also dimerize with JUN to form AP-1 transcription factor complexes [24]. The subunit composition determines the affinity of the AP-1 factor for the respective DNA sequence. Heterodimers formed by FOS and JUN bind with the highest affinity to a symmetric heptanucleotide recognition sequence TGA(C/G) TCA, referred to as AP-1/TPA responsive element (TRE) and with lower affinity to the symmetric octanucleotide CRE sequence. The c-JUN/c-JUN homodimer has a higher affinity for the AP-1 sequence, whereas the heterodimer c-JUN/ATF2 has a higher affinity for the CRE sequence. Differential expression of AP-1 proteins in response to extracellular stimuli was suggested to be one of the major mechanisms that modulate AP-1 activity. Phosphorylation of AP-1 proteins by MAP kinases further influences their activities and provides another route for extracellular stimuli to regulate the activity of AP-1 transcription factors.

AP-1 is activated by a multitude of effectors, ranging from growth factors, cytokines, hormones and mechanical and osmotic stress to hypoxia, ultraviolet radiation and oxidative stress. IR gives rise to multiple reactive oxygen species (ROS) including superoxide radicals ($O_2 \bullet^-$) and hydroxyl radicals (•OH), as well as hydrogen peroxide ($H_2O_2$) and organic hydroperoxides (ROOH). ROS activate AP-1 through the JNK pathway, which modifies the c-JUN and ATF-2 constituents of the AP-1 complex and promotes the induction of the transcription factor ATF-3. Because a number of AP-1 binding sites are located in the promoter region of the *c-JUN* gene, the phosphorylation and the subsequent activation of c-*JUN* result in its autoactivation. Such regulation of c-JUN activity leads to long-term activation of AP-1 and to a steady increase in the expression levels of its target genes under oxidative stress conditions [25].

## Nuclear Factor Kappa B (NFκB)

The NFκB pathway is generally thought to be the primary oxidative stress-response pathway in which ROS act as second messengers. NFκB is a member of the ubiquitously-expressed family of Rel-related transcription factors. It acts as a key regulator of numerous genes involved in inflammatory processes, stress response and programmed cell death. NFκB orchestrates the rapid cellular response to a myriad of seemingly-unrelated exogenous and endogenous stress-inducing agents such as bacterial cell walls, viral infections, pro-inflammatory cytokines, etc. The NFκB transcription factor consists of two subunits, NFκB1 (p50) and RelA (p65). According to the classical paradigm, NFκB is sequestered in the cytoplasm together with its inhibitor IκBα in the form of an inactive complex. Exposure to a variety of stimuli results in the activation of IκB kinases which phosphorylate IκBα on Ser32 and Ser36. The phosphorylated form of IκBα is ubiquitinylated and degraded, unmasking the nuclear localization sequence on NFκB, which then translocates into the nucleus, where it binds to the consensus sequence 5`-GGGACTTTCC-3` in the promoters of its target genes.

NFκB is a well-known radiation-responsive transcription factor. An insult by IR activates NFκB already 2–4 h after exposure, with its activity returning to basal levels by 8 h [26–28]. Activation of NFκB by oxidative stress and IR appears to proceed through a common cascade involving ROS generation, but the exact mechanism that activates NFκB is not completely understood [29]. Lee et al. [30] reported that the regulation of NFκB is impaired in cells with the human genetic disease ataxia telangiectasia (AT) and that the ataxia-telangiectasia mutated (ATM) kinase phosphorylates IκBα in vitro, suggesting an important role for ATM in the induction of NFκB by radiation. Li and Karin [31] showed that IR activates IKK and that IR-induced IκBα degradation is phosphorylation-dependent. Furthermore, inhibition of IκBα phosphorylation on Ser32 and Ser36 was shown to sensitize human glioma cells to DNA damaging agents and inhibition of NFκB activity increased the radiosensitivity of several human ovarian carcinoma cell lines. Furthermore, blocking radiation-induced NFκB activation increased the apoptotic response and decreased the growth and clonogenic survival of irradiated colorectal cancer cells [32]. Ectopic expression of mutated IκB in human malignant glioma MO54 and T98 cells led to their sensitization to IR. This finding confirms the radiosensitizing role of NFκB [33, 34]. Recent experiments in the human glioblastoma U251 and SH539 cell lines performed by Russel and Tofilon [28] indicated that the IR-sensitive pool of IκBα/NFκB is located at the plasma membrane. The membrane-association of IκBα is consistent with earlier experiments carried out by the same team, showing that a single chain antibody fragment targeted to the RAS protein inhibited IR-induced NFκB activation in U251 cells [35]. They propose a scenario in which activated RAS protein recruits IκBα/NFκB complexes to the cell membrane, which leads to the selective degradation of IκBα and the consequent translocation of NFκB into the nucleus. The above evidence shows the importance of NFκB activation in defraying the toxicity of IR, but it is also evident that NFκB activation can be accomplished by several distinct mechanisms and that some important links of the activation still remain to be elucidated.

## Early Growth Response Factor Egr-1

The immediate early gene *Egr-1* (also known as *NGFI-A*, *Zif268*, *Tis8* and *Krox24*) encodes a transcription factor containing a DNA binding domain formed by three zinc finger motifs. Egr-1 preferentially binds to the GC-rich consensus sequence GCGGGGGCG. This sequence is found in the regulatory regions of many genes such as tumor necrosis factor-α (*TNF*-α), interleukin-1 (*IL*-1), platelet-derived growth factor-α (*PDGF*–α) and basic fibroblast growth factor (*bFGF*). In response to radiation injury, cytokine and growth factor products participate in the late response that will lead to the survival of the tissue or that will drive cells to cell death.

Expression of *Egr-1* is transiently induced by a broad spectrum of extracellular stimuli such as mitogens (PDGF, FGF, EGF) and stress signals (hypoxia, shear stress, bacterial lipopolysaccharides, wound healing), but also by stimuli such as anisomycin and X-rays. Transcription of the *Egr-1* gene is rapidly and transiently induced by IR in a variety of cell types. The response occurs within 15 min and lasts for at most 3 h after exposure [20]. In order to understand the rapid transient induction of this gene in response to radiation, molecular studies of the enhancer/repressor regulatory elements on the *Egr-1* promoter were performed. The initial steps in the induction of expression are not completely understood, although several signal transduction pathways involved in activation of this gene have been characterized. Functional dissection of the human *EGR-1* promoter sequence revealed that it contains at least five copies of the SRE element [36]. By deletion analysis, Datta et al. [12] identified the SRE binding site as the radiation-responsive element in the *EGR-1* promoter and proved that the three distal SRE elements confer its X-ray inducibility. Moreover, exposure of HL-525 human leukaemia cells to ROS-induced *EGR-1* transcription through the SRE element [37]. As for the induction of the *c-Fos* gene by extracellular stimuli [15], SRF and the ternary complex factors Elk-1, Sap1 or Sap2 are required for SRE-mediated activation of the *Egr-1* promoter. As discussed above, Elk-1 is phosphorylated by MAP kinases, which leads to its enhanced DNA-binding activity and ternary complex-forming ability and thus to an enhanced SRE-mediated transcription. It has been previously shown that, upon exposure to various stress agents such as heat shock, anisomycin or UV light, the two stress kinases p38 and JNK1, but not ERK2, become activated by phosphorylation and induce *Egr-1* promoter activity through modification of Elk-1 [38]. Elk-1 was also found to be activated by IR [39]. It is therefore most likely that radiation modulates the binding of the phosphorylated activated complex SRF/Elk-1 to the SRE element in the *Egr-1* promoter through activation of the p38 and JNK/SAPK pathways, and that this ultimately leads to the transactivation of the *Egr-1* gene [40].

Another intracellular pathway, this time activated by PKC, appears to contribute to the regulation of the *EGR-1* gene by IR. Prolonged stimulation with TPA, known to deplete PKC, was shown to block X-ray inducibility of *EGR-1* in the SQ20B squamous carcinoma cell line. In addition, pre-treatment of SQ20B or 293 cells with H7, a non-specific inhibitor of protein kinases, markedly attenuated X-ray inducibility of *EGR-1* [20]. It is thus likely that activation of PKC contributes to the phosphorylation of Elk-1 and therefore to the induction of *Egr-1* expression in response to IR.

The architecture of human *EGR-1* revealed that the full-length promoter (700 bp) includes several types of binding sites. A JNK/SAPK-dependent AP-1/thiophorbol ester-responsive element (AP-1/TRE) site is located 600 bp upstream from the TATA box. Through binding to two Egr-1 binding sites (CGCCCCCGC) the Egr-1 protein down-regulates the transcription of its own gene. The fact that forskolin, an activator of adenylate cyclase, does not stimulate E*gr-1* promoter activity [40] indicates that the CRE consensus sequence in the promoter does not function as a cAMP-inducible enhancer element as described for other genes, such as *c-fos*. Whether or not CRE sites contribute to radio-inducibility of the *egr-1* promoter is not yet clear. However, upon genotoxic stress, i.e. anisomycin treatment, the SAPK/JNK and p38/MAPK pathways become activated. This activation triggers the phosphorylation of the CREB and ATF-1 proteins. These phosphorylated proteins form a specific complex on the CRE site of the *egr-1* promoter and cause transient induction of the Egr-1 protein.

In the recent experiments of Meyer et al. [40], a core *egr-1* promoter of 490 bp (nucleotides −425 to +65 relative to the transcription start site) containing the five SRE sequences, Sp1 sites and two CRE elements was described to be sufficient for radio-induction of a luciferase reporter gene.

## Radiogenetic Therapy

Radiotherapy is the primary treatment modality for many solid tumors. In recent years, the improved targeting of radiation and innovations, such as conformal radiotherapy and intensity-modulated radiation therapy, have increased the precision of dose delivery to the tumor volume, while also limiting exposure to surrounding normal tissues. However, curative radiotherapy for certain tumor types still remains challenging, especially where local control is the predominant issue. Consequently, several successful pharmacologically based approaches have been combined with radiation treatment to reduce or modify intrinsic radioresistance [41]. Strategies involving radiosensitizing drugs or inhibitors of cellular repair processes and/or tumor cell proliferation are well established and have proven efficacy in many instances. More recently, the problem of intrinsic radiosensitivity has been addressed using methods that exploit contemporary molecular biology techniques. These approaches are designed to modify tumor sensitivity using methods that alter the 'genetic profile' of a tumor or introduce foreign genes that kill tumor cells when expressed [42, 43]. Although still in its infancy, a number of clinical gene therapy trials have already been conducted [44]. As was found with pharmacological approaches, initial attempts at using the technology *in vivo* have demonstrated some practical difficulties. For gene therapy these include a number of efficacy issues, mainly with regard to the gene delivery systems [45].

Ionizing Radiation (IR) upregulates the expression of a number of genes; many of them are involved in immediate early responses to mitogenic stimulation or cellular stress [46-49]. In 1994, Boothman proposed that 'promoter' sequences of radiation-inducible genes could be used for the controlled expression of therapeutic genes. However, for cancer gene therapy, IR-inducible genes that are p53 dependent (e.g., *Waf-1* [50] and *Gadd-45* [51, 52]) are not ideal, since mutations in the p53 gene are common in many tumors and their promoters may not function efficiently in this context. Consequently, attention has focused on the p53-independent radiation-inducible early growth response (*Egr*)-1 gene promoter for anti-tumor gene therapy [53-55].

The therapeutic potential of *Egr-1* radiation-inducibility was demonstrated by positioning the E425 region upstream of the cDNA of the tumoricidal cytokine tumor necrosis factor (TNF)α [56]. This DNA construct was delivered to human epidermoid carcinoma xenografts (SQ-20B) with cell carriers [56], liposomes [53] or adenoviral vectors (Ad5, [57- 59]). The combination of a fractionated radiation dose schedule of 40 Gy (5 Gy fractions twice a day for 4 days) and intratumorally delivered Ad5-E425-TNF-α resulted in increased tumor regression by up to 90% of control values compared with maxima of 50% for vector or radiation alone [55, 57]. Similarly, Joki *et al.* [60] and Takahashi *et al.* [61] used the E425 enhancer for radio-induced expression of the herpes simplex virus thymidine kinase (HSVtk) suicide gene. Glioma cells containing this vector were sensitized to the antiviral agent ganciclovir (GCV), a substrate for HSVtk, after exposure to a single radiation dose of 20 Gy. *In vivo*, human hepatoma Huh-7 cells xenografted into nude mice regressed significantly after liposome delivery of an E425- HSVtk construct, followed by 20 Gy γ-irradiation and GCV administration, but not after IR alone [62].

To create gene therapy vectors that can be activated by clinically relevant doses of IR, synthetic enhancers containing isolated CArG elements were manufactured [63]. These promoters consisted of an enhancer region, containing tandemly arranged CArG2 elements, immediately upstream from the cytomegalovirus (CMV) immediate early gene basal promoter [63]. The synthetic promoters therefore lacked binding sites for the potentially antagonistic transcription factors seen in the native *Egr-1* promoter that could restrict radioresponsiveness. Indeed, the synthetic enhancers were more responsive to IR than the parental *Egr-1* gene [63, 64]. An enhancer containing 4 isolated copies of the CArG2 element (E4) showed 3.1-fold (± 0.25) induction after IR compared with 1.86-fold (± 0.2) for the native human *Egr-1* counterpart after 3 Gy activation dose [63]. Multiple doses of 3 Gy resulted in greater levels of induced expression than after a single dose and the synthetic promoters responded to radiation doses as low as 1 Gy [63]. Promoters containing different numbers, sequences and arrangements of CArG elements were also radioresponsive [64]. Increasing the number of CArG2 elements from four to six and then nine (E4, E6 and E9 enhancers) improved the specific Irresponsiveness and reduced basal expression. The alteration of CArG element core sequences substantially affected the response, either positively or negatively, with CArG1 being the most IR-responsive.

The HSVtk/GCV gene-directed enzyme prodrug therapy (GDEPT) system has proven efficacy in a number of tumor models, including glioma, and particularly in combination with radiation treatment [65, 66]. The system potentiates radiation cytotoxicity, as the GCV prodrug becomes incorporated into radiation-damaged DNA at strand breaks, preventing further strand synthesis. HSVtk/GCV also produces a 'bystander effect' [67], by which the HSVtk activated prodrug is able to kill non-vector-containing tumor cells adjacent to those expressing the suicide gene. HSVtk GDEPT has been used to demonstrate the anti-tumor potential of the synthetic radiation responsive promoters.

The anti-tumor potential of this GDEPT system was also demonstrated when the synthetic radiation-responsive CArG promoters were used to regulate HSVtk expression *in vitro* [63] and *in vivo* [64]. In the latter study, systemic GCV administration produced a significantly greater tumor regrowth delay for irradiated E9HSVtk-modified (9 CArG elements) U87-MG xenografts. To increase the bystander effect of GDEPT, The use of the Herpes Simplex Virus (HSV) intercellular transport viral protein 22 (VP22) was investigated for radiogenetic therapy. During the normal HSV replication cycle, this tegument protein is exported from virus-infected cells and localizes in the nucleus of neighboring, noninfected cells [68]. Importantly, intercellular VP22 transport is independent of the presence of intercellular gap junctions, which can limit other bystander systems. Fusion proteins, expressed from chimeric VP22 genes, have been shown to be similarly transported and maintain their inherent function using plasmid [68] or viral delivery systems [69] and in a wide range of cell types [70] as well as *in vivo* [71]. A typical example of the intercellular transport of a green fluorescent protein (GFP)-VP22 fusion from plasmid-transfected U87 MG glioma cells to non-transfected recipients. Incorporating a VP22-HSVtk fusion to enhance HSVtk bystander effect produced a fivefold increase in tumor cell growth control compared with HSVtk alone [72]. As tumor cells often display poor cell-cell communication,

VP22 has obvious advantages in anti-tumor therapy. The use of VP22 transport protein has the potential to address the current limitations of efficient gene delivery in the therapy of proliferating and terminally differentiated tissues [69, 73-77].

Gene therapy has been combined with experimental radiotherapy by a number of groups. A high therapeutic potential was shown by delivering a replication-competent oncolytic adenovirus expressing a cytosine deaminase *(CD)/HSVtk* fusion gene to an irradiated tumor (single 8-10 Gy dose) in mice, given the corresponding prodrugs 5- fluorocytosine (5-FC) and GCV intraperitoneally (i.p.) [78]. This trimodal treatment produced significant tumor radiosensitization and regression in the experimental C33A tumor xenograft model. Radiolabeled antibodies that target ligands expressed by tumor cells have been shown to be an attractive method for tumor selective drug expression [79]. A similar radiolabeling approach is the use of nonimmunogenic molecules that are specifically incorporated into tumor cells with high affinity. One example is the specific uptake of $^{131}$I-meta-iodobenzylguanidine ($^{131}$IMIBG) by the noradrenaline transporter [80, 81] that is over expressed by some tumors of the neural crest. The system has been experimentally exploited for gene therapy by Boyd and colleagues, who have specifically elevated NAT (noradrenaline transporter) expression of tumor cells using a telomerase promoter, which is differentially more active in tumor cells [82-85]. Similar results were obtained using the sodium/iodide symporter (NIS) combined with ionic $^{131}$Iadministration [86].

In contrast, gene therapy has also been exploited to decrease the side effects of radiation-induced damage in normal tissue. For example, intratracheal injection of a vector carrying the human superoxide dismutase (SOD-2) transgene prior to irradiation prevented radiation-induced damage of transduced tissues. This resulted in decreased radiation-induced oesophageal stricture [87] or decreased late pulmonary fibrosis [88]. These examples of combining radiotherapy and gene therapy illustrate the breadth of ideas being investigated; moreover they highlight the benefit of adopting a combinational treatment approach that can be tailored to address individual situations.

## HYPOXIA TARGETED GENE THERAPY

### Tumor Hypoxia

The micromilieu of solid tumors plays a fundamental role in the response to therapy. In particular, much attention has been recently focused on the pathophysiology of vasculature and blood flow. Blood vessels within the tumor mass are highly irregular, tortuous, and elongated, with blind ends, incomplete endothelial linings, increased vascular permeability, and irregular blood flow [89-91]. This abnormal vascular system results in reduced or even abolished $O_2$ delivery to the neoplastic and stromal cells. In addition, anemia and the formation of methemoglobin or carboxyhemoglobin can reduce $O_2$ transport capacity [92]. Hypoxia is usually defined by biochemists as $O_2$-limited electron transport; by clinicians as a state of reduced $O_2$ availability or $O_2$ partial pressure below critical values [93, 94]; radiobiologists refer to the proportion of clonogenic cells in tumors which exhibit maximal radioresistance, often described in animal models by the paired survival curve assay [95]. The inadequate vascular geometry relative to the volume of oxygen consuming tumor cells creates diffusion-limited $O_2$ delivery (chronic hypoxia) [96]. Moreover, the dynamic changes in microregional blood flow in tumors have been related to the formation of areas of perfusion-limited $O_2$ delivery (acute or transient hypoxia) [97-99]. Both chronic and transient hypoxia has been detected in animal tumor models and clinical data confirm that they occur in human cancers as well [100-102]. Low oxygen tension in tumors is frequently associated with low glucose concentration, high lactate levels, and low extracellular pH [103].

A variety of invasive and non-invasive methods have been developed to measure the oxygenation status of solid malignancies [104]. Hypoxia in human tumors has been estimated indirectly by measuring tumor vascularization (e.g., intercapillary distance, vascular density) [105]; the degree of DNA damage after radiation [106]; the expression of hypoxia-regulated genes [107,108]; and by hypoxia marker techniques (misonidazole) [109]; pimonidazole [110]; the 2-nitroimidazole drug EF5 [111]. Direct measurements of tissue oxygen partial pressure ($pO_2$) have been obtained by utilizing oxygen sensitive polarographic electrodes [112] and luminescence- based optical sensors [113]. Using oxygen electrodes, it has been observed that the majority of solid tumors present median$pO_2$ levels lower than their normal tissue of origin. For example, measurements carried out in normal breast revealed a median $pO_2$ of 65 mmHg (8.6% $O_2$), whereas in breast carcinomas of stages pT1–4 the median $pO_2$ was 28 mmHg (3.9% $O_2$). More than 30% of the breast cancers investigated exhibited $pO_2$ values between 0 and 2.5 mmHg (0.3% $O_2$). In contrast, values <12.5 mmHg (1.6% $O_2$) could not be detected in the normal breast. In several tumor types, high heterogeneity in the hypoxic distribution has been observed both within the tumor mass and between tumors of same clinical stage and grade [114]. In metastatic lesions, as in primary tumors, red cell flux was found to be anisotropic and compromised compared to surrounding normal tissue [115]. In metastases of carcinomas of the head and neck, breast and rectal cancers, lower median $pO_2$ values and higher hypoxic fractions were recorded, compared not only with the normal surrounding tissue, but also the primary tumors [116].

## Effects on Cancer Treatment

The relevance of tumor oxygenation to radiocurability was first proposed by Gray et al. [117] and its role in the response to radiation has since been recognized both in experimental and clinical systems. Anoxic cells are~3-fold more radioresistant than normoxic cells, with a steep increase in radiosensitivity between 2 and 10 mmHg. This phenomenon, known as the "oxygen effect," is observed when oxygen is present during or within milliseconds after radiation exposure, and results from the reaction of $O_2$ with ionized target molecules, generating poorly repairable peroxide lesions (oxygen-fixation hypothesis) [95]. A correlation between the presence of hypoxia and response to therapy has been shown in a range of human tumor sites. Studies performed in patients with soft tissue sarcomas [118,119], carcinomas of the uterine cervix [120-122], and of the head and neck [123-125] indicated that the presence of hypoxic regions adversely affects locoregional control and/or disease-free survival after primary radiotherapy. Radiation resistance induced by the oxygen effect is unlikely to be the only explanation, since tumor oxygen status has been observed to be the most important prognostic factor for treatment outcome and metastatic free survival in cervical carcinoma after radiotherapy as well as surgery. Hypoxia-driven cellular modifications may contribute to this poor prognostic outlook, giving rise to more aggressive locoregional disease, invasive capacity, and angiogenesis [126-128].

Oxygen dependency has been shown for some chemotherapeutic agents both in vitro and in vivo [129-131]. A number of factors may be involved. Firstly, hypoxic cells slow down or even arrest their rate of progression through the cell division cycle [132]. Experiments conducted in mammalian cells of different origin showed that prolonged hypoxia causes accumulation in the G1-phase of the cell cycle and inhibition of DNA replication, effects reversible upon reoxygenation [133-136]. In experimental tumors, the fraction of proliferating cells and/or the rate of cell proliferation decreased as the distance from the vasculature increased [137-139]. This can result in a loss of efficacy of most anticancer agents, which are primarily effective against rapidly dividing cells. Secondly, because of drug metabolism by the cells in the intermediate layers, the limited penetration of plasma-borne agents determines a reduction in the dose of drug reaching the hypoxic population. Also, the extracellular pH is lower in hypoxic than in well-oxygenated areas, while the intracellular pH is kept constant [140]. This leads to the uptake and activity of weak acids such as chlorambucil to be increased, while that of weak bases like vinblastine to be decreased [141]. Finally, hypoxia can induce the production of stress proteins responsible for resistance to doxorubicin, etoposide and methotrexate [142-144]. Clinical studies have demonstrated a correlation between hypoxia mediated gene expression and response to chemotherapy.

## Molecular Effects

The hypoxic microenvironment in solid tumors, which affects neoplastic cells and non-neoplastic stromal cells such as macrophages and fibroblasts, is likely to have profound effects on tumor propagation if one considers the molecular changes demonstrated in vitro and in vivo under hypoxic conditions. The pathophysiological microenvironment of tumors is generally considered to be mutagenic. Point mutations, deletions, and gene amplification after hypoxia/reoxygenation may occur as a result of errors in DNA repair and/or replication, oxidative damage leading to DNA strand breakage and impaired activity of enzymes such as topoisomerases, helicases, and ligases [145-147]. Experimental evidence suggests that low oxygen levels cause apoptosis in normal and neoplastic cells [148, 149]. p53 accumulated under hypoxia and was required for induction of apoptosis. However, although reduced, hypoxia-induced apoptotic death was also detected in p53 null cells, indicating the presence of p53-independent pathways [150]. Involvement of Apaf-1, caspase-9, and genes of the bcl-2 family has also been reported [151, 152]. Moreover, hypoxia can select for tumor cells that have acquired p53 mutations and have lost their apoptotic potential, providing them with a growth advantage [153]. However, clinical data are conflicting. Squamous cell carcinomas of the uterine cervix, characterized by pronounced hypoxia and low apoptotic index, showed a high probability for lymphatic spread and recurrence, despite adjuvant treatment with radiation or chemotherapy in addition to radical surgery. Also, in cervix carcinomas a significant correlation between hypoxia and functionally impaired p53 was demonstrated

[154]. p53 status and hypoxia had no independent prognostic impact on overall survival, but the combination of these two parameters was a significant prognostic factor. On the other hand, in patients with primary soft tissue sarcoma, no association was found between median $pO_2$ and p53 status. In squamous cell carcinoma of the cervix, the pre-radiotherapy apoptotic index did not correlate with pre-treatment oxygenation (both hypoxic fraction and median $pO_2$), but correlated significantly with the change in oxygenation post-treatment, ascribed by the authors to reduced interstitial fluid pressure as a result of cell loss via apoptosis [155].

Hypoxia-related tumor progression and metastatic spread has been related to the up-regulation of gene products that may promote tumor progression, by enabling tumor cells to adapt to nutritional deprivation or to escape a hostile environment. To facilitate tumor cell detachment, migration and invasion, hypoxia can down-regulate cell adhesion molecules such as integrins [156], and upregulate the urokinase-type plasminogen activator receptor (uPAR) [157] and the autocrine motility factor (AMF) [158]. An association between primary tumor oxygenation and the likelihood of distant metastasis has been reported in clinical studies involving patients with high-grade soft tissue sarcoma and advanced squamous cell carcinoma of the uterine cervix [159]. Also, a positive correlation has been observed between tumor lactate concentration and the presence of metastatic deposits in cervix and head and neck squamous cell carcinomas [160], while ATP and glucose concentration did not show significant correlation. When murine tumor models are employed, acute rather than chronic hypoxia appears to be responsible for metastatic spread [161].

In summary, hypoxia not only provides an environment directly facilitating chemo- and radio-resistance, but also encourages the evolution of phenotypic changes inducing permanent resistance to treatment. The main strategies adopted to overcome the resistance of hypoxic tumors to therapy include increasing the delivery of oxygen (or oxygen-mimetic drugs), and exploiting the tumor hypoxia's unique physiological nature for targeted cancer treatment. One of the first attempts to improve tumor oxygenation in the clinic was the use of hyperbaric oxygen in combination with radiotherapy [162]. Multicenter clinical trials showed a significant increase in locoregional control and survival in patients with cervix or advanced head and neck carcinoma treated with radiation and hyperbaric oxygen, compared with radiotherapy given in air [163]. However, these studies were discontinued primarily because of problems with patient compliance. Subsequently, chemical radiosensitizers, in particular electron-affinic radiosensitizers, were introduced by Adams et al. [164, 165]. The rationale for their use is that they can diffuse out of the tumor blood supply and, not being metabolized in cellular respiration, can reach hypoxic areas and radiosensitize hypoxic cells in an oxygenmimicking fashion. Of these drugs, misonidazole, a 2- nitroimidazole, showed remarkable results in laboratory studies [166], but the clinical experience was disappointing because of dose limitations due to high neurotoxicity [167]. New nitroimidazole compounds were then developed, and the 5-nitroimidazole nimorazole was reported to significantly improve the effect of radiotherapy in some head and neck cancers, with only mild associated toxicity [168].

In order to overcome both chronic and transient hypoxia, the combination of carbogen (95% $O_2$ and 5% $CO_2$), effective against the former, and the vitamin B derivative nicotinamide, which is believed to prevent transient blood-flow fluctuation [169], has been successfully tested in animal models [170]. In clinical studies, the treatment was given in combination with standard or accelerated radiotherapy (ARCON). Phase I, II, and III trials indicated feasibility and some therapeutic efficacy, in particular in the treatment of bladder and head and neck carcinoma, albeit limited by the gastro-intestinal toxicity of nicotinamide [171-175].

Bioreductive drugs, such as the indolequinones mitomycin C and EO9, SR 4233 (later known as tirapazamine, TPZ), RSU 1069, AQ4N, and CB1954, have been extensively utilized as hypoxia-selective cytotoxins [176]. In order for bioreductive drugs to be activated, the cells need to be hypoxic and to produce the appropriate set of reductase enzymes. By contrast, bioactivation is restricted by the presence of oxygen in normal tissue. The concentration of bioreductive drug required to induce the same level of killing in hypoxic vs. normoxic cells (hypoxic cytotoxicity ratio, HCR) may vary depending on the cell type and the level of hypoxia. HCR values for the prototype bioreductive drug mitomycin C did not exceed 10 [177], to be compared with values in the 7–300 range for TPZ [178], 10–200 for nitroimidazoles [179-181], and up to 5,000 for E08 and E09 [182]. Nevertheless, clinical evaluation of mitomycin C in combination with radiotherapy for the treatment of squamous cell carcinoma of the head and neck indicated significant improvement in locoregional control and survival, compared with radiation treatment alone [183]. In the case of TPZ, an improvement in survival was observed in conjunction with radiotherapy, but it did not reach statistical significance [184]. However, the combination of TPZ, cisplatin and radiotherapy resulted in acceptable levels of toxicity [185] and remarkably good and durable clinical responses in patients with advanced head and neck cancers [186].

## Hypoxia-Targeted Gene Therapy

Hypoxia is an independent stimulus of gene expression that can to some extent be mimicked by carbon monoxide, the iron chelator desferrioxamine, cobalt, nickel, and manganese, but not by zinc, iron, or cadmium. The exact molecular mechanism by which cells detect $O_2$ concentration has for long been unclear. Potassium channels have been implicated in $O_2$ sensing by carotid body type I cells and a number of different vascular cells [187]. On the other hand, studies on hypoxia-regulated erythropoietin (Epo) gene expression suggested that the $O_2$ sensor is a heme-containing protein that exists in different conformations (oxy, deoxy) dependent on $O_2$ binding. Carbon monoxide could simulate hypoxic induction by irreversibly substituting for oxygen, while hypoxia-mimicking metals are thought to displace iron in the porphyrin ring and their low affinity for oxygen would lock the heme protein in the deoxy conformation, triggering the generation of reactive oxygen species (ROS). ROS were also found to increase in mitochondria after hypoxia, and the inhibition of the mitochondrial electron transport chain blocked the induction of hypoxia-dependent transcription factors [188]. It has recently been suggested that a prolyl hydroxylase may act as a cellular oxygen sensor [189, 190]. The signal is then transduced through an interactive network rather than a linear pathway involving both tyrosine phosphorylation and redox regulation, which is not surprising given the importance of $O_2$ homeostasis.

Several genes regulated by hypoxia have been described, and the number is rapidly increasing, especially with the advent of array technology. The most studied encode for proteins such as: 1. Transcription factors, including activator protein (AP)-1 [191], hypoxia-inducible factor (HIF) [192], nuclear factor (NF)-κB [193], and p53 [194], which regulate genes for proteins governing growth control, apoptosis, differentiation, and metastasis; 2. Metabolic enzymes, like aldolase (ALD)-A and –C [195], carbonic anhydrase (CA)-9 [196], enolase (Eno)-1 [197], glucose transporter (Glut)-1 and -3 [198], lactate dehydrogenase (LDH)-A, phosphofructokinase (PFK)-L and -C, phosphoglycerate kinase (PGK)-1 [199], and pyruvate kinase (PK)-M; 3. Cytokines, growth factors, and other proteins that regulate angiogenesis, vascular permeability, and inflammation, including Epo [200, 201], endothelin-1 [202], inducible nitric oxide synthase (iNOS) [203], plateletderived growth factor-B, vascular endothelial growth factor (VEGF) [204], and its receptors (VEGFR-1 and -2) [205]; 4. Stress proteins, such as the heat shock proteins (HSPs) and cellular redox regulators [206].

The control of Epo, the main regulator of red blood cell production, was used as a model to gain an understanding of how cells sense and respond to changes in oxygen tension. Madan and Curtin [201] defined the minimal DNA region necessary for hypoxia response of the Epo gene as a 24 bp sequence, able to regulate transcription regardless of the orientation of, and distance from, the coding region. Beck et al. [207] identified a 120 kDa protein that is upregulated by hypoxia and binds to the Epo hypoxia enhancer sequence. This nuclear transcription factor was defined as HIF-1 and found to be common to a variety of Epo-producing and non-producing mammalian cells. Affinity purification and molecular cloning of HIF-1 showed it to function as a heterodimer, consisting of two basic-helix-loop-helix proteins from the Per-aryl hydrocarbon receptor nuclear translocator (ARNT)-Sim (PAS) family of transcription factors: HIF-1α (120 kDa) and HIF-1β (91–94 kDa) [208]. More recently, the endothelial PASdomain protein (EPAS)-1 has been reported to show close sequence homology and similar properties to HIF-1α, and therefore has been renamed HIF-2α or HIF-1 alike factor [209]. A third HIFα subunit, HIF-3α, shares sequence identity with that of HIF-1α and HIF-2α (57% and 53% identity at the N-terminal bHLH-PAS domain, respectively [210]. Of the three HIFα subunits, HIF-1α has been the most extensively characterized, although little redundancy has been observed in the functions of HIF-1α and HIF-2α. HIF is expressed in a number of cell types and human tissues [211-213], and has an important pathophysiological role within solid tumors. Mouse Hepa-1 hepatomas from HIF-1β-deficient cells exhibited reduced hypoxia-mediated gene expression, vascularity and growth rate, compared with the wild type tumors [214]. Analogously, HIF-1$\beta^{-/-}$ knockout embryonic stem (ES) cells failed to activate hypoxia responsive genes and to respond to a decrease in glucose concentration [215]. HIF-1$\beta^{-/-}$ embryos were not viable past embryonic day 10 and showed defective angiogenesis of the yolk sac, stunted development, and embryo wasting. Similar effects were seen in HIF-1α-deficient embryos [216]. In subcutaneously (s.c.) implanted HIF-1$\alpha^{-/-}$ ES cells, vessel perfusion, oxygenation and VEGF expression were significantly reduced [217]. Tumor growth rate and apoptosis were increased in one instance, decreased in another. In a third report, VEGF mRNA levels and the growth rate of HIF-1$\alpha^{-/-}$ ES teratocarcinomas were reduced, compared with tumors derived from HIF-1$\alpha^{t/t}$ ES cells [218]. Moreover, no difference could be detected in VEGF protein levels, blood flow, vessel density, and apoptosis. Disruption of the interaction between HIF-1α and p300/CBP, a co-activator required for initiation of HIF-1-mediated transcription, led to attenuation of hypoxia-inducible gene expression and tumor growth [219]. In breast cancer cells in vitro, the cumulative induction of HIF-1α and HIF-2α protein levels was inversely related to clonogenic survival under hypoxia [220].

HIF-1 was stabilized after inactivation of the von Hippel-Lindau (VHL) tumor suppressor gene, and amplified by other oncogenic mutations [221,222]. Increased levels of HIF-1α protein in human prostate cancer cell lines correlated with increased metastatic potential [223]. More importantly, the HIF-1α subunit was overexpressed in 68% of different clinical tumors and not in non-malignant tumors such as breast fibroadenoma and uterine leiomyoma [224]. In patients undergoing chemotherapy, radiotherapy, and/or surgery, HIF-1α production was a strong independent prognostic marker in cancer of the oropharynx [225], of the esophagus [226] and the head and neck [227], in lymph node-positive breast cancer [228], in early stage [229] but not in locally advanced cervical carcinoma [230], nor in patients with ovarian cancer [231]. However, a significant reduction in overall survival after platinum-based chemotherapy was observed in ovarian cancer patients with overexpression of both p53 and HIF-1α. In early operable nonsmall- cell lung cancer, HIF-2α but not HIF-1α protein levels were significantly associated with poor prognosis [232].

Hypoxia-mediated gene regulation occurs at different levels, including transcription, mRNA stability, translation and post-translational modification. Of the two HIF subunits, $HIF_β$ is not oxygen sensitive, while $HIF_α$ is regulated at post-translational levels [233], and in some cells at the mRNA level. HIFα protein levels increase during hypoxia and the protein are degraded within 3–5 min during reoxygenation [234]. HIFα is polyubiquinated in air, by targeting it to the ubiquitinproteasome degradation pathway, a process mediated by the VHL protein [235,236]. Binding of HIFα to the VHL protein requires the hydroxylation of a $HIF_α$ praline residue in its oxygen-dependent degradation domain by a prolyl-4-hydroxylase, and is followed by the activation of the ubiquitin-E3 ligase. $HIF_α$ hydroxylation is strictly dependent on the presence of oxygen as a co-substrate and iron as a cofactor. Therefore, under hypoxia, HIFα remains stable and complexes with the β-subunit to form the functional transcription factor. To induce gene expression, HIF binds to an enhancer sequence named the hypoxia regulatory element (HRE), containing the core sequence 50-(A/G)CGT(G/C)(G/C)-30. HREs have been found at varying distances from and orientations to the coding sequence region of hypoxia-regulated genes.

The HIF/HRE transcription machinery is a powerful tool to target the hypoxic areas of solid tumors with gene therapy. In the first report on hypoxia-regulated gene therapy, a trimer of the murine PGK-1 HRE was inserted in the human 9-27 promoter to regulate the expression of the gene for the enzyme cytosine deaminase (CD) [237]. This enzyme is not toxic per se, but is able to convert the prodrug 5-fluorocytosine (5-FC) into a cytotoxic agent (gene-directed enzyme/ prodrug therapy, GDEPT) [238]. In human fibrosarcoma HT1080 cells transfected with the HRE-CD construct, a 16 h incubation under anoxia triggered HIF binding to the HREs and resulted in a 5.4-fold increase in sensitivity to 5-FC (IC50 ratio), compared with cells incubated with the prodrug in air. In vivo, HRE-mediated transgenic expression was localized adjacent to areas of pyknotic cells and necrosis. Over the last years, a number of different promoter constructs have been engineered to optimize hypoxia-mediated gene expression for gene therapy [239]. In general, the hypoxic regulation system appears to be affected by the cellular background, since cell lines of diverse origin are characterized by different responses. Moreover, different reporter assays may result in different induction levels of identical promoter constructs. For example, compared with fluorescence protein assays or immunological detection, the conversion by an enzyme of multiple substrate molecules into detectable units further amplifies any increase in transcription. In survival assays, other GDEPT paradigms have been tested, such as the Herpes Simplex Virus thymidine kinase (HSVtk) and its prodrug ganciclovir (GCV), the Escherichia coli (E. coli) nitroreductase (NTR) with CB1954, the human redox-sensitive flavoprotein NADPH: cytochrome P450 reductase (P450R) and RSU1069, the human cytochrome P450 2B6 (CYP 2B6) with the prodrug cyclophosphamide (CP), and the horseradish peroxidase (HRP)/indole-3-acetic acid (IAA) combination.

The HSVtk/GCV system is certainly the most characterized enzyme/prodrug strategy in cancer GDEPT, and is currently used in a number of clinical trials, in particular in combination with radiation [240, 241]. GCV is specifically phosphorylated by HSVtk to its monophosphate, which is subsequently converted to the di- and tri-phosphate forms by guanylate kinase and other cellular kinases. GCV-triphosphate can be incorporated into elongating DNA, causing inhibition of DNA replication and single strand breaks. Koshikawa et al. [242] constructed a retroviral vector in which the HSVtk coding sequence (CDS) was controlled by the murine VEGF promoter. After a 16 h promoter induction under anoxia, Lewis lung carcinoma A11 cell monolayers transduced with the VEGF-HSVtk retrovirus were significantly more sensitive to GCV, compared with cells transduced with an identical virus lacking the HSVtk CDS. The HSVtk CDS was replaced with the marker gene green fluorescent protein (GFP), VEGF-GFP, and VEGF-HSVtk stable lines established and implanted s.c. in the flank of syngenic C57BL/6 mice. In the VEGF-GFP tumors, upregulation of GFP expression was limited to poorly vascularized regions. Moreover, administration of 30 mg/kg GCV intraperitoneally (i.p.) twice daily for 5 days resulted in the regression of VEGF-HSVtk-lung tumors, although there was no direct evidence that GCV-mediated toxicity was due to hypoxia-regulated overexpression of HSVtk. Interestingly, another study showed that the use of a hypoxia-responsive promoter can also reduce the normal tissue toxicity of HSVtk/GCV gene therapy [243]. Mice bearing human breast carcinoma MDA-MB468 xenografts transduced with an adenovirus containing the HSVtk CDS under the control of the constitutive cytomegalovirus (CMV) showed significant weight loss and increased hepatic cellular injury and death, when treated with 25 mg/kg daily GCV. On the other hand, when the CMV promoter was replaced with the OBHRE promoter (containing a murine PGK-1 HRE trimer upstream of the minimal SV40 promoter) [244], transgene expression was limited to the tumor areas and neither weight loss nor liver abnormalities were observed. The low basal activity of the OBHRE promoter did not compromise its therapeutic potential, as shown with the CYP 2B6/CP GDEPT system.

NTR is a versatile flavoenzyme that has proven efficacy in a number of GDEPT systems in combination with nitroaromatic, nitroheterocyclic and quinone based substrates. The majority of the studies involve the prodrug CB1954, 5-(aziridin-1-yl)-2, 4-dinitrobenzamide, which can be converted by NTR, via an oxygen independent mechanism, to the difunctional alkylator 5-(aziridin-1-yl)-4-hydroxylamino-2-nitrobenzamide.

The latter compound is able to form poorly repairable DNA interstrand cross-links after further reactions with cellular thioesters, such as acetyl coenzyme-A. The NTR/CB1954 combination was tested for hypoxia gene therapy, by exploiting the transcriptional control of five copies of the human VEGF HRE in the basal CMV promoter [245,246]. In vitro, HT1080 cells stably transfected with the VEGF-NTR construct and primed by a 24 h anoxic incubation showed a 40–50-fold decrease in IC50, compared with oxic controls. In vivo, however, two injections of 50 mg/kg CB1954 failed to induce a significant growth delay of VEGF-NTR xenografts. This lack of response appeared to be due to the oxygenation status of the experimental tumors, as tumor growth delay reached significance when the animals were breathing 10% $O_2$ for 4 h prior to prodrug treatment, and the median $pO_2$ levels were reduced from 7.1 to 1.0mmHg.

For GDEPT, hypoxia can be exploited not only for selective gene expression, but also for prodrug activation, by adopting a bioreductive agent and its corresponding reductase enzyme. The redox-sensitive flavoprotein NADPH: cytochrome P450 reductase (P450R) is an important endogenous bioactivator of many nitroaromatic, aromatic N-oxide and quinone ''triggered'' hypoxia selective cytotoxins. P450R overexpression in human fibrosarcoma (HT1080) or breast cancer (MDA231) cells conferred increased sensitivity to the bioreductive drugs tirapazamine, RSU1069 (1-3-aziridinyl-2-hydroypropyl-2-nitroimidazole), mitomycin C, and porfiromycin [247,248]. In HT1080 cells transfected with the P450RCDS under the control of a murine PGK- 1 HRE trimer upstream of the SV40 minimal promoter, 18 h anoxic incubation produced a 30-fold enhancement of in vitro hypoxic cytotoxicity of RSU1069. HT1080 tumor xenografts treated with a combination of a single 10 Gy X-ray dose and RB6145 (250 mg/kg), a precursor of RSU1069, displayed a 50% cure rate at 100 days after therapy. A hypoxia-inducible GFP control was refractory to 10 Gy, RB6145 alone, or the combination, with 100% mortality at 100 days.

## Hypoxia/Radiation Dual Responsive Gene Therapy

The combination of different enhancer elements in chimeric promoters for gene therapy presents the potential advantage of targeting a wide range of cancer types, without losing specificity. An example of endogenous transcriptional co-operation between an HRE and a CArG element (CArG4) has been observed in the 5′ enhancer of the murine *Glut-1* gene [249]. CArG4 was shown to be responsible for HIF-1-independent hypoxic activation of the c-*fos* gene, via a mitogen-activated protein kinase (MAPK) pathway, involving the ternary complex factor Elk-1 [250]. However, this specific CArG4 element was found to respond poorly to IR. We have shown that combination of HREs and CArG elements can act as gene enhancers, responding to hypoxic and radiation stimuli, and can effectively control GDEPT [251]. A549 lung carcinoma cells were transiently transfected with plasmid vectors, containing either the GFP reporter or a suicide gene under control of these condition-specific gene promoters. The synthetic promoters contained either nine radiation-responsive CArG elements, or five hypoxia responsive elements derived from *PGK-1*, *Epo* or *VEGF*, or combinations of both. As expected, all HREs were significantly induced by hypoxia, with hypoxic gene expression as high as that seen for the strong CMV promoter. The *PGK-1* and *VEGF* enhancers were also activated by exposure to 2 Gy X-rays. The radiation inducibility of HREs had not been observed before, and the molecular mechanisms involved require further study.

However, it is known that enhanced VEGF production is seen after IR stimulation in tumor cells *in vitro* and *in vivo*, with a ~2-fold increase in VEGF levels 24 h after 5 Gy [252]. Moreover, ROI have been shown to play a role in the expression of *Epo*, *PGK-1* and *VEGF* in response to hypoxia, by stabilizing HIF-1 [253]. Differentiated C2C12 myoblasts and endothelial cells exposed to ROI-producing agents also exhibited a concentration dependent increase in VEGF production *in vitro* and *in vivo* [254-256]. Also, the flavoprotein diphenylene iodonium, which blocks ROI generation by NADP oxidase, abolished the hypoxic induction of HIF-1-regulated genes [257]. However, $H_2O_2$ was shown to inhibit HIF-1 binding and *Epo* induction under hypoxia [258] but this may be due to cellular damage that overwhelms the antioxidant defenses, since low $H_2O_2$ levels induce of the *Epo* and *Glut-1* HREs [259].

CArG promoters were not only activated by IR, but they also showed some response to hypoxia [252]. This effect is likely to be the result of a hypoxic stress associated pathway rather than a direct response to a change in ambient oxygen levels. Reoxygenation and hypoxia itself [254, 255] increase the intracellular levels of ROI, involved in IR- and $H_2O_2$-mediated CArG activation [260]. Indeed, it has been noted that *Egr-1* mRNA accumulated in mouse and rat kidney after ischemia/ reperfusion [261]. Rapid transcriptional inducibility of the *Egr-1* gene after hypoxia has been observed in the lung of mice breathing ~6% $O_2$ *in vivo* [262] and in endothelial cells [264] and mononuclear phagocytes *in vitro* [263, 265].

Mutational analysis indicated that the distal Egr-1 binding site (EBS)-CArG1 elements were critical for hypoxia-responsiveness [262]. We have demonstrated that chimeric HRE/CArG promoters produced the most selective and robust control of GFP expression following radiation, hypoxia or dual treatments, with the HRE/CArG combination proving the best across treatments and cell types [266]. The E9, Epo, Epo/E9 and CMV promoters were also tested in a suicide gene assay, using the novel horseradish peroxidase (HRP)/indole-3-acetic acid (IAA) GDEPT system [265]. The use of HRP/IAA confirmed the GFP data, and demonstrated that the Epo/E9 promoter could drive GDEPT at least as well as the strong, CMV IE promoter.

Despite the ability to control and target expression of therapeutic genes using radiation- and hypoxia-responsive gene promoters, the levels of expression may be low for therapeutic purposes. Furthermore transgene expression will only continue with constant stimulation by the corresponding trigger and may in part be transient. In order to address these problems, Scott SD et al. have devised a system to enable long-term, high-level expression of therapeutic genes following the modest radiation-induction of the CArG promoters. The strategy utilizes a novel 'molecular switch' based on the *Cre/loxP* recombination system of bacteriophage P1 [267]. Using this approach the radiation-responsive promoter drives the expression of the *Cre* recombinase gene, which in turn activates a transcriptionally silenced tumor-sensitizing gene following *loxP* site-mediated recombination. The therapeutic gene is then placed under the control of a strong constitutive promoter, such as the one derived from the CMV IE gene.

Scott SD et al. employed the GFP reporter to quantify the amplification of gene expression via this scheme [268]. First, a plasmid, containing a 4 CArG2 element promoter (E4) regulating *Cre* expression, was used to establish a stable MCF-7 cell line. This line was then transfected with a plasmid bearing the silenced GFP CDS. For comparison, MCF-7 cells were transfected with a construct in which E4 controlled GFP expression directly. Following a single 5 Gy dose of γ-rays, the number of fluorescent cells increased ~3-fold for E4GFP and over 8-fold for the 'switch'. In addition, the median intensity of fluorescence was ~15 times greater in the latter, extrapolating to an approximately 40-fold signal amplification using the promoter transfer compared with direct E4 control. Furthermore, tumor cell killing assays using HSVtk in place of GFP, produced a growth inhibition of 27% after 2 Gy (a typical radiation fraction value used clinically) using the switch, compared with 8% for the direct expression plasmid (E4HSVtk), a >3-fold increase. To avoid the necessity to deliver two separate vectors to each target cell, this system has now been engineered to function in a single vector. The single "molecular switch" vector has been successfully tested using the GFP reporter (in the E9CreStopGFP plasmid) and in tumor cell growth inhibition assays (with E9CreStopHSVtk) in transiently transfected MCF-7 cells. A single 3 Gy radiation dose led to a mean of 32% growth inhibition of tumor cells for E9CreStopHSVtk-transfectants, compared with 20% for E9HSVtk and 12% for radiation alone (with a cell transfection efficiency of ~12-20%). Since this system involves two controlling gene promoters, the secondary CMV promoter used above could be replaced by, for example, tumor-, tissue-, condition or microenvironment specific promoters [269, 270] if these allowed the production of sufficient therapeutic product. Thus, greater specificity, selectivity and indeed safety may be achieved.

The efficient delivery of DNA to tumor sites remains a formidable task, but progress has been made in recent years using both viral and non-viral methods. Vehicles, such as retro- and adenoviruses, liposomes and naked DNA injection, have been regularly adopted in clinical studies. Nevertheless, new therapeutic modalities are also being explored in order to overcome the limitation of poor gene transfer, including macrophages and bacteria. The ability of anaerobic bacteria to selectively germinate and replicate in necrotic and hypoxic regions of human solid tumors makes them a promising tumor-selective vehicle for gene therapeutics. In the clinic, wild type anaerobic bacteria were administered to cancer patients with little or no associated toxicity, but also no therapeutic gain [271, 272]. However, because of their large genome size, bacteria can be genetically engineered to express multiple therapeutic transgenes, and, if necessary, their spread can be controlled with antibiotics. Examples of prokaryotic vectors include anaerobic bacteria of the genera *Clostridium* [273-275], *Bifidobacterium* [276] and tumor-invasive *Salmonella* auxotroph [277]. Spores of *C. beijerinckii* genetically engineered to produce the *E. coli* enzyme, NTR, have been intravenously (i.v.) injected into tumor-bearing mice, and NTR protein was detected in all tumors tested but not in normal tissues. *In vitro* conversion of the prodrug CB1954 into a cytotoxic agent by *Clostridia*-produced NTR demonstrated the therapeutic potential of this approach. *In vivo*, i.v. injection of spores of CD-transfected *C. sporogens* followed by systemic administration of the prodrug 5-FC induced significant antitumor activity [275].

Tumor selective spore germination was also observed in rhabdomyosarcoma-bearing rats injected with five different bacterial strains, the most efficient species being *C. acetobutylicum* and *C. oncolyticum* [278]. Further tumor selectivity could be achieved by utilizing the radiation responsive prokaryotic promoter from the *recA* gene to control TNF-α expression [279]. After 2 Gy γ-rays, recombinant *C. acetobutylicum* produced levels of TNF-α 44% higher than unirradiated bacteria, and a further 42% increase was observed after a repeated 2 Gy exposure [279].

## CONCLUSION

Combining conventional cancer treatments with gene therapy offers exciting prospects for improved lung cancer control. Novel strategies that specifically target damage to tumor cells, while sparing normal tissue, will be particularly effective. We outlined two new approaches for targeting anti-tumor therapy. The first uses clinically relevant radiation doses to activate gene therapy vectors, via radiation-responsive gene promoters, following delivery to the tumor volume. This system could be applied to the wide range of tumors currently treated by radiotherapy, especially those that are highly resistant to current cancer treatments.

The second approach exploits the physiological condition of hypoxia, which occurs commonly in solid tumors but is rarely seen in normal tissues. Hypoxia-regulated gene promoters can be used to drive expression of therapeutic genes in intratumoral areas of low oxygen. Furthermore, gene therapy vectors that respond both to radiation and hypoxia stimulation have recently been developed, allowing more tumor cell populations to be targeted. An additional scheme to marry these two approaches has been to utilize attenuated anaerobic bacteria as a method of gene delivery. These bacteria carry the transgenes controlled by radiation responsive promoters to areas of hypoxia where they replicate. Such tailoring of gene therapy vectors to tumor treatment and environment, in combination with an efficient delivery system, is likely to produce significantly more efficacious clinical treatments in the near future.

## ACKNOWLEDGEMENT

This work was supported by National Natural Science Fund of China (No.3030097).

## REFERENCES

[1] Emal A, Murray T, Samuels A, Ghafoor A, Ward E, Thun M. Cancer statistics, 2003. *CA Cancer J. Clin.* 2003; 53:5–26.

[2] Schiller, JH, Harrington, D, Belani, CP, et al Comparison of four chemotherapy regimens for advanced non-small-cell lung cancer. *N. Engl. J. Med.* 2002;346:92-98.

[3] Mountain, CF Revisions in the International System for Staging Lung Cancer. *Chest.* 1997; 111:1710-1717.

[4] Kim SH, Kim JH, Djordjevic B. Effects of X-irradiation on RNA and protein synthesis in HeLa cells, *Radiat. Res.* 1970;42: 577–589.

[5] Weichselbaum RR, Hallahan D, Fuks Z, Kufe D. Radiation induction of immediate early genes: effectors of the radiation-stress response, *Int. J. Radiat. Oncol. Biol. Phys.* 1994; 30:229–234.

[6] Greenberg ME, Ziff EB. Stimulation of 3T3 cells induces transcription of the c-fos proto-oncogene, *Nature.* (1984:311; 433–438.

[7] Amundson SA, Fornace AJ. Gene expression profiles for monitoring radiation exposure, *Radiat. Prot. Dosim.* 2001; 97:11–16.

[8] Prasad AV, Mohan N, Chandrasekar B, Meltz ML. Induction of transcription of "immediate early genes" by low-dose ionizing radiation, *Radiat. Res.* 1995; 143: 263–272.

[9] Sherman ML, Datta R, Hallahan DE, Weichselbaum RR, Kufe DW. Ionizing radiation regulates expression of the c-jun protooncogene, *Proc. Natl. Acad. Sci. U.S.A.* 1990; 87: 5663–5666.

[10] Janknecht R. Regulation of the c-fos promoter, *Immunobiology.* 1995;193: 137–142.

[11] Treisman R. Transient accumulation of c-fos RNA following serum stimulation requires a conserved 5_ element and c-fos 3_ sequences, *Cell.* 1985;42: 889–902.

[12] Datta R, Rubin E, Ukhatme V, Qureshi S, Hallahan D, Weichselbaum RR, Kufe DW. Ionizing radiation activates transcription of the EGR1 gene via CArG elements, *Proc. Natl. Acad. Sci. U.S.A.* 1992; 89: 10149–10153.

[13] Chai J, Tarnawski AS. Serum response factor: discovery, biochemistry, biological roles and implications for tissue injury healing, *J. Physiol. Pharmacol.* 2002; 53 :147–157.

[14] Hazzalin C, Mahadevan LC. MAPK-regulated transcription: a continuously variable gene switch? *Nat. Rev. Mol. Cell Biol.* 2002;3: 30–40.

[15] Sharrocks AD. Complexities in ETS-domain transcription factor function and regulation: lessons from the TCF (ternary complex factor) subfamily. *The Colworth Medal Lecture, Biochem. Soc. Trans.* 2002; 30:1–9.

[16] Choi EK, Rhee YH, Park HJ, Ahn SD, Shin KH, Park KK. Effect of protein kinase C inhibitor (PKCI) on radiation sensitivity and c-fos transcription, *Int. J. Radiat. Oncol. Biol. Phys.* 2001;49:397–405.

[17] Hausser A, Storz P, Hubner S, Braendlin I, Martinez-Moya M, Link G, Johannes FJ. Protein kinase C mu selectively activates the mitogen-activated protein kinase (MAPK) p42 pathway, *FEBS Lett.* 2001;492: 39–44.

[18] Amorino GP, Hamilton VM, Valerie K, Dent P, Lammering G, Schimdt-Ullrich RK. EGF-R dependence of radiation-induced transcription factor activation in human breast carcinoma cells, *Mol. Cell Biol.* 2002;13 :2233–2244.

[19] Datta R, Hallahan DE, Kharbanda SM, Rubin E, Sherman ML, Huberman E, Weichselbaum RR, Kufe DW. Involvement of reactive oxygen intermediates in the induction of c-jun gene transcription by ionizing radiation, *Biochemistry.* 1992;31: 8300–8306.

[20] Hallahan DE, Sukhatme VP, Sherman ML, Virudachalam S, Kufe D, Weichselbaum RR. Protein kinase C mediates X-ray inducibility of nuclear signal transducers EGR1 and JUN, *Proc. Natl. Acad. Sci. U.S.A.* 1991; 88: 2156–2160.

[21] Kool J, Hamdi M, Cornelissen-Steijger P, van der Eb AJ, Terleth C, van Dam H. Induction of ATF3 by ionizing radiation is mediated via a signaling pathway that includes ATM, Nibrin1, stress-induced MAPkinases and ATF-2, *Oncogene.* 2003;22: 4235– 4242.

[22] Raingeaud J, Whitmarsh AJ, Barrett T, Derijard B, Davis RJ. MKK3- and MKK6-regulated gene expression is mediated by the p38 mitogen-activated protein kinase signal transduction pathway, *Mol. Cell Biol.* 1996;16:1247–1255.

[23] Hallahan DE, Dunphy E, Kuchibhotla J, Kraft A, Unlap T, Weichselbaum RR Prolonged c-jun expression in irradiated ataxia telangiectasia fibroblasts, *Int. J. Radiat. Oncol. Biol. Phys.* 1996;36:355–360.

[24] Angel P, Karin M. The role of Jun, Fos and the AP-1 complex in cell-proliferation and transformation, *Biochim. Biophys. Acta.* 1991; 1072 :129–157.

[25] Turpaev KT. Reactive oxygen species and regulation of gene expression, *Biochem.* (Mosc.) 2002;67:281–292.

[26] Brach MA, Hass R, Sherman ML, Gunji H, Weichselbaum RR, Kufe D. Ionizing radiation induces expression and binding activity of the nuclear factor kappa B, *J. Clin. Invest.* 1991;88:691–695.

[27] Prasad AV, Mohan N, Chandrasekar B, Meltz ML. Activation of nuclear factor kappa B in human lymphoblastoid cells by low-dose ionizing radiation, *Radiat. Res.* 1994;138:367–372.

[28] Russell JS, Tofilon PJ. Radiation-induced activation of nuclear factor-kappaB involves selective degradation of plasma membrane-associated I(kappa) B(alpha), *Mol. Biol. Cell.* 2002;13 :3431–3440.

[29] Mohan N, Meltz ML Induction of nuclear factor kappa B after low-dose ionizing radiation involves a reactive oxygen intermediate signaling pathway, *Radiat. Res.* 1994;140:97–104.

[30] Lee SJ, Dimtchev A, Lavin MF, Dritschilo A, Jung M. A novel ionizing radiation-induced signaling pathway that activates the transcription factor NF-_B, *Oncogene.* 1998;17:1821–1826.

[31] Li N, Karin M. Ionizing radiation and short wavelength UV activate NF-kappaB through two distinct mechanisms, *Proc. Natl. Acad. Sci. U.S.A.* 1998;95: 13012–13017.

[32] Wang T, Zhang X, Li JJ. The role of NF-kappaB in the regulation of cell stress responses, *Int. Immunopharmacol.* 2002;2 :1509– 1520.

[33] Honda N, Yagi K, Ding GR, Miyakoshi J. Radiosensitization by overexpression of the nonphosphorylation form of IkappaB-alpha in human glioma cells, *J. Radiat. Res.* (Tokyo) 2002;43:283–292.

[34] Ding GR, Honda N, Nakahara T, Tian F, Yoshida M, Hirose H, Miyakoshi J. Radiosensitization by inhibition of IkappaB-alpha phosphorylation in human glioma cells, *Radiat. Res.* 2003;160: 232–237.

[35] Russell JS, Raju U, Gumin GJ, Lang FF, Wilson DR, Huet T, Tofilon P.J. Inhibition of radiation-induced nuclear factor-kappaB activation by an anti-Ras single-chain antibody fragment: lack of involvement in radiosensitization, *Cancer Res.* 2002;62:2318– 2326.

[36] Schwachtgen JL, Campbell CJ, Braddock M. Full promoter sequence of human early growth response factor-1 (EGR-1): demonstration of a fifth functional serum response element, *DNA Seq.* 2000;10: 429–432.

[37] Datta R, Taneja N, Sukhatme V., Qureshi SA, Weichselbaum R, Kufe DW. Reactive oxygen intermediates target CC(A/T)6GG sequences to mediate activation of the early growth response 1 transcription factor gene by ionizing radiation, *Proc. Natl. Acad. Sci. U.S.A.* 1993;90: 2419–2422.

[38] Lim CP, Jain N, Cao X. Stress-induced immediated-early gene, egr-1, involves activation of p38/JNK1, *Oncogene.* 1998; 16: 2915– 2926.

[39] Suzuki K, Kodama S, Watanabe M. Extremely low-dose ionizing radiation causes activation of mitogen-activated protein kinase pathway and enhances proliferation of normal human diploid cells, *Cancer Res.* 2001; 61: 5396–5401.

[40] Meyer RG, Kupper JH, Kandolf R, Rodemann HP. Early growth response-1 gene (Egr-1) promoter induction by ionizing radiation in U87 malignant glioma cells in vitro, *Eur. J. Biochem.* 2002;269: 337–346.

[41] Brown JM. Therapeutic targets in radiotherapy. *Int. J. Radiat. Oncol. Biol. Phys.* 2001; 49: 319-26.

[42] Harrington KJ, Melcher AA, Bateman AR, Ahmed A, Vile RG. Cancer gene therapy: Part 2. Candidate transgenes and their clinical development. *Clin. Oncol.* (*R. Coll. Radiol.*) 2002; 14: 148-69.

[43] Harrington KJ, Bateman AR, Melcher AA, Ahmed A, Vile RG. Cancer gene therapy: Part 1. Vector development and regulation of gene expression. *Clin. Oncol.* (*R. Coll. Radiol.*) 2002; 14: 3-16.

[44] Human Gene Marker/Therapy Clinical Protocols. *Hum. Gene Ther.* 2000; 11: 2543-617.

[45] Greco O, Scott SD, Marples B, Dachs GU. Cancer gene therapy: 'delivery, delivery, delivery'. *Front Biosci.* 2002; 7: d1516-24.

[46] Boothman DA, Bouvard I, Hughes EN. Identification and characterization of X-ray-induced proteins in human cells. *Cancer Res.* 1989; 49: 2871-2878.

[47] Fornace AJ. Mammalian genes induced by radiation; activation of genes associated with growth control. *Annu. Rev. Genet.* 1992; 26: 507-526.

[48] Boothman DA, Majmudar G, Johnson T. Immediate X-ray-inducible responses from mammalian cells. *Radiation Research.* 1994; 138(1 Suppl):S44-6.

[49] Amundson SA, Do KT, Fornace AJ. Jr. Induction of stress genes by low doses of gamma rays. *Radiat. Res.* 1999; 152: 225-231.

[50] el-Deiry WS, Tokino T, Velculescu VE, Levy DB, Parsons R, Trent JM, et al. WAF1, a potential mediator of p53 tumor suppression. *Cell.* 1993; 75: 817-25.

[51] Kastan MB, Zhan Q, el-Deiry WS, Carrier F, Jacks T, Walsh WV, et al. A mammalian cell cycle checkpoint pathway utilizing p53 and GADD45 is defective in ataxia-telangiectasia. *Cell.* 1992; 71: 587-97.

[52] Zhan Q, Lord KA, Alamo IJ, Hollander MC, Carrier F, Ron D, et al. The gadd and MyD genes define a novel set of mammalian genes encoding acidic proteins that synergistically suppress cell growth. *J. Mol. Cell Biol.* 1994; 14: 2361-2371.

[53] Seung LP, Mauceri HJ, Beckett MA, Hallahan DE, Hellman S, Weichselbaum RR. Genetic radiotherapy overcomes tumor resistance to cytotoxic agents. *Cancer Res.* 1995; 55: 5561-5.

[54] Buchsbaum DJ, Raben D, Stackhouse MA, Khazaeli MB, Rogers BE, Rosenfeld ME, et al. Approaches to enhance cancer radiotherapy employing gene transfer methods. *Gene Ther.* 1996; 3: 1042-68.

[55] Staba MJ, Mauceri HJ, Kufe DW, Hallahan DE, Weichselbaum RR. Adenoviral TNF-alpha gene therapy and radiation damage tumor vasculature in a human malignant glioma xenograft. *Gene Ther.* 1998; 5: 293-300.

[56] Weichselbaum RR, Hallahan DE, Beckett MA, Mauceri HJ, Lee H, Sukhatme VP, et al. Gene therapy targeted by radiation preferentially radiosensitizes tumor cells. *Cancer Res.* 1994; 54: 4266-9.

[57] Hallahan DE, Mauceri HJ, Seung LP, Dunphy EJ, Wayne JD, Hanna NN, et al. Spatial and temporal control of gene therapy using ionizing radiation. *Nat. Med.* 1995; 1: 786-91.

[58] Mauceri HJ, Hanna NN, Wayne JD, Hallahan DE, Hellman S, Weichselbaum RR. Tumor necrosis factor alpha (TNF-alpha) gene therapy targeted by ionizing radiation selectively damages tumor vasculature. *Cancer Res.* 1996; 56: 4311-4.

[59] Mauceri HJ, Seung LP, Grdina WL, Swedberg KA, Weichselbaum RR. Increased injection number enhances adenoviral genetic radiotherapy. *Radiat. Oncol. Investig.* 1997; 5: 220-6.

[60] Joki T, Nakamura M, Ohno T. Activation of the radiosensitive EGR-1 promoter induces expression of the herpes simplex virus thymidine kinase gene and sensitivity of human glioma cells to ganciclovir. *Hum. Gene Ther.* 1995; 6: 1507-13.

[61] Takahashi T, Namiki Y, Ohno T. Induction of the suicide HSV-TK gene by activation of the Egr-1 promoter with radioisotopes. *Hum. Gene Ther.* 1997; 8: 827-833.

[62] Kawashita Y, Ohtsuru A, Kaneda Y, Nagayama Y, Kawazoe Y, Eguchi S, et al. Regression of hepatocellular carcinoma in vitro and in vivo by radiosensitizing suicide gene therapy under the inducible and spatial control of radiation. *Hum. Gene Ther.* 1999; 10: 1509-19.

[63] Marples B, Scott SD, Hendry JH, Embleton MJ, Lashford LS, Margison GP. Development of synthetic promoters for radiation-mediated gene therapy. *Gene Ther.* 2000; 7: 511-517.

[64] Scott SD, Joiner MC, Marples B. Optimizing radiation-responsive gene promoters for radiogenetic cancer therapy. *Gene Ther.* 2002; 9: 1396-1402.

[65]

[66] Kim JH, Kim SH, Brown SL, Freytag SO. Selective enhancement by an antiviral agent of the radiation-induced cell killing of human glioma cells transduced with HSV-tk gene. *Cancer Res.* 1994; 54: 6053-6.

[67] Kim JH, Kim SH, Kolozsvary A, Brown SL, Kim OB, Freytag SO. Selective enhancement of radiation response of herpes simplex virus thymidine kinase transduced 9L gliosarcoma cells in vitro and in vivo by antiviral agents. *Int. J. Radiat. Oncol. Biol. Phys.* 1995; 33: 861-8.

[68] Freeman SM, Abboud CN, Whartenby KA, Packman CH, Koeplin DS, Moolten FL, et al. The "bystander effect": tumor regression when a fraction of the tumor mass is genetically modified. *Cancer Res.* 1993; 53: 5274-83.

[69] Elliott G, O'Hare P. Intercellular trafficking and protein delivery by a herpesvirus structural protein. *Cell.* 1997; 88: 223-33.

[70] Lai Z, Han I, Zirzow G, Brady RO, Reiser J. Intercellular delivery of a herpes simplex virus VP22 fusion protein from cells infected with lentiviral vectors. *Proc. Natl. Acad. Sci. USA.* 2000; 97: 11297-302.

[71] Wybranietz WA, Gross CD, Phelan A, O'Hare P, Spiegel M, Graepler F, et al. Enhanced suicide gene effect by adenoviral transduction of a VP22-cytosine deaminase (CD) fusion gene. *Gene Ther.* 2001; 8: 1654-64.

[72] Zender L, Kock R, Eckhard M, Frericks B, Gosling T, Gebhardt T, et al. Gene therapy by intrahepatic and intratumoral trafficking of p53-VP22 induces regression of liver tumors. *Gastroenterology.* 2002; 123: 608-18.

[73] Marples B, Greco O, Joiner MC, Scott SD. Molecular approaches to chemo-radiotherapy. *Eur. J. Cancer.* 2002; 38: 231-9.

[74] Luft FC. Can VP22 resurrect gene therapy? *J. Mol. Med.* 1999; 77: 575-6.

[75] Derer W, Easwaran HP, Knopf CW, Leonhardt H, Cardoso MC. Direct protein transfer to terminally differentiated muscle cells. *J. Mol. Med.* 1999; 77, 609-13.

[76] Lai Z, Brady RO. Gene transfer into the central nervous system in vivo using a recombinanat lentivirus vector. *J. Neurosci. Res.* 2002; 67: 363-71.

[77] Wills KN, Atencio IA, Avanzini JB, Neuteboom S, Phelan A, Philopena J, et al. Intratumoral spread and increased efficacy of a p53-VP22 fusion protein expressed by a recombinant adenovirus. *J. Virol.* 2001; 75: 8733-41.

[78] Cheng WF, Hung CF, Hsu KF, Chai CY, He L, Polo JM, et al. Cancer immunotherapy using Sindbis virus replicon particles encoding a VP22-antigen fusion. *Hum. Gene Ther.* 2002; 13: 553-68.

[79] Rogulski KR, Wing MS, Paielli DL, Gilbert JD, Kim JH, Freytag SO. Double suicide gene therapy augments the antitumor activity of a replication-competent lytic adenovirus through enhanced cytotoxicity and radiosensitization. *Hum. Gene Ther.* 2000; 11: 67-76.

[80] Press OW, Rasey J. Principles of radioimmunotherapy for hematologists and oncologists. *Semin. Oncol.* 2000; 27: 62-73.

[81] Mairs RJ, Cunningham SH, Boyd M, Carlin S. Applications of gene transfer to targeted radiotherapy. *Curr. Pharm. Des.* 2000; 6: 1419-32.

[82] Mairs RJ. Neuroblastoma therapy using radiolabelled [131I]meta-iodobenzylguanidine ([131I]MIBG) in combination with other agents. *Eur. J. Cancer.* 1999; 35: 1171-3.

[83] Boyd M, Mairs RJ, Cunningham SH, Mairs SC, McCluskey A, Livingstone A, et al. A gene herapy/targeted radiotherapy strategy for radiation cell kill by. *J. Gene Med.* 2001 Mar-Apr;3(2):165-72. *J. Gene Med.* 2001; 3: 165-72.

[84] Boyd M, Mairs RJ, Mairs SC, Wilson L, Livingstone A, Cunningham SH, et al. Expression in UVW glioma cells of the noradrenaline transporter gene, driven by the telomerase RNA promoter, induces active uptake of [131I]MIBG and clonogenic cell kill. *Oncogene.* 2001; 20: 7804-8.

[85] Boyd M, Cunningham SH, Brown MM, Mairs RJ, Wheldon TE. Noradrenaline transporter gene transfer for radiation cell kill by 131I meta-iodobenzylguanidine. *Gene Ther.* 1999; 6: 1147-52.

[86] Cunningham S, Boyd M, Brown MM, Carlin S, McCluskey A, Livingstone A, et al. A gene therapy approach to enhance the targeted radiotherapy of neuroblastoma. *Med. Pediatr. Oncol.* 2000; 35: 708-11.

[87] Carlin S, Cunning SH, Boyd M, McCluskey AG, Mairs RJ. Experimental targeted radioiodide therapy following transfection of the sodium iodide symporter gene: effect on clonogenicity in both two-and three-dimensional models. *Cancer Gene Ther.* 2000; 7: 1529-1536.

[88] Epperly MW, Gretton JA, DeFilippi SJ, Greenberger JS, Sikora CA, Liggitt D, et al. Modulation of radiation-induced cytokine elevation associated with esophagitis and esophageal stricture by manganese superoxide dismutase-plasmid/liposome (SOD2-PL) gene therapy. *Radiat. Res.* 2001; 155: 2-14.

[89] Epperly MW, Defilippi S, Sikora C, Gretton J, Kalend A, Greenberger JS. Intratracheal injection of manganese superoxide dismutase (MnSOD) plasmid/liposomes protects normal lung but not orthotopic tumors from irradiation. *Gene Ther.* 2000; 7: 1011-8.

[90] Jain RK. Transport of molecules in the tumor interstitium: A review. 1987;47:3039–3051.

[91] Brown JM. Selective radiosensitization of the hypoxic cells of mouse tumours with the nitroimidazoles metronidazole and Ro 7- 0582. *Radiat. Res.* 1975;64:633–647.

[92] Vaupel P, Hockel M. 1998. Oxygenation of human tumours. In: Molls M, Vaupel P, editors. *Blood perfusion and microenvironment of human tumours.* Berlin: Springer-Verlag. pp 63–72.

[93] Fyles AW, Milosevic M, Wong R, Kavanagh MC, Pintilie M, Sun A, Chapman W, Levin W, Manchul L, Keane TJ, Hill RP. Oxygenation predicts radiation response and survival in patients with cervix cancer. *Radiother. Oncol.* 1998;48:149–156.

[94] Boyer P, Chance B, Ernester L, Mitchell P, Racker E, Slater EC. Oxidative phosphorylation and photo phosphorylation. Annu Rev Biochem 1977;46:955–1026.

[95] Zander R, Vaupel P. Proposal for using a standardized terminology on oxygen transport to tissue. *Adv. Exp. Med. Biol.* 1985;191:965–970.

[96] Hall EJ. 2000. Radiobiology for the radiologist. Philadelphia: Lippincott Williams and Wilkins. Pp 588.

[97] Thomlinson RH, Gray LH. The histological structure of some human lung cancers and the possible implications for radiotherapy. *Br. J. Cancer.* 1955;9:539–549.

[98] Brown JM. Evidence for autely hypoxic cells in mouse tumours and a possible mechanism of reoxygenation. 1979;52:650–656.

[99] Chaplin DJ, Olive PL, Durand RE. Intermittent blood flow in a murine tumor: Radiobiological effects. *Cancer Res.* 1987;47:597–601.

[100] Kimura H, Braun RD, Ong ET, Hsu R, Secomb TW, Papahadjopoulos D, Hong K, Dewhirst MW. Fluctuations in red cell flux in tumormicrovessels can lead to transient hypoxia and reoxygenation in tumor parenchyma. *Cancer Res.* 1996;56:5522–5528.

[101] Hill SA, Pigott KH, Saunders MI, Powell ME, Arnold S, Obeid A,Ward G, Leahy M, Hoskin PJ, Chaplin DJ. Microregional blood flow in murine and human tumours assessed using laser Doppler microprobes. *Br. J. Cancer.* 1996;Suppl 27:S260–S263.

[102] Brizel DM, Sibley GS, Prosnitz LR, Scher RL, Dewhirst MW. Tumor hypoxia adversely affects the prognosis of carcinoma of the head and neck. *Int. J. Radiat. Oncol. Biol. Phys.* 1997;38:285–289.

[103] Raleigh JA, Calkins-Adams DP, Rinker LH, Ballenger CA, Weissler MC, Fowler WC, Jr., Novotny DB, Varia MA. Hypoxia and vascular endothelial growth factor expression in human squamous cell carcinomas using pimonidazole as a hypoxia marker. *Cancer Res.* 1998;58:3765–3768.

[104] Vaupel P, Kallinowski F, Okunieff P. Blood flow, oxygen and nutrient supply, and metabolic microenviroment of human tumors: A review. 1989;49:6449–6465.

[105] Stone HB, Brown JM, Phillips TL, Sutherland RM. Oxygen in human tumors: Correlations between methods of measurement and response to therapy. *Radiat. Res.* 1993;136:422–434.

[106] West CM, Cooper RA, Loncaster JA, Wilks DP, Bromley M. Tumor vascularity: A histological measure of angiogenesis and hypoxia. *Cancer Res.* 2001;61:2907–2910.

[107] Partridge SE, Aquino-Parsons C, Luo C, Green A, Olive PL. A pilot study comparing intratumoral oxygenation using the comet assay following 2.5% and 5% carbogen and 100% oxygen. *Int. J. Radiat. Oncol. Biol. Phys.* 2001;49:575–580.

[108] Airley R, Loncaster J, Davidson S, Bromley M, Roberts S, Patterson A, Hunter R, Stratford I, West C. Glucose transporter glut-1 expression correlates with tumor hypoxia and predicts metastasisfree survival in advanced carcinoma of the cervix. *Clin. Cancer Res.* 2001;7:928–934.

[109] Airley RE, Loncaster J, Raleigh JA, Harris AL, Davidson SE, Hunter RD, West CM, Stratford IJ. GLUT-1 and CAIX as intrinsic markers of hypoxia in carcinoma of the cervix: Relationship to pimonidazole binding. *Int. J. Cancer.* 2003;104:85–91.

[110] Chapman JD, Baer K, Lee J. Characteristics of the metabolisminduced binding of misonidazole to hypoxic mammalian cells. *Cancer Res.* 1983;43:1523–1528.

[111] Arteel GE, Thurman RG, Yates JM, Raleigh JA. Evidence that hypoxia markers detect oxygen gradients in liver: Pimonidazole and retrograde perfusion of rat liver. *Br. J. Cancer.* 1995;72:889–895.

[112] Evans SM, Hahn SM, Magarelli DP, Zhang PJ, Jenkins WT, Fraker DL, Hsi RA, McKenna WG, Koch CJ. Hypoxia in human intraperitoneal and extremity sarcomas. *Int. J. Radiat. Oncol. Biol. Phys.* 2001;49:587–596.

[113] Vaupel P, Schlenger K, Knoop C, Hockel M. Oxygenation of human tumors: Evaluation of tissue oxygen distribution in breast cancers by computerized O2 tension measurements. *Cancer Res.* 1991;51:3316–3322.

[114] Collingridge DR, Young WK, Vojnovic B, Wardman P, Lynch EM, Hill SA, Chaplin DJ. Measurement of tumor oxygenation: A comparison between polarographic needle electrodes and a timeresolved luminescence-based optical sensor. *Radiat. Res.* 1997;147:329– 334.

[115] Nordsmark M, Loncaster J, Chou SC, Havsteen H, Lindegaard JC, Davidson SE, Varia M, West C, Hunter R, Overgaard J, Raleigh JA. Invasive oxygen measurements and pimonidazole labeling in human cervix carcinoma. *Int. J. Radiat. Oncol. Biol. Phys.* 2001;49:581–586.

[116] Pigott KH, Hill SA, Chaplin DJ, Saunders MI. Microregional fluctuations in perfusion within human tumours detected using laser Doppler flowmetry. *Radiother. Oncol.* 1996;40:45–50.

[117] Becker A, Hansgen G, BlochingM,Weigel C, Lautenschlager C, Dunst J. Oxygenation of squamous cell carcinoma of the head and neck: Comparison of primary tumors, neck node metastases, and normal tissue. *Int. J. Radiat. Oncol. Biol. Phys.* 1998;42:35–41.

[118] Gray LH, Conger AO, Ebert M, Hornsey S, Scott OCA. The concentration of oxygen dissolved in tissues at the time of irradiation as a factor in radiotherapy. *Br. J. Radiol.* 1953;26:638–648.

[119] Brizel DM, Scully SP, Harrelson JM, Layfield LJ, Bean JM, Prosnitz LR, Dewhirst MW. Tumor oxygenation predicts for the likelihood of distant metastases in human soft tissue sarcoma. *Cancer Res.* 1996;56:941–943.

[120] Nordsmark M, Alsner J, Keller J, Nielsen OS, Jensen OM, Horsman MR, Overgaard J. Hypoxia in human soft tissue sarcomas: Adverse impact on survival and no association with p53 mutations. *Br. J. Cancer.* 2001;84:1070–1075.

[121] Hockel M, Schlenger K, Aral B, Mitze M, Schaffer U, Vaupel P. Association between tumor hypoxia and malignant progression in advanced cancer of the uterine cervix. *Cancer Res.* 1996;56:4509–4515.

[122] Knocke TH, Weitmann HD, Feldmann HJ, Selzer E, Potter R. Intratumoral $pO_2$-measurements as predictive assay in the treatment of carcinoma of the uterine cervix. *Radiother. Oncol.* 1999;53:99–104.

[123] Fyles A, Milosevic M, Hedley D, Pintilie M, Levin W, Manchul L, Hill RP. Tumor hypoxia has independent predictor impact only in patients with node-negative cervix cancer. *J. Clin. Oncol.* 2002;20:680–687.

[124] Nordsmark M, Overgaard M, Overgaard J. Pretreatment oxygenation predicts radiation response in advanced squamous cell carcinoma of the head and neck. *Radiother. Oncol.* 1996;41:31–39.

[125] Brizel DM, Dodge RK, Clough RW, Dewhirst MW. Oxygenation of head and neck cancer: Changes during radiotherapy and impact on treatment outcome. *Radiother. Oncol.* 1999;53:113–117.

[126] Nordsmark M, Overgaard J. A confirmatory prognostic study on oxygenation status and loco-regional control in advanced head and neck squamous cell carcinoma treated by radiation therapy. *Radiother. Oncol.* 2000;57:39–43.

[127] Sundfor K, Lyng H, Rofstad EK. Tumour hypoxia and vascular density as predictors of metastasis in squamous cell carcinoma of the uterine cervix. *Br. J. Cancer.* 1998;78:822–827.

[128] Graham CH, Forsdike J, Fitzgerald CJ, Macdonald-Goodfellow S. Hypoxia-mediated stimulation of carcinoma cell invasiveness via upregulation of urokinase receptor expression. *Int. J. Cancer.* 1999;80:617–623.

[129] Walenta S, Wetterling M, Lehrke M, Schwickert G, Sundfor K, Rofstad EK, Mueller-Klieser W. High lactate levels predict likelihood of metastases, tumor

recurrence, and restricted patient survival in human cervical cancers. *Cancer Res.* 2000;60:916–921.

[130] Teicher BA, Lazo JS, Sartorelli AC. Classification of antineoplastic agents by their selective toxicities toward oxygenated and hypoxic tumor cells. *Cancer Res.* 1981;41:73–81.

[131] Grau C, Overgaard J. Effect of cancer chemotherapy on the hypoxic fraction of a solid tumor measured using a local tumor control assay. *Radiother. Oncol.* 1988;13:301–309.

[132] Chaplin DJ, Acker B, Olive PL. Potentiation of the tumor cytotoxicity of melphalan by vasodilating drugs. *Int. J. Radiat. Oncol. Biol. Phys.* 1989;16:1131–1135.

[133] Durand RE, Raleigh JA. Identification of nonproliferating but viable hypoxic tumor cells in vivo. *Cancer Res.* 1998;58:3547–3550.

[134] Amellem O, Pettersen EO. Cell inactivation and cell cycle inhibition as induced by extreme hypoxia: The possible role of cell cycle arrest as a protection against hypoxia-induced lethal damage. *Cell Prolif.* 1991;24:127–141.

[135] Giaccia AJ. Hypoxic stress proteins: Survival of the fittest. *Semin. Radiat. Oncol.* 1996;6:46–58.

[136] Krtolica A, Ludlow JW. Hypoxia arrests ovarian carcinoma cell cycle progression, but invasion is unaffected. *Cancer Res.* 1996;56:1168–1173.

[137] Schmaltz C, Hardenbergh PH, Wells A, Fisher DE. Regulation of proliferation-survival decisions during tumor cell hypoxia. *Mol. Cell Biol.* 1998;18:2845–2854.

[138] Tannock IF. The relation between cell proliferationand the vacular system in a transplanted mouse mammary tumour. *Br. J. Cancer.* 1968;22:258–273.

[139] Minchinton AI, Durand RE, Chaplin DJ. Intermittent blood flow in the KHT sarcoma-flow cytometry studies using Hoechst 33342. *Br. J. Cancer.* 1990;62:195–200.

[140] Rodriguez R, Ritter MA, Fowler JF, Kinsella TJ. Kinetics of cell labeling and thymidine replacement after continuous infusion of halogenated pyrimidines in vivo. *Int. J. Radiat. Oncol. Biol. Phys.* 1994;29:105–113.

[141] Griffiths JR. Are cancer cells acidic? *Br. J. Cancer.* 1991;64:425–427.

[142] Chaplin DJ, Horsman MR, Trotter M, Siemann D. 1998. Therapeutic significance of microenvironmental factors. In: Molls M, Vaupel P, editors. Blood perfusion and microenvironment of human tumours. Berlin: Springer-Verlag, pp 133–143.

[143] Shen J, Hughes C, Chao C, Cai J, Bartels C, Gessner T, Subjeck J. Coinduction of glucose-regulated proteins and doxorubicin resistance in Chinese hamster cells. *Proc. Natl. Acad. Sci. USA.* 1987;84:3278–3282.

[144] Hughes CS, Shen JW, Subjeck JR. Resistance to etoposide induced by three glucose-regulated stresses in Chinese hamster ovary cells. *Cancer Res.* 1989;49:4452–4454.

[145] Sanna K, Rofstad EK. Hypoxia-induced resistance to doxorubicin and methotrexate in human melanoma cell lines in vitro. *Int. J. Cancer.* 1994;58:258–262.

[146] Janssen YM, Van Houten B, Borm PJ, Mossman BT. Cell and tissue responses to oxidative damage. *Lab. Invest.* 1993;69:261–274.

[147] Russo CA, Weber TK, Volpe CM, Stoler DL, Petrelli NJ, Rodriguez- Bigas M, Burhans WC, Anderson GR. An anoxia inducible endonuclease and enhanced DNA breakage as contributors to genomic instability in cancer. *Cancer Res.* 1995;55:1122–1128.

[148] Reynolds TY, Rockwell S, Glazer PM. Genetic instability induced by the tumor microenvironment. *Cancer Res.* 1996;56:5754–5757.

[149] Yao KS, Clayton M, O'Dwyer PJ. Apoptosis in human adenocarcinoma HT29 cells induced by exposure to hypoxia. *J. Natl. Cancer Inst.* 1995;87:117–122.

[150] Graeber TG, Osmanian C, Jacks T, Housman DE, Koch CJ, Lowe SW, Giaccia AJ. Hypoxia-mediated selection of cells with diminished apoptotic potential in solid tumours. *Nature.* 1996; 379:88–91.

[151] Kim CY, Tsai MH, Osmanian C, Graeber TG, Lee JE, Giffard RG, DiPaolo JA, Peehl DM, Giaccia AJ. Selection of human cervical epithelial cells that possess reduced apoptotic potential to low-oxygen conditions. *Cancer Res.* 1997;57:4200–4204.

[152] Shimizu S, Eguchi Y, Kosaka H, KamiikeW,Matsuda H, Tsujimoto Y. Prevention of hypoxia-induced cell death by Bcl-2 and Bcl-xL. *Nature.* 1995;374:811–813.

[153] Soengas MS, Alarcon RM, Yoshida H, Giaccia AJ, Hakem R, Mak TW, Lowe SW. Apaf-1 and caspase-9 in p53-dependent apoptosis and tumor inhibition. *Science.* 1999;284:156–159.

[154] Alarcon RM, Rupnow BA, Graeber TG, Knox SJ, Giaccia AJ. Modulation of c-Myc activity and apoptosis in vivo. *Cancer Res.* 1996;56:4315–4319.

[155] Haensgen G, Krause U, Becker A, Stadler P, Lautenschlaeger C, WohlrabW, Rath FW, Molls M, Dunst J. Tumor hypoxia, p53, and prognosis in cervical cancers. *Int. J. Radiat. Oncol. Biol. Phys.* 2001;50:865–872.

[156] Sheridan MT, West CM, Cooper RA, Stratford IJ, Logue JP, Davidson SE, Hunter RD. Pretreatment apoptosis in carcinoma of the cervix correlates with changes in tumour oxygenation during radiotherapy. *Br. J. Cancer.* 2000;82:1177–1182.

[157] Hasan NM, Adams GE, Joiner MC, Marshall JF, Hart IR. Hypoxia facilitates tumour cell detachment by reducing expression of surface adhesion molecules and adhesion to extracellular matrices without loss of cell viability. *Br. J. Cancer.* 1998;77:1799–1805.

[158] Rofstad EK, Rasmussen H, Galappathi K, Mathiesen B, Nilsen K, Graff BA. Hypoxia promotes lymph node metastasis in human melanoma xenografts by up-regulating the urokinase-type plasminogen activator receptor. *Cancer Res.* 2002;62:1847–1853.

[159] Niizeki H, Kobayashi M, Horiuchi I, Akakura N, Chen J, Wang J, Hamada JI, Seth P, Katoh H, Watanabe H, Raz A, Hosokawa M. Hypoxia enhances the expression of

autocrine motility factor and the motility of human pancreatic cancer cells. *Br. J. Cancer.* 2002;86: 1914–1919.

[160] Pitson G, Fyles A, Milosevic M, Wylie J, Pintilie M, Hill R. Tumor size and oxygenation are independent predictors of nodal diseases in patients with cervix cancer. *Int. J. Radiat. Oncol. Biol. Phys.* 2001;51:699–703.

[161] Brizel DM, Schroeder T, Scher RL, Walenta S, Clough RW, Dewhirst MW, Mueller-Klieser W. Elevated tumor lactate concentrations predict for an increased risk of metastases in head-and-neck cancer. *Int. J. Radiat. Oncol. Biol. Phys.* 2001;51:349–353.

[162] Cairns RA, Kalliomaki T, Hill RP. Acute (cyclic) hypoxia enhances spontaneous metastasis of KHT murine tumors. *Cancer Res.* 2001.61:8;903–8908.

[163] Churchill-Davidson I. Hyperbaric oxygen and radiotherapy: Clinical experiences. *Front Radiat. Ther. Oncol.* 1968;1:156–161.

[164] Overgaard J, Horsman MR. 1997. Overcoming hypoxic cell radioresistance. In: Steel GG, editor. *Basic clinical radiobiology.* London: Arnold. pp 141–151.

[165] Adams GE, Cooke MS. Electron-affinic sensitization. A structural basis for chemical radiosensitizers in bacteria. *Int. J. Radiat. Biol.* 1969;15:457–471.

[166] Adams GE, Asquith JC, Watts ME, Smithen CE. Radiosensitization of hypoxic cells in vitro: A water-soluble derivative of paranitroacetophenone. *Nat. New Biol.* 1972; 239:23–24.

[167] Sheldon PW, Foster JL, Fowler JF. Radiosensitisation of C3H mouse mammary tumours by a 2-nitroimidazole. *Br. J. Cancer.* 1974;30:560–565.

[168] Dische S. Chemical sensitizers for hypoxic cells: A decade of experience in clinical radiotherapy. *Radiother. Oncol.* 1985;3:97–115.

[169] Overgaard J, Hansen HS, Overgaard M, Bastholt L, Berthelsen A, Specht L, Lindelov B, Jorgensen K. A randomized doubleblind phase III study of nimorazole as a hypoxic radiosensitizer of primary radiotherapy in supraglottic larynx and pharynx carcinoma. Results of the Danish Head and Neck Cancer Study (DAHANCA) Protocol 5-85. *Radiother. Oncol.* 1998;46:135–146.

[170] Chaplin DJ, HorsmanMR, Trotter MJ. Effect of nicotinamide on the microregional heterogeneity of oxygen delivery within a murine tumor. *J. Natl. Cancer Inst.* 1990;82:672–676.

[171] Kjellen E, Joiner MC, Collier JM, Johns H, Rojas A. A therapeutic benefit from combining normobaric carbogen or oxygen with nicotinamide in fractionated X-ray treatments. *Radiother. Oncol.* 1991;22:81–91.

[172] Hoskin PJ, Saunders MI, Phillips H, Cladd H, Powell ME, Goodchild K, Stratford MR, Rojas A. Carbogen and nicotinamide in the treatment of bladder cancer with radical radiotherapy. *Br. J. Cancer.* 1997;76:260–263.

[173] Hoskin PJ, Saunders MI, Dische S. Hypoxic radiosensitizers in radical radiotherapy for patients with bladder carcinoma: Hyperbaric oxygen, misonidazole, and accelerated radiotherapy, carbogen, and nicotinamide. *Cancer.* 1999;86:1322–1328.

[174] Miralbell R, Mornex F, Greiner R, Bolla M, Storme G, Hulshof M, Bernier J, Denekamp J, Rojas AM, Pierart M, van Glabbeke M, Mirimanoff RO. Accelerated radiotherapy, carbogen, and nicotinamide in glioblastoma multiforme: Report of European Organization for Research and Treatment of Cancer Trial 22933. *J. Clin. Oncol.* 1999;17:3143–3149.

[175] Bernier J, Denekamp J, Rojas A, Minatel E, Horiot J, Hamers H, Antognoni P, Dahl O, Richaud P, van Glabbeke M, Pierart M. ARCON: Accelerated radiotherapy with carbogen and nicotinamide in head and neck squamous cell carcinomas. The experience of the co-operative group of radiotherapy of the european organization for research and treatment of cancer (EORTC). *Radiother. Oncol.* 2000;55: 111–119.

[176] Kaanders JH. Pop LA, Marres HA, Bruaset I, van den Hoogen FJ, Merkx MA, van der Kogel AJ. ARCON: Experience in 215 patients with advanced head-and-neck cancer. *Int. J. Radiat. Oncol. Biol. Phys.* 2002;52:769–778.

[177] Stratford IJ, Workman P. Bioreductive drugs into the next millennium. *Anticancer Drug Des.* 1998;13:519–528.

[178] Rauth AM, Mohindra JK, Tannock IF. Activity of mitomycin C for aerobic and hypoxic cells in vitro and in vivo. *Cancer Res.* 1983;43:4154–4158.

[179] Brown JM, Wang LH. Tirapazamine: Laboratory data relevant to clinical activity. *Anticancer Drug Des.* 1998;13:529–539.

[180] Mohindra JK, Rauth AM. Increased cell killing by metronidazole and nitrofurazone of hypoxic compared to aerobic mammalian cells. *Cancer Res.* 1976;36:930–936.

[181] Hill RP, Gulyas S, Whitmore GF. Studies of the in vivo and in vitro cytotoxicity of the drug RSU-1069. *Br. J. Cancer.* 1986;53:743–751.

[182] Stratford IJ, O'Neill P, Sheldon PW, Silver AR, Walling JM, Adams GE. RSU 1069, a nitroimidazole containing an aziridine group. Bioreduction greatly increases cytotoxicity under hypoxic conditions. *Biochem. Pharmacol.* 1986;35:105–109.

[183] Jaffar M, Naylor MA, Robertson N, Lockyer SD, Phillips RM, Everett SA, Adams GE, Stratford IJ. 5-Substituted analogues of 3- hydroxymethyl-5-aziridinyl-1-methyl-2-1H-indole-4,7-dioneprop-2- en-1-ol (EO9, NSC 382459) and their regioisomers as hypoxiaselective agents: Structure-cytotoxicity in vitro. *Anticancer Drug Des.* 1998;13:105–123.

[184] Haffty BG, Son YH, Papac R, Sasaki CT, Weissberg JB, Fischer D, Rockwell S, Sartorelli AC, Fischer JJ. Chemotherapy as an adjunct to radiation in the treatment of squamous cell carcinoma of the head and neck: Results of the Yale mitomycin randomized trials. *J. Clin. Oncol.* 1997;15:268–276.

[185] Del Rowe J, Scott C, Werner-Wasik M, Bahary JP, Curran WJ, Urtasun RC, Fisher B. Single-arm, open-label phase II study of intravenously administered tirapazamine

and radiation therapy for glioblastoma multiforme. *J. Clin. Oncol.* 2000;18:1254–1259.

[186] Craighead PS, Pearcey R, Stuart G. A phase I/II evaluation of tirapazamine administered intravenously concurrent with cisplatin and radiotherapy in women with locally advanced cervical cancer. *Int. J. Radiat. Oncol. Biol. Phys.* 2000;48:791–795.

[187] Rischin D, Peters L, Hicks R, Hughes P, Fisher R, Hart R, Sexton M, D'Costa I, von Roemeling R. Phase I trial of concurrent tirapazamine, cisplatin, and radiotherapy in patients with advanced head and neck cancer. *J. Clin. Oncol.* 2001;19:535–542.

[188] Wang GL, Semenza GL. Oxygen sensing and response to hypoxia by mammalian cells. *Redox Report.* 1996;2:89–96.

[189] Chandel NS, Maltepe E, Goldwasser E, Mathieu CE, Simon MC, Schumacker PT. Mitochondrial reactive oxygen species trigger hypoxia-induced transcription. *Proc. Natl. Acad. Sci. USA.* 1998;95:11715–11720.

[190] Ivan M, Kondo K, Yang H, Kim W, Valiando J, Ohh M, Salic A, Asara JM, Lane WS, Kaelin WG, Jr. HIFalpha targeted for VHLmediated destruction by proline hydroxylation: Implications for O2 sensing. *Science.* 2001;292:464–468.

[191] Jaakkola P, Mole DR, Tian YM, Wilson MI, Gielbert J, Gaskell SJ, Kriegsheim A, Hebestreit HF, Mukherji M, Schofield CJ, Maxwell PH, Pugh CW, Ratcliffe PJ. Targeting of HIF-alpha to the von Hippel-Lindau ubiquitylation complex by $O_2$-regulated prolyl hydroxylation. *Science.* 2001;292:468–472.

[192] Yao KS, Xanthoudakis S, Curran T, O'Dwyer PJ. Activation of AP-1 and of a nuclear redox factor, Ref-1, in the response of HT29 colon cancer cells to hypoxia. *Mol. Cell Biol.* 1994;14:5997–6003.

[193] Semenza GL, Wang GL. A nuclear factor induced by hypoxia via de novo protein synthesis binds to the human erythropoietin gene enhancer at a site required for transcriptional activation. *Mol. Cell Biol.* 1992; 12:5447–5454.

[194] Koong AC, Chen EY, Giaccia AJ. Hypoxia causes the activation of nuclear factor kappa B through the phosphorylation of I kappa B alpha on tyrosine residues. *Cancer Res.* 1994;54:1425–1430.

[195] Graeber TG, Peterson JF, Tsai M, Monica K, Fornace AJ, Jr., Giaccia AJ. Hypoxia induces accumulation of p53 protein, but activation of a G1-phase checkpoint by low-oxygen conditions is independent of p53 status. *Mol. Cell Biol.* 1994;14:6264–6277.

[196] Semenza GL, Roth PH, Fang HM, Wang GL. Transcriptional regulation of genes encoding glycolytic enzymes by hypoxiainducible factor 1. *J. Biol. Chem.* 1994;269:23757–23763.

[197] Wykoff CC, Beasley NJ, Watson PH, Turner KJ, Pastorek J, Sibtain A, Wilson GD, Turley H, Talks KL, Maxwell PH, Pugh CW, Ratcliffe PJ, Harris AL. Hypoxia-

inducible expression of tumorassociated carbonic anhydrases. *Cancer Res.* 2000;60:7075–7083.

[198] Semenza GL, Jiang BH, Leung SW, Passantino R, Concordet JP, Maire P, Giallongo A. Hypoxia response elements in the aldolase A, enolase 1, and lactate dehydrogenase A gene promoters contain essential binding sites for hypoxia-inducible factor 1. *J. Biol. Chem.* 1996;271:32529–32537.

[199] Sivitz WI, Lund DD, Yorek B, Grover-McKay M, Schmid PG. Pretranslational regulation of two cardiac glucose transporters in rats exposed to hypobaric hypoxia. *Am. J. Physiol.* 1992;263:E562–E569.

[200] Firth JD, Ebert BL, Pugh CW, Ratcliffe PJ. Oxygen-regulated control elements in the phosphoglycerate kinase 1 and lactate dehydrogenase A genes: Similarities with the erythropoietin 30 enhancer. *Proc. Natl. Acad. Sci. USA.* 1994;91:6496–6500.

[201] Goldberg MA, Glass GA, Cunningham JM, Bunn HF. The regulated expression of erythropoietin by two human hepatoma cell lines. *Proc. Natl. Acad. Sci. USA.* 1987;84:7972–7976.

[202] Madan A, Curtin PT. A 24-base-pair sequence 30 to the human erythropoietin gene contains a hypoxia-responsive transcriptional enhancer. *Proc. Natl. Acad. Sci. USA.* 1993;90:3928–3932.

[203] Kourembanas S, Hannan RL, Faller DV. Oxygen tension regulates the expression of the platelet-derived growth factor-B chain gene in human endothelial cells. *J. Clin. Invest.* 1990;86:670–674.

[204] Melillo G, Musso T, Sica A, Taylor LS, Cox GW, Varesio L. A hypoxia-responsive element mediates a novel pathway of activation of the inducible nitric oxide synthase promoter. *J. Exp. Med.* 1995;182: 1683–1693.

[205] Shweiki D, Itin A, Soffer D, Keshet E. Vascular endothelial growth factor induced by hypoxia may mediate hypoxia-initiated angiogenesis. *Nature.* 1992;359:843–845.

[206] Veikkola T, Karkkainen M, Claesson-Welsh L, Alitalo K. Regulation of angiogenesis via vascular endothelial growth factor receptors. *Cancer Res.* 2000;60:203–212.

[207] Benjamin IJ, Kroger B, Williams RS. Activation of the heat shock transcription factor by hypoxia in mammalian cells. *Proc. Natl. Acad. Sci. USA.* 1990;87:6263–6267.

[208] Beck I, Weinmann R, Caro J. Characterization of hypoxiaresponsive enhancer in the human erythropoietin gene shows presence of hypoxia-inducible 120-kDa nuclear DNA-binding protein in erythropoietin-producing and nonproducing cells. *Blood.* 1993;82:704– 711.

[209] Wang GL, Jiang BH, Rue EA, Semenza GL. Hypoxia-inducible factor 1 is a basic-helix-loop-helix-PAS heterodimer regulated by cellular O2 tension. *Proc. Natl. Acad. Sci. USA.* 1995;92:5510–5514.

[210] Wenger RH, Gassmann M. Oxygen(es) and the hypoxiainducible factor-1. *Biol. Chem.* 1997;378:609–616.

[211] Gu YZ, Moran SM, Hogenesch JB, Wartman L, Bradfield CA. Molecular characterization and chromosomal localization of a third alpha-class hypoxia inducible factor subunit, HIF3alpha. *Gene Expr.* 1998;7:205–213.

[212] Maxwell PH, Pugh CW, Ratcliffe PJ. Inducible operation of the erythropoietin enhancer in multiple cell lines: Evidence for a widespread oxygen-sensing mechanism. *Proc. Natl. Acad. Sci. USA.* 1993;90:2423–2427.

[213] Wiener CM, Booth G, Semenza GL. In vivo expression of mRNAs encoding hypoxia-inducible factor 1. *Biochem. Biophys. Res. Commun.* 1996;225:485–488.

[214] Wiesener MS, Turley H, Allen WE, Willam C, Eckardt KU, Talks KL, Wood SM, Gatter KC, Harris AL, Pugh CW, Ratcliffe PJ, Maxwell PH. Induction of endothelial PAS domain protein-1 by hypoxia: Characterization and comparison with hypoxia-inducible factor-1alpha. *Blood.* 1998;92:2260–2268.

[215] Maxwell PH, Dachs GU, Gleadle JM, Nicholls LG, Harris AL, Stratford IJ, Hankinson O, Pugh CW, Ratcliffe PJ. Hypoxiainducible factor-1 modulates gene expression in solid tumors and influences both angiogenesis and tumor growth. *Proc. Natl. Acad. Sci. USA.* 1997;94:8104–8109.

[216] Maltepe E, Schmidt JV, Baunoch D, Bradfield CA, Simon MC. Abnormal angiogenesis and responses to glucose and oxygen deprivation in mice lacking the protein ARNT. *Nature.* 1997;386:403–407.

[217] Ryan HE, Lo J, Johnson RS. HIF-1 alpha is required for solid tumor formation and embryonic vascularization. *EMBO J.* 1998;17:3005–3015.

[218] Carmeliet P, Dor Y, Herbert JM, Fukumura D, Brusselmans K, DewerchinM, Neeman M, Bono F, Abramovitch R, Maxwell P, Koch CJ, Ratcliffe P, Moons L, Jain RK, Collen D, Keshert E, Keshet E. Role of HIF-1alpha in hypoxia-mediated apoptosis, cell proliferation and tumour angiogenesis. *Nature.* 1998;394:485–490.

[219] Hopfl G, Wenger RH, Ziegler U, Stallmach T, Gardelle O, Achermann R, Wergin M, Kaser-Hotz B, Saunders HM, Williams KJ, Stratford IJ, Gassmann M, Desbaillets I. Rescue of hypoxia-inducible factor-1alpha-deficient tumor growth by wild-type cells is independent of vascular endothelial growth factor. *Cancer Res.* 2002;62:2962–2970.

[220] Kung AL, Wang S, Klco JM, Kaelin WG, Livingston DM. Suppression of tumor growth through disruption of hypoxiainducible transcription. *Nat. Med.* 2000;6:1335–1340.

[221] Blancher C, Moore JW, Talks KL, Houlbrook S, Harris AL. Relationship of hypoxia-inducible factor (HIF)-1alpha and HIF- 2alpha expression to vascular endothelial growth factor induction and hypoxia survival in human breast cancer cell lines. *Cancer Res.* 2000;60:7106–7113.

[222] Jiang BH, Agani F, Passaniti A, Semenza GL. V-SRC induces expression of hypoxia-inducible factor 1 (HIF-1) and transcription of genes encoding vascular endothelial growth factor and enolase 1: Involvement of HIF-1 in tumor progression. *Cancer Res.* 1997;57:5328–5335.

[223] Maxwell PH, Wiesener MS, Chang GW, Clifford SC, Vaux EC, Cockman ME, Wykoff CC, Pugh CW, Maher ER, Ratcliffe PJ. The tumour suppressor protein VHL targets hypoxia-inducible factors for oxygen-dependent proteolysis. *Nature.* 1999;399:271–275.

[224] Zhong H, Agani F, Baccala AA, Laughner E, Rioseco-Camacho N, Isaacs WB, Simons JW, Semenza GL. Increased expression of hypoxia inducible factor-1alpha in rat and human prostate cancer. *Cancer Res.* 1998;58:5280–5284.

[225] Zhong H, De Marzo AM, Laughner E, Lim M, Hilton DA, Zagzag D, Buechler P, Isaacs WB, Semenza GL, Simons JW. Overexpression of hypoxia-inducible factor 1alpha in common human cancers and their metastases. *Cancer Res.* 1999;59:5830–5835.

[226] Aebersold DM, Burri P, Beer KT, Laissue J, Djonov V, Greiner RH, Semenza GL. Expression of hypoxia-inducible factor-1alpha: A novel predictive and prognostic parameter in the radiotherapy of oropharyngeal cancer. *Cancer Res.* 2001;61:2911–2916.

[227] KoukourakisMI, Giatromanolaki A, Skarlatos J, Corti L, Blandamura S, Piazza M, Gatter KC, Harris AL. Hypoxia inducible factor (HIF-1a and HIF-2a) expression in early esophageal cancer and response to photodynamic therapy and radiotherapy. *Cancer Res.* 2001;61:1830–1832.

[228] Koukourakis MI, Giatromanolaki A, Sivridis E, Simopoulos C, Turley H, Talks K, Gatter KC, Harris AL. Hypoxia-inducible factor (HIF1A and HIF2A), angiogenesis, and chemoradiotherapy outcome of squamous cell head-and-neck cancer. *Int. J. Radiat. Oncol. Biol. Phys.* 2002;53:1192–1202.

[229] Schindl M, Schoppmann SF, Samonigg H, Hausmaninger H, Kwasny W, Gnant M, Jakesz R, Kubista E, Birner P, Oberhuber G. Overexpression of hypoxia-inducible factor 1alpha is associated with an unfavorable prognosis in lymph node-positive breast cancer. *Clin. Cancer Res.* 2002;8:1831–1837.

[230] Birner P, Schindl M, Obermair A, Plank C, Breitenecker G, Oberhuber G. Overexpression of hypoxia-inducible factor 1alpha is a marker for an unfavorable prognosis in early-stage invasive cervical cancer. *Cancer Res.* 2000; 60:4693–4696.

[231] Haugland HK, Vukovic V, Pintilie M, Fyles AW, Milosevic M, Hill RP, Hedley DW. Expression of hypoxia-inducible factor-1alpha in cervical carcinomas: Correlation with tumor oxygenation. *Int. J. Radiat. Oncol. Biol. Phys.* 2002;53:854–861.

[232] Birner P, Schindl M, Obermair A, Breitenecker G, Oberhuber G. Expression of hypoxia-inducible factor 1alpha in epithelial ovarian tumors: Its impact on prognosis and on response to chemotherapy. *Clin. Cancer Res.* 2001;7:1661–1668.

[233] Giatromanolaki A, Koukourakis MI, Sivridis E, Turley H, Talks K, Pezzella F, Gatter KC, Harris AL. Relation of hypoxia inducible factor 1 alpha and 2 alpha in operable non-small cell lung cancer to angiogenic/molecular profile of tumours and survival. *Br. J. Cancer.* 2001;85:881–890.

[234] Pugh CW, O'Rourke JF, Nagao M, Gleadle JM, Ratcliffe PJ. Activation of hypoxia-inducible factor-1; definition of regulatory domains within the alpha subunit. *J. Biol. Chem.* 1997;272:11205–11214.

[235] Huang LE, Arany Z, Livingston DM, Bunn HF. Activation of hypoxia-inducible transcription factor depends primarily upon redox-sensitive stabilization of its alpha subunit. *J. Biol. Chem.* 1996;271: 32253–32259.

[236] Huang LE, Gu J, Schau M, Bunn HF. Regulation of hypoxiainducible factor 1alpha is mediated by an O2-dependent degradation domain via the ubiquitin-proteasome pathway. *Proc. Natl. Acad. Sci. USA.* 1998;95:7987–7992.

[237] Kallio PJ, Wilson WJ, O'Brien S, Makino Y, Poellinger L. Regulation of the hypoxia-inducible transcription factor 1alpha by the ubiquitin-proteasome pathway. *J. Biol. Chem.* 1999;274:6519–6525.

[238] Dachs GU, Patterson AV, Firth JD, Ratcliffe PJ, Townsend KM, Stratford IJ, Harris AL. Targeting gene expression to hypoxic tumor cells. *Nat. Med.* 1997;3:515–520.

[239] Greco O, Dachs GU. Gene directed enzyme/prodrug therapy of cancer: Historical appraisal and future prospectives. *J. Cell Physiol.* 2001;187:22–36.

[240] Shalev M, Kadmon D, Teh BS, Butler EB, Aguilar-Cordova E, Thompson TC, Herman JR, Adler HL, Scardino PT, Miles BJ. Suicide gene therapy toxicity after multiple and repeat injections in patients with localized prostate cancer. *J. Urol.* 2000;163:1747–1750.

[241] Teh BS, Aguilar-Cordova E, Kernen K, Chou CC, Shalev M, Vlachaki MT, Miles B, Kadmon D, Mai WY, Caillouet J, Davis M, Ayala G, Wheeler T, Brady J, Carpenter LS, Lu HH, Chiu JK, Woo SY, Thompson T, Butler EB. Phase I/II trial evaluating combined radiotherapy and in situ gene therapy with or without hormonal therapy in the treatment of prostate cancer—A preliminary report. *Int. J. Radiat. Oncol. Biol. Phys.* 2001;51:605–613.

[242] Freytag SO, Khil M, Stricker H, Peabody J, Menon M, DePeralta-Venturina M, Nafziger D, Pegg J, Paielli D, Brown S, Barton K, Lu M, Aguilar-Cordova E, Kim JH. Phase I study of replicationcompetent adenovirus-mediated double suicide gene therapy for the treatment of locally recurrent prostate cancer. *Cancer Res.* 2002;62:4968–4976.

[243] Koshikawa N, Takenaga K, Tagawa M, Sakiyama S. Therapeutic efficacy of the suicide gene driven by the promoter of vascular endothelial growth factor gene against hypoxic tumor cells. *Cancer Res.* 2000;60:2936–2941.

[244] Binley K, Askham Z, Martin L, Spearman H, Day D, Kingsman S, Naylor S. Hypoxia-mediated tumour targeting. *Gene Ther.* 2003;10:540–549.

[245] Boast K, Binley K, Iqball S, Price T, Spearman H, Kingsman S, Kingsman A, Naylor S. Characterization of physiologically regulated vectors for the treatment of ischemic disease. *Hum. Gene Ther.* 1999;10:2197–2208.

[246] Shibata T, Giaccia AJ, Brown JM. Development of a hypoxiaresponsive vector for tumor-specific gene therapy. *Gene Ther.* 2000;7:493–498.

[247] Shibata T, Giaccia AJ, Brown JM. Hypoxia-inducible regulation of a prodrug-activating enzyme for tumor-specific gene therapy. *Neoplasia.* 2002;4:40–48.

[248] Patterson AV, Saunders MP, Chinje EC, Talbot DC, Harris AL, Strafford IJ. Overexpression of human NADPH: Cytochrome c (P450) reductase confers enhanced sensitivity to both tirapazamine (SR 4233) and RSU 1069. *Br. J. Cancer.* 1997;76:1338–1347.

[249] Saunders MP, Patterson AV, Chinje EC, Harris AL, Stratford IJ. NADPH: Cytochrome c (P450) reductase activates tirapazamine (SR4233) to restore hypoxic and oxic cytotoxicity in an aerobic resistant derivative of the A549 lung cancer cell line. *Br. J. Cancer.* 2000;82:651–656.

[250] Ebert BL, Firth JD, Ratcliffe PJ. Hypoxia and mitochondrial inhibitors regulate expression of glucose transporter-1 via distinct Cis-acting sequences. *J. Biol. Chem.* 1995; 270: 29083-9.

[251] Muller JM, Krauss B, Kaltschmidt C, Baeuerle PA, Rupec RA. Hypoxia induces c-fos transcription via a mitogen-activated protein kinase-dependent pathway. *J. Biol. Chem.* 1997; 272: 23435-9.

[252] Wang WD, Chen ZT, Li R, Li DZ, Duan YZ, Cao ZH. Enhanced efficacy of radiation-induced gene therapy in mice bearing lung adenocarcinoma xenografts using hypoxia responsive elements. *Cancer Science.* 2005,96(12):918-924.

[253] Gorski DH, Beckett MA, Jaskowiak NT, Calvin DP, Mauceri HJ, Salloum RM, et al. Blockage of the vascular endothelial growth factor stress response increases the antitumor effects of ionizing radiation. *Cancer Res.* 1999; 59: 3374-8.

[254] Chandel NS, McClintock DS, Feliciano CE, Wood TM, Melendez JA, Rodriguez AM, et al. Reactive oxygen species generated at mitochondrial complex III stabilize hypoxia-inducible factor-1alpha during hypoxia: a mechanism of O2 sensing. *J. Biol. Chem.* 2000; 275: 25130-8.

[255] Kuroda T, Mikawa K, Mishima H, Kishimoto A. H1 histone stimulates limited proteolysis of protein kinase C subspecies by calpain II. *J. Biochem.* 1991; 110: 364-368.

[256] Chua CC, Hamdy RC, Chua BH. Upregulation of vascular endothelial growth factor by H2O2 in rat heart endothelial cells. *Free Radic. Biol. Med.* 1998; 25: 891-7.

[257] Kosmidou I, Xagorari A, Roussos C, Papapetropoulos A. Reactive oxygen species stimulate VEGF production from C(2)C(12) skeletal myotubes through a PI3K/Akt pathway. *Am. J. Physiol. Lung Cell Mol. Physiol.* 2001; 280: L585-92.

[258] Gleadle JM, Ebert BL, Ratcliffe PJ. Diphenylene iodonium inhibits the induction of erythropoietin and other mammalian genes by hypoxia. Implications for the mechanism of oxygen sensing. *Eur. J. Biochem.* 1995; 234: 92-9.

[259] Fandrey J, Frede S, Ehleben W, Porwol T, Acker H, Jelkmann W. Cobalt chloride and desferrioxamine antagonize the inhibition of erythropoietin production by reactive oxygen species. *Kidney Int.* 1997; 51: 492-6.

[260] Gonzalez-Flecha B, Reides C, Cutrin JC, Llesuy SF, Boveris A. Oxidative stress produced by suprahepatic occlusion and reperfusion. *Hepatology.* 1993; 18: 881-9.

[261] Datta R, Hallahan DE, Kharbanda SM, Rubin E, Sherman ML, Huberman E, et al. Involvement of reactive oxygen intermediates in the induction of c-jun gene transcription by ionizing radiation. *Biochemistry.* 1992; 31: 8300-6.

[262] Bonventre JV, Sukhatme VP, Bamberger M, Ouellette AJ, Brown D. Localization of the protein product of the immediate early growth response gene, Egr-1, in the kidney after ischemia and reperfusion. *Cell Regul.* 1991; 2: 251-60.

[263] Yan SF, Lu J, Zou YS, Soh-Won J, Cohen DM, Buttrick PM, et al. Hypoxia-associated induction of early growth response-1 gene expression. *J. Biol. Chem.* 1999; 274: 15030-40.

[264] Lo LW, Cheng JJ, Chiu JJ, Wung BS, Liu YC, Wang DL. Endothelial exposure to hypoxia induces Egr-1 expression involving PKCalpha-mediated Ras/Raf-1/ERK1/2 pathway. *J. Cell Physiol.* 2001; 188: 304-12.

[265] Yan SF, Lu J, Zou YS, Kisiel W, Mackman N, Leitges M, et al. Protein kinase C-beta and oxygen deprivation. A novel Egr-1-dependent pathway for fibrin deposition in hypoxemic vasculature. *J. Biol. Chem.* 2000; 275: 11921-8.

[266] Greco O, Folkes LK, Wardman P, Tozer GM, Dachs GU. Development of a novel enzyme/prodrug combination for gene therapy of cancer: horseradish peroxidase/indole-3-acetic acid. *Cancer Gene Ther.* 2000; 7: 1414-20.

[267] Wang WD, Chen ZT, Li DZ, Duan YZ, Wang ZX, Cao ZH. Oncostatin M gene therapy in mice bearing lung adenocarcinoma xenograft using a hypoxia/radiation dual-sensitive promoter. *Zhonghua Jie He He Hu Xi Za Zhi.* 2004;27(4):240-3.

[268] Scott SD, Marples B. Comment on the use of the cre/loxP recombinase system for gene therapy vectors. *Gene Ther.* 2000; 7: 1706.

[269] Scott SD, Marples B, Hendry JH, Lashford LS, Embleton MJ, Hunter RD, et al. A radiation-controlled molecular switch for use in gene therapy of cancer. *Gene Ther.* 2000; 7: 1121-1125.

[270] Lohr F, Hu K, Huang Q, Zhang L, Samulski TV, Dewhirst MW, et al. Enhancement of radiotherapy by hyperthermia-regulated gene therapy. *Int. J. Radiat. Oncol. Biol. Phys.* 2000; 48: 1513-8.

[271] Nettelbeck DM, Jerome V, Muller R. Gene therapy: designer promoters for tumour targeting. *Trends Genet.* 2000; 16: 174- 81.

[272] Malmgren RA, Flanigan CC. Localization of the vegetative form of Clostridium tetani in mouse tumors following intravenous spore administration. *Cancer Res.* 1955; 15: 473-478.

[273] Carey RW, Holland JF, Sheehe PR, Graham S. Association of cancer of the breast and acute myelocytic leukemia. *Cancer.* 1967;20(7):1080-8.

[274] Fox ME, Lemmon MJ, Mauchline ML, Davis TO, Giaccia AJ, Minton NP, et al. Anaerobic bacteria as a delivery system for cancer gene therapy: in vitro activation of 5-fluorocytosine by genetically engineered clostridia. *Gene Ther.* 1996; 3: 173-8.

[275] Lemmon MJ, van Zijl P, Fox ME, Mauchline ML, Giaccia AJ, Minton NP, et al. Anaerobic bacteria as a gene delivery system that is controlled by the tumor microenvironment. *Gene Ther.* 1997; 4: 791-6.

[276] Liu SC, Minton NP, Giaccia AJ, Brown JM. Anticancer efficacy of systemically delivered anaerobic bacteria as gene therapy vectors targeting tumor hypoxia/necrosis. *Gene Ther.* 2002; 9: 291-6.

[277] Yazawa K, Fujimori M, Amano J, Kano Y, Taniguchi S. Bifidobacterium longum as a delivery system for cancer gene therapy: selective localization and growth in hypoxic tumors. *Cancer Gene Ther.* 2000; 7: 269-74.

[278] Pawelek JM, Low KB, Bermudes D. Tumor-targeted Salmonella as a novel anticancer vector. *Cancer Res.* 1997; 57: 4537- 44.

[279] Lambin P, Theys J, Landuyt W, Rijken P, van der Kogel AJ, Van der Schueren E, et al. Colonisation ofClostridiumin the body is restricted to hypoxic and necrotic areas of tumours. *Anaerobe.* 1998; 4: 183-188.

[280] Nuyts S, Van Mellaert L, Theys J, Landuyt W, Bosmans E, Anne J, et al. Radio-responsive recA promoter significantly increases TNFalpha production in recombinant clostridia after 2 Gy irradiation. *Gene Ther.* 2001; 8: 1197-201.

In: Lung Cancer in Women
Editor: Varetta N. Torres, pp. 45-71
ISBN: 978-1-60021-659-6


*Chapter II*

# Novel Pathways and Targets for the Development of Anti-Cancer Therapeutics 1: Glucose Transport and Metabolism in Cancer

***Rachel E. Airley[1] and Ali Mobasheri*[2]***

[1] Department of Developmental and Molecular Biology, Chanin Institute, Albert Einstein College of Medicine of Yeshiva University, Bronx, N.Y., USA

[2] Division of Veterinary Medicine, School of Veterinary Medicine and Science, University of Nottingham, Sutton Bonington Campus, Sutton Bonington, UK

## Abstract

Accelerated glycolysis is one of the biochemical characteristics of cancer. Tumor cells require a steady source of metabolic energy in the form of adenosine tri-phosphate (ATP) in order to continue their uncontrolled growth and proliferation. Glucose transport and metabolism are important determinants of post-treatment survival in tumor cells, leading to poor prognosis. Glycolytic breakdown of glucose is preceded by the transport of glucose across the cell membrane, a rate-limiting process mediated by facilitative glucose transporter proteins (GLUTs). Tumors frequently exhibit over-expression of GLUTs, especially the hypoxia-responsive GLUT1 and GLUT3 proteins. Significant associations between GLUT expression and proliferative indices have been reported suggesting that GLUT expression may be of prognostic significance. Here we review the recent clinical and basic research on glucose metabolism in cancer. We explore the involvement of GLUT proteins as potential coordinators of metabolic processes in the tumour microenvironment. With the discovery of the oxygen-sensitive transcription factor hypoxia-inducible factor (HIF) has come a new understanding of the molecular link between hypoxia and deregulated glucose metabolism. HIF induces a number of

* Corresponding author. Tel: +44 115 951 6449; fax: +44 115 951 6415; E-mail address: ali.mobasheri@nottingham.ac.uk (A. Mobasheri)

genes integral to angiogenesis, e.g. vascular endothelial growth factor (VEGF), a process intimately involved with metastatic spread. We discuss the links between HIF, glucose transporters, angiogenic factors and tumour development. This knowledge may enhance existing chemotherapeutic strategies so that treatment can be more rationally applied and personalized for cancer patients.

**Keywords:** Cancer; Glucose metabolism; Glucose transport; GLUT1; GLUT3; Hypoxia; Hypoxia-inducible factor 1 alpha; Anaerobic metabolism; Angiogenesis; 2-Deoxy-D-glucose; Fluoro-2-deoxy-D-glucose; Tumor progression; Metastasis; Prognostic indicator; Anticancer therapeutics.

## Introduction

It has been known, for more than 70 years, that one of the most fundamental characteristics of cancer cells is increased levels of glucose uptake and glycolysis despite reduced levels of oxygen consumption [1]. The primary metabolic characteristic of malignant cells is an increased uptake of glucose and its anaerobic metabolism. Malignant cells have been shown to utilize more glucose than normal cells *in vitro* and *in vivo*. These cells exhibit increased rates of glucose utilization, poor perfusion and areas of low oxygenation. Therefore, glucose is a vital energy source of tumors, and glucose transporter isoform 1 (GLUT1) and hexokinase are key rate-limiting factors in the transport and metabolism of glucose in cancer cells. GLUT1 expression is largely undetectable in normal epithelial tissues and benign epithelial tumors. However, GLUT1 is over-expressed in a significant proportion of a variety of human carcinomas [2-4] and correlates with aggressive tumor behavior such as high grade (poorly differentiated) invasion and metastasis [5-7]. Furthermore, oncogene transformation, loss of functional tumor suppressor genes and mitogen stimulation all increase rates of glucose uptake [8]. Many investigators have hypothesized that elevated GLUT1 expression by human carcinomas indicates an increased metabolic state, increased utilization of energy, and an associated increase in aggressive, metastatic behavior.

## The GLUT/SLC2A Gene Family of Transport Facilitators

The facilitative glucose transporter /solute carrier GLUT/SLC2A family incorporates at least fourteen highly homologous, integral membrane transport proteins that catalyze the entry of monosaccharide sugars such as glucose into mammalian cells [9]. These proteins are characterized by the presence of 12 membrane spanning helices and several conserved sequence motifs [10]. The GLUT/SLC2A proteins are expressed in a tissue- and cell-specific manner and exhibit distinct kinetic and regulatory properties that reflect their functional and tissue specific roles. The sequence similarities of the GLUT/SLC2A family members are now well defined and the family now divided into three subclasses (figure 1). Class I contains the originally identified, well characterized glucose transporters GLUT1-4. These proteins are distinguishable by their tissue distribution, kinetic properties, and regulation by hormones, especially insulin. GLUT1 is found in very low levels in most tissues, but is especially abundant in erythrocytes, and blood-tissue endothelial and epithelial borders, such as the blood-brain barrier, retina, and placenta. GLUT2 is a low affinity, high $K_m$ isoform expressed in the liver, gut and pancreatic islets [11, 12]. GLUT3 is primarily expressed in the brain where it is localized exclusively to neurons, but other sites of expression include placenta, sperm, and human platelets [13-15]. GLUT4 is an "insulin-responsive" isoform expressed in skeletal muscle, heart, white and brown adipose tissue, all tissues which respond to insulin or contraction by acutely increasing their rates of glucose uptake [16]. Class II consists of the fructose transporter GLUT5 and three related but as yet poorly characterized proteins, GLUT7, GLUT9 and GLUT11. Class III GLUT/SLC2A members are characterized by the lack of a glycosylation site in the extracellular loop 1, and by the presence of such a site in loop 9. The recently cloned $H^+$-myoinositol symporter (HMIT; [17]) has been included in class III, despite the fact that it does not transport glucose but is a polyol transporter. GLUT14, which was thought to be a pseudogene has been shown to be a duplicon of GLUT3 and is specifically expressed in testis with alternative splice forms [18]. Functional glucose transport has been demonstrated for GLUT6 (formerly known as GLUT9) and GLUT8 (formerly known as GLUTX1). It should be emphasized that the designation of the family as "glucose transporters" does not necessarily reflect the substrate specificity of individual members, which may transport hexose sugars or polyols other than glucose (e.g. GLUT5 transports fructose; HMIT1 (GLUT13) transports myoinositol, other GLUTs may transport galactose or sugar-derived compounds).

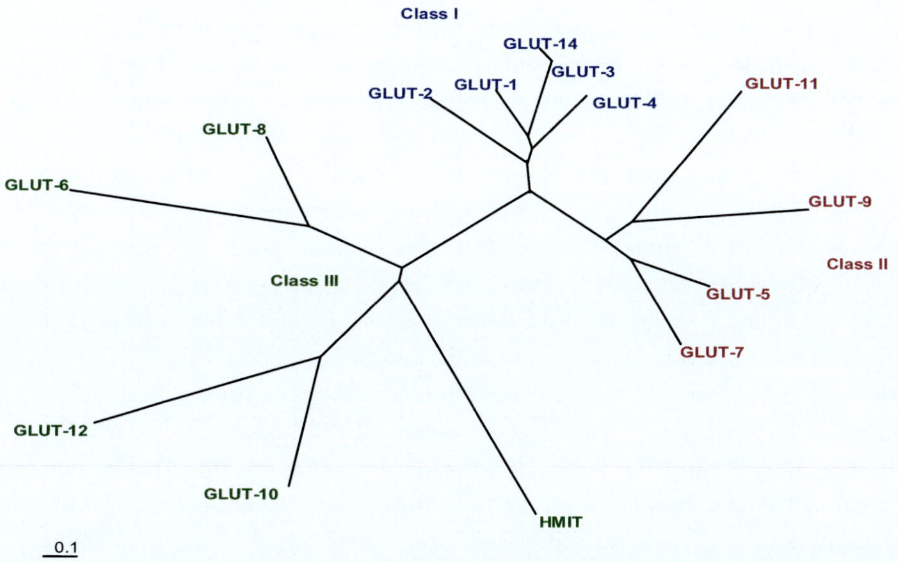


Figure 1. Members of the extended GLUT/SLC2A family of glucose/polyol transporter facilitators. Unrooted radial phylogram drawn from a multiple sequence alignment of all fourteen known members of the human GLUT/SLC2A family. There are three classes of GLUT proteins: class I, class II and class III. The tree was constructed using neighbor-joining analysis of a distance matrix generated with PHYLIP software. The scale bar represents 0.1 substitutions per amino acid position. HMIT = H+-Coupled myoinositol transporter (GLUT13).

# GLUT1 Is Overexpressed in Tumors

The expanding knowledge base now available describing the structure, regulation and functionality of glucose transporters has led to a renewed interest in tumor glucose transport, and in particular, how this may be mediated through particular glucose transporters [4, 19, 20]. The genomic era has led to a desire for inexpensive, minimally invasive and reproducible prognostic markers which will enable the individualization of medicines in the clinic, according to the predicted response to treatment and overall survival. A proliferation of translational studies, which have investigated the over-expression of glucose transporters in a wide variety of tumor types, has firmly placed GLUT1, in particular, amongst such prognostic markers. The over-expression of these glucose transporters alone may have an application as markers of malignancy, as they are frequently associated with poor prognosis, along with putative prognostic indicators such as invasiveness, proliferation and grade in many tumors [2],[4], they may also assist in the selection of patients for more aggressive therapy.

The expression of the glucose transporters GLUT1 to GLUT4 has been investigated in various cell lines and tissue samples, and an upregulation of GLUT1 transcription or protein expression, relative to benign type, is apparent for virtually all cell lines tested [3]. One example is the over-expression of GLUT1 that occurs in breast tumors where there is a higher expression of GLUT1 in breast cancer cells compared with the healthy breast tissue [21, 22]. This has been associated with invasive ability [6],[23] and markers of poor prognosis such as higher grade and proliferative activity. However, this latter study also suggests that glucose transport in the majority of breast cancers may be mediated by glucose transporters other than GLUT1 [24]. This notion has been confirmed by other investigators who found that human MCF-7 and MDA-468 breast cancer cell lines transport fructose and express the fructose transporter GLUT5 [25]. More recent observations suggest that the novel GLUT12 glucose transporter is expressed in MCF-7 breast cancer cells [26]. Other studies have suggested that 43% of breast cancer tissues express the insulin responsive GLUT4 isoform and functional evidence for GLUT4 has been demonstrated by insulin-responsiveness experiments [3]. However, other studies have failed to detect GLUT4 in breast cancer [6]. In colorectal tumors, GLUT1 expression is associated with poor prognosis after surgical resection [27], [28] where it is found at the sites of deepest invasion, and after radiotherapy [29]. The expression of GLUT1 in head and neck cancers was first observed in 1994 [30], and has now been described in a number of head and neck tumor subtypes. Among these, GLUT1 predicts poor prognosis in hypopharyngeal [31], oesophageal [32], and oral squamous carcinomas treated with surgery [5, 33]. Over-expression of GLUT1 is also associated with poor survival in non-small cell lung carcinoma [34] and adenocarcinoma of the lung [35], and with tumor aggressiveness and poor survival in transitional cell carcinoma of the bladder [36] and gallbladder [37]. The association of GLUT1 with metastasis has been shown in studies involving patients with gastric carcinoma [38], and advanced carcinoma of the cervix [39]. As it may be inferred that poor outcome in lung and colorectal cancers is most likely due to metastatic spread, the effect of GLUT1 on survival in these cancers also offers evidence that increased GLUT-mediated glucose transport confers metastatic potential. The over-expression of GLUT1, and links with parameters conferring more aggressive behavior have been further demonstrated in tumors of the thyroid [40]. Tumors of the pancreas [41], endometrium, gliomas [42] and human penile proliferative lesions [43] over-express GLUT1, and we have recently found that the paediatric cancers neuroblastoma and rhabdomyosarcoma express GLUT1 in around one fifth of cases studied. Curiously, although GLUT1 predicts malignant progression, invasion and prognosis in ovarian carcinoma [44-46], over-expression of GLUT1 also predicted a better response to chemotherapy in one study [46].

## GLUT3 Is over-Expressed in Tumors

Although GLUT3 mRNA is elevated in a variety of human cancers, including tumors of the head and neck [30], colon and pancreas [47], investigations of GLUT3 protein have found it to be not as ubiquitous as GLUT1. This suggests the need for additional post-transcriptional regulation to express increased levels of GLUT3 protein . For example, in one investigation of GLUT3 protein expression across a wide range of tumor types, it was only detectable in non-small cell lung, stomach, ovary and testicular tumors, the latter of which also showed GLUT3 expression in the corresponding normal tissue [48]. However, the prognostic effect of GLUT3 has been demonstrated in laryngeal tumors [49], and where it is co-expressed with GLUT1 in non-small cell lung tumors, the prognostic effect of GLUT1 is more significant.

## Glucose Metabolism and Tumor Hypoxia

Cancer cells have the ability to sense diminishing glucose and oxygen supplies as the pace and intensity of tumor growth outstrips the capacity for vascularization. In response they can make appropriate adjustments to their metabolism to adapt to the new conditions. Normal cells require glucose and sufficient oxygen, i.e. normoxia, to survive and proliferate. Too much oxygen or no oxygen (i.e. hyperoxia and anoxia respectively) are incompatible with life (figure 2). Hyperoxia results in oxygen toxicity and anoxia causes necrosis and tissue atrophy. However, living cells have the capacity to adapt to low oxygen tensions (i.e. hypoxia) and this adaptation involves the hypoxia inducible transcription factor (HIF) oxygen sensing pathway and a number of key downstream regulated genes (figure 3). Tumor cells appear to have taken advantage of this pathway to condition their metabolism to low oxygen tensions and reduced glucose levels (figure 4).

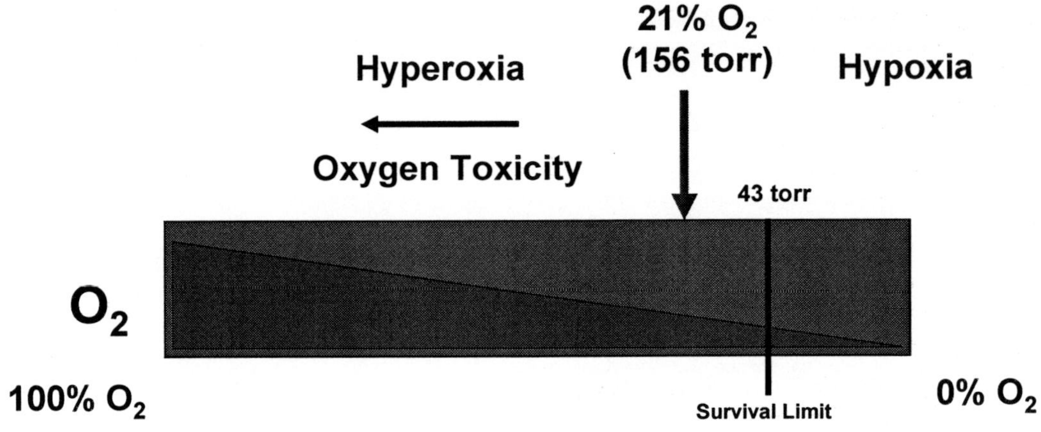


Figure 2. Spectrum of tissue oxygenation. Hyperoxia and anoxia are lethal to all cells whereas most cells have the varied capacity to adapt to low oxygen tension hypoxia.

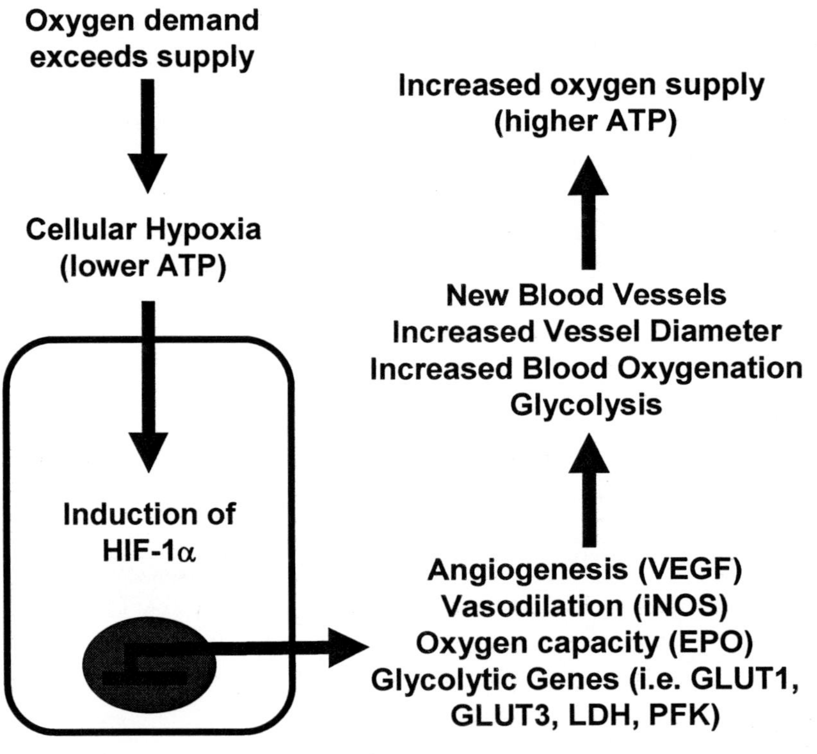


Figure 3. Molecular responses to hypoxia. When oxygen demand exceeds supply, the HIF-1 oxygen-sensing pathway results in activation of key genes involved in angiogenesis, vasodilatation, oxygen delivery and glycolysis in order to increase tissue oxygenation.

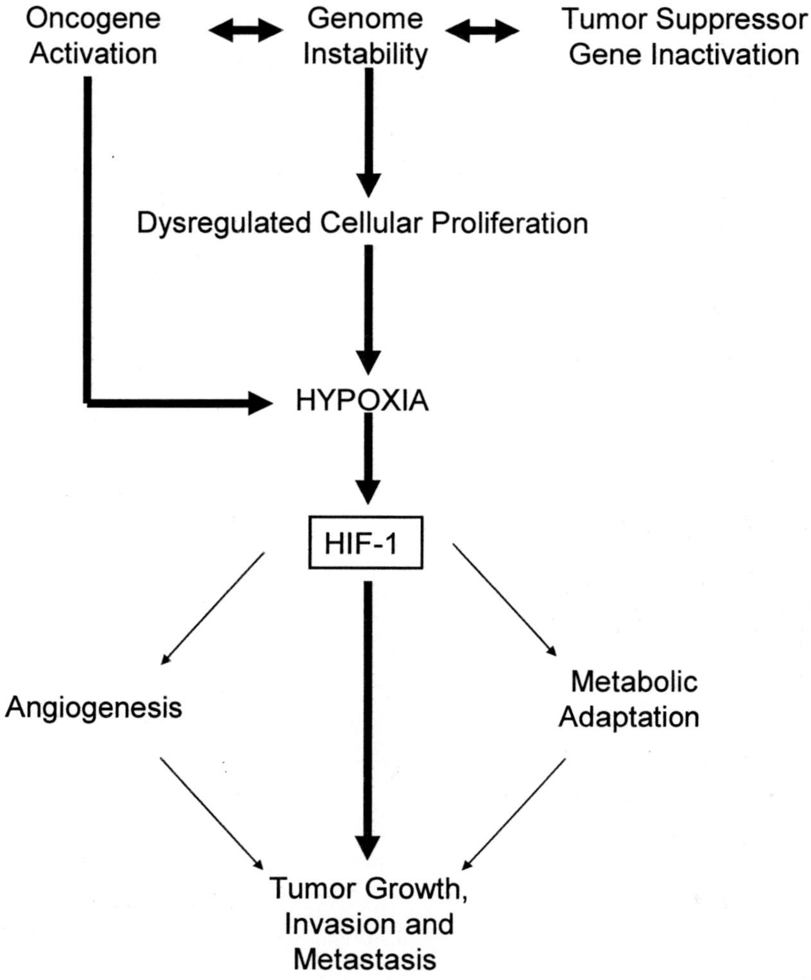


Figure 4. The role of HIF-1 in promoting angiogenesis and metabolic adaptation of tumor cells.

## Glucose Analogues and Conjugates for the Treatment of Cancer

This strategy involved the use of 2-deoxyglucose and 5-thioglucose as anti-metabolites that would interfere with the increased metabolic requirements of tumor cells. The rationale here was that selective toxicity might be achieved through the increased uptake of a glucose analogue into tumor cells, which would then act as glycolytic inhibitors. Early experiments showed that these compounds were indeed more toxic to hypoxic cells *in vitro* [50, 51], since under these conditions glycolysis would be a major source of energy. However, the development of this approach was compromised by normal tissue toxicity in mice, presumably due to non-specific inhibition of glycolysis [51]. Other approaches have included the use of 2-deoxyglucose as a radiosensitizer [52,53,54] its effects being brought about through reduced DNA repair or through inhibition of anaerobic glycolysis by resistant hypoxic cells [55]. More recent work has employed the use of glucose conjugates, where selective uptake of conventional cytotoxic drugs is achieved through conjugation with glucose . Examples of this approach include 2-GluSNAP [56], a glucose-conjugated nitric oxide donor, which has shown promise in ovarian carcinomas. Further, glucose-conjugated inhibitors of O[6] methyl-guanine DNA methyl transferase, a major determinant of resistance to alkylating anti-tumor agents [57] and the cyclophosphamide- glucose conjugate gluphosphamide [58]. More recently gluphosphamide has been the subject of phase III trials for the treatment of glioblastoma multiforme [59]. Although this agent originally received fast track status by the US FDA and entered phase I/II trials for the treatment of pancreatic cancer in combination with gemcitabine, this line of research was recently halted.

The re-emerging interest in glucose transport in basic and translational cancer biology can arguably be attributed to both the discovery of glucose transporters, an area that has been growing steadily since the cloning and molecular of GLUT1 by Mueckler in 1985 [60], and the explosion of interest in hypoxia-driven processes instrumental to the malignant progression, proliferation and survival of tumors. Tumor hypoxia was traditionally a problem of interest to radiobiologists, owing to the pronounced radio-resistance experienced in extremely low oxygen tensions (below 1% $O_2$). Hypoxic tumors are known to be more malignant, more likely to metastasize, and to have a poor prognosis [61-64]. Hypoxic tumors are also radio- and chemo-resistant. To be effective, radiation therapy depends upon the 'fixation' of radiation-induced DNA damage, which occurs following 'ionisation', when molecular oxygen stabilizes the free radical products formed by either DNA or surrounding intracellular water molecules. This phenomenon, termed the oxygen effect, results in the formation of organic peroxides, which give rise to non-restorable changes in the chemical composition of the target material. In the absence of oxygen, the target molecules may repair themselves and resume normal function, and the oxygen enhancement ratio (OER), which describes the relative radiation dose necessary to kill normoxic versus anoxic cells for X-rays and $\chi$-rays is 3 [65, 66]. Oxygen itself is a potent radiosensitizer. However, compounds such as the 2-nitroimidazoles, which share the property of a lone pair of electrons within the molecule, may act as oxygen mimetics, and have been also been described as radiosensitizers [67]. However, this strategy, which includes the use of agents such as misonidazole, doranidazole and etanidazole has met with little success so far [68-70]. The oxygen status of a tumor also exerts a drug-dependent effect on the response to chemotherapy [71]. For example, the active species of bleomycin depends upon the formation of a DNA-bleomycin-ferrous ion-dioxygen complex in the presence of molecular oxygen [72]. However, the characteristic tumor architecture and hypoxia-regulated molecular and biochemical pathways accompanying tumor hypoxia offer a substantial and more generalized contribution to the poor chemosensitivity observed in these tumors.

## ALTERATIONS IN THE TUMOR MICROENVIRONMENT

Tumor hypoxia occurs when aggressively growing tumors rapidly outgrow their blood supply, thus forming an adverse microenvironment that is characteristic of solid tumors, where tissue is oxygen and nutrient starved, and at low pH. A rapidly growing tumor eventually surpasses the host-tissue-derived vascularization that can only provide microcirculatory functions in selected parts of the tumor. Where the tumor must depend upon tumor-derived neovascularization, the delivery of oxygen and nutrients is severely compromised by the formation of elongated, dilated and twisted vessels that may be heterogeneously distributed, resulting in avascular areas and increased diffusion distances (see figure 5). Perfusion is consequently restricted and unstable, and vasculature is fragile, giving rise to chronic or diffusion-limited hypoxia. This is exacerbated by deterioration of blood rheology, platelet aggregation and increased interstitial pressure within the tumor. Morphological changes in tumor vasculature might also cause vasospasm, which will affect downstream capillary blood flow. This will give rise to acute or perfusion limited hypoxia. Tumors therefore contain both highly perfused areas, which support rapid cell growth and infiltration into surrounding tissue, and areas of necrosis that are associated with compromised perfusion. Chronically hypoxic tissue will exist in peri-necrotic areas [65, 73-75]. The resulting poor delivery of drugs to these areas will result in chemo-resistance. Within areas that are dependent upon tumor-derived neovascularization, blood flow will be transiently interrupted, giving rise to spatially and temporally shifting acute hypoxia. It is now believed that radio-sensitivity is determined chiefly by acute falls in tumor oxygenation, so that acute hypoxia is the over-riding problem in radiation therapy [76]. Both DNA-damaging radiation therapy and chemotherapeutic agents that target DNA are compromised by hypoxia due to cell cycle changes: hypoxic cells have a larger $G_0$ fraction that remains refractory to treatment and hypoxia-induced cell cycle arrest will confer resistance to cell-cycle dependent drugs such as methotrexate. Further, hypoxia-induced resistance to drugs such as etoposide, may be due to the induction of glucose-regulated proteins that ultimately reduces the level of DNA topoisomerase II, its cellular target [71]. There is also evidence that hypoxia, via HIF-1 may induce multi-drug resistance efflux transporters [77].

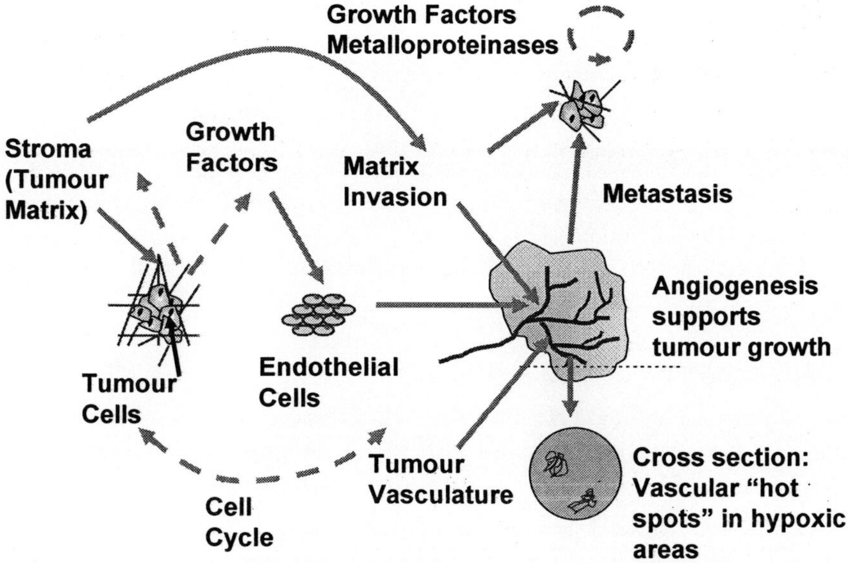


Figure 5. Dynamic interplay between hypoxia, angiogenesis and tumor-promoting factors such as growth factors and matrix metalloproteinases.

The use of hypoxia-selective bioreductive drugs was a natural progression from the use of radio-sensitizers: whereas radio-sensitizers act as oxygen mimetics to help 'fix' radiation-induced damage, bio-reductive drugs are themselves cytotoxic towards hypoxic cells. Bio-reductive drugs show differential toxicity towards hypoxic cells in tumors. There are several classes of agent in various stages of pre-clinical and clinical development, the most advanced being tirapazamine (SR 4233) [78, 79], an aromatic benztriazine-di-N-oxide, and AQ4N, an aliphatic N-oxide [80], in phase III and phase I clinical trials respectively. New variations on 2-nitroimidazoles, having been investigated thoroughly as radio-sensitizers over the years, are now also being studied for their potential as bio-reductive cytotoxics [81, 82]. The aim of bio-reductive drugs is not only to overcome the chemo- and radio-resistance caused by hypoxia, but also to exploit this feature by using agents that selectively kill these cells. Therefore, when used in combination with radiotherapy or conventional chemotherapy, the relatively chemosensitive normoxic cell populations are eradicated, and residual hypoxic cells, which might otherwise lead to local or distant metastasis, may be targeted and killed by bio-reductive agents. Differential toxicity of bio-reductive drugs is defined by the *hypoxic cytotoxicity ratio*, i.e. the ratio of drug concentrations under normoxic and hypoxic conditions to give the same level of cell kill [83-85]. The cytotoxicity of these agents depends upon a 1- or 2-electron reduction, activated in hypoxic conditions, to a cytotoxic species. For example, the active species of tirapazamine is a toxic intermediate tirapazamine radical produced via a 1-electron reduction, which DNA by hydrogen abstraction, causing single strand breaks [86]. The activity of hypoxia-selective bio-reductive drugs depends upon the depth and duration of hypoxia within the tumor[87] and the level of reducing enzymes: for example, activation of tirapazamine is by the reducing enzyme NADPH cytochrome P450 reductase [88].

The adverse effect of tumor hypoxia on treatment response and outcome has stimulated a proliferation of interest in how hypoxia influences the molecular biology of tumors. In particular, research has focused on hypoxia as a survival signal. The discovery of the HIFs (HIF-1, HIF-2, HIF-3) has formed an integral part of what is now understood about the mechanism by which cells sense the level of oxygenation within a tissue. The first, HIF-1, is the best characterized, but two further transcription factors, HIF-2 (EPAS-1) [89] and HIF-3 [90] are now known to exist and studies being carried out to assess their functionality. HIF-1 is part of a family of heterodynamic basic helix-loop-helix (bHLH proteins, composed of two subunits- HIF-1 and HIF-1, the latter of which is also designated as the aryl hydrocarbon receptor nuclear translocator (ARNT), which is involved in the xenobiotic metabolism of drugs and environmental toxins [91]. HIF-1 activation is dependent on the stabilization of the HIF-1 subunit, most likely post-translational, as the subunit is rapidly degraded in normoxic conditions [91-93]. Stabilization and subsequent dimerization with the HIF-1 subunit leads to complex formation with the hypoxia response element (HRE), an enhancer sequence found in the promoter regions of hypoxia-regulated genes, such as the glucose transporters GLUT1 and GLUT3, and the glycolytic enzymes, as well as the angiogenic growth factor vascular endothelial growth factor (VEGF), erythropoietin and the tumor associated carbonic anhydrases CAIX and CAXII [94-98]. The transcription factor HIF-1 is an important mediator of hypoxic adaptation of tumor cells and controls several genes that have been implicated in tumor growth. Constitutive up-regulation of HIF-1 has been observed in the majority of clear cell renal carcinomas leading to more widespread accumulation of this transcription factor than hypoxic stimulation [99]. Increased expression of HIF-1 is associated with alterations in gene expression patterns that are likely to contribute to tumor phenotype and progression.

Studies suggest that HIF-1 expression in tumor cells may be increased by both genetic alterations and physiological induction (hypoxia). HIF-1 may thus play important roles in the major processes of tumor progression (figures 3 and 4): (a) HIF-1 mediates hypoxia-induced angiogenesis via activation of VEGF gene transcription, which is necessary for both establishment of the primary tumor and the generation of metastases. (b) HIF-1 mediates increased glycolytic generation of ATP and possibly other intracellular metabolic adaptations to hypoxia that are essential for progression to the phenotype i.e. invasiveness and metastasis (3). Tissue invasion, which is normally a property of only vascular endothelial and placental trophoblastic cells, can be considered an adaptive response to hypoxia that may therefore also require the involvement of HIF-1. HIF-1 may have a protective role in adaptation to the tumor micro-environment. Indeed HIF-1-deficient tumor cells are less tumorigenic than wild-type cells. HIF-1-deficient tumors lack focal expression of GLUT1 in hypoxic tumor regions. Compromised glucose uptake and metabolic adaptation to the tumor micro-environment may form the basis of the reduced tumorigenicity [100]. Reduced tumorigenicity and enhanced sensitivity to apoptosis and growth inhibition by glucose or oxygen deprivation also been observed using xenografts generated from dominant negative HIF-1 mutants, which also exhibit a marked decrease in GLUT1 over-expression [101].

## HIF Is Actively Induced in Tumor Cells

The role of HIF in the growth, survival and radiation response of tumors has been extensively studied using tumor cell lines, and xenografts derived from tumor cell lines lacking either the HIF-1α or HIF-1B subunit. ARNT (HIF-1B)-deficient mouse C4 hepatoma cells demonstrate markedly reduced induction of VEGF mRNA in response to hypoxic culture conditions [102-104]. When injected into nude mice, C4 cells form tumors at a reduced rate relative to wild-type Hepa 1 cells, whereas partially revertant RB13 cells with intermediate levels of HIF-1 expression demonstrate an intermediate rate of tumor growth [105]. Capillary density is increased in tumors derived from Hepa 1 cells compared with C4 cells, and necrotic areas of Hepa 1 tumors are surrounded by high levels of VEGF and mRNA expression which are not detected in corresponding areas of C4-derived tumors [98].

## Control of Glucose Transporter Expression and Function in Malignancy

Even for non-transformed cells, glucose is required for progression through the cell cycle, particularly through the G1-S boundary, in order to progress to the DNA synthetic stage [106]. GLUT1 expression is stimulated by serum growth factors, such as platelet-derived growth factor and fibroblast growth factor, which, owing to their ability to render quiescent cells competent to synthesize DNA, implies the relevance of increased glucose transport during serum-induced mitogenesis [107, 108]. Early transformation experiments undertaken using murine cells infected with sarcoma virus showed increased uptake of natural sugars, such as glucose, mannose and galactose; the increased sugar transport occurring simultaneously with the appearance of transformed cells. The fact that increased glucose uptake by tumor cells was due to increased numbers of membrane bound glucose transporters was confirmed by studies involving the use of the glucose transporter binding inhibitor cytochalasin B [109].

The expression and functionality of glucose transporters in tumors is related to a number of factors, although the widespread over-expression and prognostic effects of GLUT1 is likely to be a down stream consequence of an interaction between oncogenic and hypoxia-inducible pathways. The role of oncogenes in tumor metabolism has been investigated with particular emphasis on the expression of the oncogenes myc, ras and src. The promoter sequence of lactate dehydrogenase, which is upregulated in response to glucose deprivation contain both the HRE and a c-myc/max binding site. It is proposed that activation of the c-myc oncogene results in an oncogenic transcription factor that activates transcription of genes through either the carbohydrate response element (ChoRE) or the hypoxia response element (HRE) enhancer sequence. Meanwhile, other oncogenes, such as ras, src and bcr-abl tyrosine kinases, may activate the HIF-1 pathway, as well as increase c-myc activity, thus leading directly or indirectly to the increased transcription of hypoxia-regulated genes [110] (figure 4). Over-expression of c-myc leads to elevation of GLUT1 expression, alongside the upregulation of further HIF-1/ChoRE regulated glycolytic enzymes such as GAPDH and enolase [111]. H-ras mutations also deregulate glucose transporter expression, causing increased expression of GLUT1 and GLUT3, and down-regulation of GLUT4 [112, 113]. The upregulation of GLUT1, at least, may occur directly or through HIF-1 binding [114].

One of the earliest observations in the study of cellular adaptations to hypoxia was the demonstration of the Pasteur Effect, where a decreased rate of oxidative phosphorylation became concomitant with increased activity of the glycolytic pathway. In fact, in xenografts derived from ras-transformed cell lines, it has been shown that the reduction of tissue oxygen levels is accompanied by a 30% elevation of glucose metabolic rate [115]. This metabolic switch to anaerobic glycolysis is regulated by HIF-1 transcription factor, substantiated by observations that cells lacking HIF-1 show decreased growth rates, lactic acid production and acidosis during periods of hypoxia [116]. HIF-1 also mediates upregulation of the glycolytic enzymes and GLUT3 [95, 96]. GLUT1 expression is dually controlled in hypoxic conditions in response to inhibitors of oxidative phosphorylation, and directly by hypoxia through the HRE/HIF-1 binding complex. In fact, the region lying 5’ to the GLUT1 gene codes for the response to both mitochondrial inhibitors such as rotenone and the response to hypoxia *per se*. However, these effects are mediated through distinct sequences [117]. The stimulation of GLUT1-mediated glucose transport by hypoxia occurs in three stages (reviewed by Behrooz and Ismail-Beigi 1999 [118], and Zhang et al., 1999 [119]). Initially, acute hypoxia stimulates the activation, or of glucose transporters pre-existing on the plasma membrane. In anoxic conditions, and in the presence of metabolic inhibitors, stimulation of glucose transport occurs due to de-suppression of GLUT1 [120]. In normoxic conditions, or in the absence of metabolic inhibitors, GLUT1 is a facilitative transporter (i.e. it facilitates the exchange of extracellular for intracellular sugar). Metabolic inhibition converts GLUT1 to a uniport mechanism, ensuring a hypoxia-induced increase of glucose uptake. GLUT1 is an ATP-binding protein, where ATP modifies transport functionality by an allosteric, rather than a hydrolysis-dependent mechanism [121]. To function as a uniporter, GLUT1 requires a loss of intracellular ATP, conditions that occur as a result of reduced oxidative phosphorylation and that may be required to effect the conformational changes necessary to achieve the antiport/uniport switch [122]. Acute hypoxia induces translocation of both GLUT1 and GLUT4 from intracellular vesicles to the plasma membrane in a number of tissues [123, 124], although variations in glucose concentration, metabolic inhibition and insulin may be involved in the response. More chronically, hypoxic tumor cells will ultimately increase glucose transport via *de novo* synthesis of GLUT1 (and possibly GLUT3). The stimulation of glucose transport by inhibition of oxidative phosphorylation is in fact biphasic. Whereas the activation and translocation of GLUT1 occurs in the early stages, the late phase (between 8 and 24 hours) delivers a doubling of GLUT1 protein content, attributed to both enhancement of GLUT1 gene transcription and to hypoxia-induced stabilization of GLUT1 mRNA [125, 126]. Finally, hypoxia (and hypoglycemia) lead to increased GLUT1 protein synthesis, due to the negative regulation of RNA binding proteins hnRNP lA2 and hnRNP L, which under normoxic, normoglycemic conditions bind an AU-rich response element in the GLUT1 3' UTR, leading to translational repression of the glucose transporter [127].

Despite the existing co-operative control through inhibition of oxidative phosphorylation, the influence of HIF-1 on GLUT1 over-expression in cancer is robust. In xenografts derived from HIF-1-deficient Chinese hamster ovary cells, and from HIF-1-deficient Hepa (mouse hepatoma) cells, no GLUT1 protein is present. However, in wild type revertants, GLUT1 is clearly observable in per-necrotic regions, the link with hypoxia confirmed by co-localization with immunohistochemical staining of adducts of the bioreductive 2-nitroimidazole marker agent, pimonidazole [100, 128]. The increased expression of GLUT1 and other HIF-1-regulated genes in constitutive HIF-1 expressing clear renal cell carcinomas also illustrates the clear influence of HIF-1 on the ultimate levels of GLUT1 [128].

## DEPRIVING NUTRIENTS FROM TUMORS

In any tumor model, it is logical that hypoxic regions will also be glucose deprived. Therefore, it is pertinent to consider possible interactions between glucose and oxygen-dependent signaling pathways. Studies of the regulation of rat L-PK (pyruvate kinase) have enabled the characterization of the glucose response element (GlRE). The GlRE is closely related to the ChoRE, having a core consensus sequence of CACGTG, which leads to transcription of glycolytic enzymes [110]. The ability of oncogenes and HIF-1 to bind to both ChoREs and HREs has been discussed. However, cross talk between the two signaling pathways, where changing oxygen concentration modulates the glucose-dependence of L-PK expression, via interaction with the GlRE, has been demonstrated [129, 130].

# GLUT1: A Marker of Tumor Hypoxia

The future use of hypoxia-selective therapies in cancer will depend upon the individualization of treatment, where patients, whether in clinical practice or in the specific treatment arms of clinical trials, are rationally selected to receive such treatment according to the hypoxic status of their tumor. As the interest in hypoxia in tumors and in other conditions such as inflammatory disease is maintained, there is also a need for a surrogate marker of hypoxia that can be used to determine hypoxia-regulated events experimentally. One prime example of the latter is in the development of hypoxia-regulated gene therapy (O2-GDEPT), where transfection with HRE's may be used to drive drug-activating enzymes [131]. Activation of bio-reductive drugs, radio-response and response to conventional chemotherapy is strongly dependent upon the level of cellular oxygenation, and pro-drugs vary in the extent and duration of hypoxia necessary for bio-reduction [132] However, there is considerable inter and intra-tumor heterogeneity of oxygenation [133]. An accurate, inexpensive and minimally invasive means of measuring tumor hypoxia is therefore highly desirable in order to facilitate the individualization of cancer treatment according to the level of hypoxia within the tumor. A surrogate marker of hypoxia also has a role in prognostication, and any clinical validation will be enhanced if the prognostic effect of tumor hypoxia measured by direct methods can also be extrapolated to the surrogate marker. Several methods exist for the measurement or prediction of tumor hypoxia, which include radiobiological measurement, tumor vascularity, direct $PO_2$ measurement using oxygen electrodes, tumor vascularity, bio-reductive markers and intrinsic markers (reviewed by Hodgkiss and Wardman 1994) [134]. Radiobiological measurement uses radio-sensitivity as a predictor of hypoxic fraction and the success of the technique lies with the detection of DNA damage in samples of cells taken from tumors. However, this method is subject to limitations due to the dose of radiation needed to generate sufficient measurable DNA damage and the risk of DNA repair occurring prior to analysis, which may compromise the end result. Direct measurement of oxygen tension within a tumor can be measured using oxygen electrodes, and its success in detecting hypoxia and predicting outcome in soft tissue sarcomas, carcinomas of the cervix and carcinomas of the head and neck rendered it the gold standard when validating other markers of hypoxia [135-138]. Their use in the clinic is limited by cost, inaccessibility of a number of tumors, and the inherent invasiveness of the procedure. However, one advantage afforded by the use of oxygen electrodes is their rapid response time, which enables the measurement of both acute and chronic hypoxia [139]. The use of tumor vascularity as an indicator of tumor hypoxia is subject to certain pitfalls. The rationale for using tumor vascularity lies with the detection of angiogenesis, which itself is a hypoxia-regulated event, owing to the HIF-1-inducible production of VEGF [98]. However, a paradox exists where increased angiogenesis may itself lead to an improvement in oxygenation, leading to an inverse relationship with hypoxia. Therefore, when using vascularity as an indicator of hypoxia-associated events such as angiogenesis, it is important to distinguish between inter-capillary distance, which correlates with tumor oxygenation and predicts poor local control in radiotherapy-treated patients with cervix carcinoma [140], and mean micro-vessel density, which is measured by counting new capillaries in vascular hot spots when angiogenesis has been induced. The latter, although it may be used as an indicator of angiogenesis, and also to predict poor prognosis in patients with carcinoma of the cervix [141],[142] does not correlate with direct oxygen measurements so is not thought to be a reliable indicator of tumor oxygenation [140]. However, angiogenesis is central to the growth of cancer. An understanding of the cellular and molecular basis of tumor angiogenesis, and a means of measuring its extent, is therefore important for clinicians who diagnose and treat cancer by whatever modalities. We would like to direct the readers to an excellent review of anti-angiogenic drugs for chemotherapeutic treatment of bladder cancer [143].

Bio-reductive markers, like the bio-reductive cytotoxic agents discussed earlier, depend upon the presence of oxygen. Therefore, the extent of reductive metabolism may be used as an indication of intracellular hypoxia. However, instead of producing a toxic metabolite which will kill the cell, the product binds covalently to cellular components, forming intracellular adducts that can be imaged using various methods. The best-known bioreductive markers are the 2-nitroimidazole class of agents [144], such as pimonidazole, an agent that is non-toxic at the appropriate dose for detection of hypoxia, and may be administered intravenously to a patient up to 18 h prior to biopsy. Upon excision, the extent of adduct formation, and therefore tumor hypoxia, can be detected by immunohistochemical techniques. Pimonidazole has been applied as a potential marker of hypoxia in carcinomas of the cervix and of the head and neck [145-147]. Analyzing the extent of pimonidazole binding, or 'scoring' the biopsy samples, has been carried out using computer-aided image analysis systems and by eye, using a semi-quantitative averaging system. Controversy exists as to the accuracy of each system. However, it may be argued that the scoring system used should reflect the setting of the study. For the assessment of hypoxia-regulated pathways in experimental systems, a more high-tech system may be warranted. However, in a clinical setting, data will be used to provide an estimate of the extent of tumor hypoxia, so that patients can be assigned to receive a particular treatment regimen. Therefore, in this case, a simple low-tech analysis, which will not give precise numerical data but is cheap and reproducible, may be more appropriate. Further, in a small series of patients with carcinoma of the cervix, data obtained using both methods strongly correlated [146]; reproducibility and experimental accuracy also being achieved through optimization of the number of biopsies taken from a patient, as well as the number of biopsies stained [148]. Comparisons between pimonidazole and oxygen electrode measurements have revealed a correlation between the two techniques in C3H mouse tumors [149]. However, further comparison in carcinoma of the cervix has failed to establish a statistically significant correlation, despite a trend where tumors with high $PO_2$ values show less pimonidazole binding [150, 151].

The use of intrinsic markers of hypoxia offer many advantages, in that, not only are they a means of detecting hypoxia at the time of biopsy, but they also provide a rapid, inexpensive and non-invasive means of detection, without addition of any exogenous agent or extra procedure. If the marker is being used to assign patients to a particular hypoxia-linked therapy, the level of hypoxia inducing expression of the marker should reflect the level of hypoxia at which the treatment is active. For the marker to be meaningful, changes in expression should be, as far as possible, a characteristic specific to hypoxia. For this reason, genes or proteins inducible via the HIF pathway are regarded as attractive candidates for use as intrinsic markers of hypoxia. Ideally, detection at the protein level should be considered, to enable detection of the marker in a clinical setting by simple protein immunohistochemistry.

The HIF-1-regulated glucose transporters GLUT1 and GLUT3 have been postulated as candidate proteins. However, due to its sporadic expression of GLUT3 [48], GLUT1 has been the subject of studies aiming to validate it clinically as a marker of hypoxia. To evaluate intrinsic markers of hypoxia in a series of human tumors, the semi-quantitative scoring system used to assess pimonidazole binding (described above) has been adopted, and found to be subject to minimal inter or intra-observer error. The first published endogenous marker of hypoxia was GLUT1, which showed a weak but significant correlation with $O_2$ measurements made using oxygen electrodes [39]. In the same series of patients, however, the HIF-1 regulated CAIX showed a better correlation with $PO_2$ [152]. However, when the two candidate markers were compared with semi-quantitative pimonidazole scores, GLUT1 correlated more closely with pimonidazole than CAIX [153]. Both HIF-1-regulated proteins predicted metastasis-free survival in a retrospective series of patients with carcinoma of the cervix, which may provide a clue as to the nature of the hypoxic sub-populations represented by these intrinsic markers of hypoxia. The acute, more transient changes in oxygenation as measured by the oxygen electrode are more likely to influence local control following treatment with radiotherapy [154]. Pimonidazole binding, however, depends upon the accumulation of pimonidazole adducts over a period of time, which may be achieved after chronic hypoxia, or several cycles of intermittent hypoxia. These conditions may be more important for influencing metastatic spread and malignancy [61, 135], [155] which in turn will influence how tumors respond to treatment with surgery, chemotherapy or hypoxia-regulated gene therapy. The co-expression of GLUT1 and CAIX in hypoxia is not surprising, as the anaerobic glycolysis facilitated by GLUT1 over-expression will induce acidosis within the tumor that may be counteracted by a pH- regulating enzyme such as carbonic anhydrase. However, it is now known that CAIX, which is a transmembrane protein with an exofacial epitope, has a role in cell to cell adhesion, evidence that this is in fact a hypoxia-mediated process [156].

## Fluorodeoxyglucose Positron Emission Tomography (FDG-PET)

The use of tumor glucose transporters to assess prognosis in cancer is not a new concept, and can be related back to the nuclear medicine technique fluorodeoxyglucose positron emission tomography (FDG-PET), which exploits the increased uptake of glucose into tumors for diagnostic purposes. This metabolic tumor imaging method has been used successfully in the differentiation of benign and malignant tumors, in the diagnosis of metastasis or recurrence, in the detection of primary unknown cancers, and in cancer screening. The degree of FDG accumulation reflects tumor glucose transport and metabolism thus quantification of FDG uptake by PET can be used in predicting biological malignancy and in monitoring treatment in both radiation and chemotherapy. Positron emission tomography (PET) is a non-invasive tumor imaging technique, which detects the uptake of radio-labeled molecules. The quantitative kinetic information obtained from PET can be applied in the diagnosis of malignancy, staging and assessment of response to therapy [157, 158]. The glucose analogue FDG (fluorodeoxyglucose) may be labeled with fluorine-18, which has a half life of 109 minutes, and like glucose, is preferentially taken up into tumors [159]. However, unlike glucose, after initial phosphorylation by hexokinase, no further catabolism may occur, and the resulting 18F-deoxyglucose-6-phpsphate is trapped in the cell. The mechanism behind FDG accumulation in tumors therefore depends upon the over-expression of glucose transporters, such as GLUT1 and GLUT3, and the relative amounts of hexokinase (reviewed by Pauwels et al. 1998 [160]). FDG accumulation correlates with GLUT1 expression in breast [161, 162], non-small cell lung [163], and pancreatic tumors [41] and with GLUT1 mRNA expression and hexokinase in rat prostate and mammary tumor models [164]. The dependence of FDG uptake on the transport and phosphorylation, as well as diffusion and perfusion through the tumor tissue, may lead to variability in uptake. In breast tumors, for example, low uptake values in lobular regions may be caused by regional differences in microvasculature, hexokinases and the number of tumor cells per volume [128]. Clinical studies aim to evaluate FDG-PET as a diagnostic and prognostic tool. The technique has proved valuable in the differential diagnosis of pancreatic [165, 166] and neuroendocrine tumors [167], though accuracy may be subject to parameters such as serum glucose levels and the degree of differentiation of the tumor. Further applications include the detection of local recurrence in soft-tissue sarcomas [168], and in breast cancer, the detection of primary and metastatic foci [169, 170], distant recurrence [171] and the response to therapy [170, 172, 173]. FDG-PET has also been used successfully to detect bone metastasis [174]. FDG-PET imaging has been evaluated in brain tumors, where a significant link between FDG uptake, tumor grade and survival following various treatment modalities has been established [175]. High FDG uptake has additional prognostic value in tumors of the head and neck, being associated with advanced disease and poor survival following radiotherapy [176, 177]. The over-expression of facilitative glucose transporters and glycolytic enzymes in tumors, and their upregulation in hypoxic conditions, may offer a means of using FDG-PET to detect hypoxia in solid tumors. Increased accumulation of FDG has been observed in human breast [178], melanoma and ovarian cancer [179, 180] and primary head and neck squamous cell carcinoma cell lines that have been exposed to anoxia [181]. *In vivo*, peri-necrotic tumor cells that may also be hypoxic also show increased FDG uptake [182]. In clinical studies of patients with head and neck [183]and brain [184] tumors, it is suggested that FDG-PET may offer an indication of the extent of tumor hypoxia. However, the merit of FDG-PET relative to the use of bioreductive tracers such as the 2-nitroimidazoles is questionable, as FDG is not always retained in hypoxic tissue in mouse models [185-188]. Further evaluation of FDG-PET in relation to intrinsic and bioreductive markers of hypoxia, and response to radiotherapy or hypoxia-dependent drugs is needed to fully assess its application as a marker of hypoxia in the clinic.

## Conclusion

Although several studies have proposed inhibition of glucose transporters as a potential therapeutic angle [6, 46, 189, 190], clinicians should be aware of a potentially important caveat to this approach: high levels of GLUT1 are expressed in a number of tissues. In addition GLUT1 is abundantly expressed in endothelial cells in normal tissues [191], in brain microvessels [192] and in other blood-tissue barriers. Thus, targeting GLUT1 will be highly toxic to cells dependent on nutrient provision at these sites and therefore the side effects of such an approach will be intolerable and potentially lethal. However, it may be possible for the pharmaceutical industry to develop diagnostic and therapeutic strategies based on targeted GLUT and HIF expression. This approach will involve identification and inhibition of HIF and specific high-affinity glucose transporters or signaling proteins involved in the regulation of glucose transporter abundance in human cancer cells. It is already known that some of the novel members of the GLUT/SLC2A family exist in several molecular forms resulting from mRNA splice variants [193], differential glycosylation and other post-translational modifications. This may create opportunities to develop novel and specific compounds to inhibit specific molecular variants of the GLUTs over-expressed in cancer.

## REFERENCES

[1] Warburg, O. (1956) *Science.* 123, 309-314.

[2] Smith, T. A. (1999) *Br. J. Biomed. Sci.* 56, 285-92.

[3] Binder, C., Binder, L., Marx, D., Schauer, A. and Hiddemann, W. (1997) *Anticancer Res.* 17, 4299-304.

[4] Medina, R. A. and Owen, G. I. (2002) *Biol. Res.* 35, 9-26.

[5] Oliver, R. J., Woodwards, R. T., Sloan, P., Thakker, N. S., Stratford, I. J. and Airley, R. E. (2004) *Eur. J. Cancer.* 40, 503-7.

[6] Grover-McKay, M., Walsh, S. A., Seftor, E. A., Thomas, P. A. and Hendrix, M. J. (1998) *Pathol. Oncol. Res.* 4, 115-20.

[7] Tateishi, U., Yamaguchi, U., Seki, K., Terauchi, T., Arai, Y. and Hasegawa, T. (2006) *Eur. J. Nucl. Med. Mol. Imaging.*

[8] Wagstaff, P., Kang, H. Y., Mylott, D., Robbins, P. J. and White, M. K. (1995) *Mol. Biol. Cell* 6, 1575-89.

[9] Wood, I. S. and Trayhurn, P. (2003) *Br. J. Nutr.* 89, 3-9.

[10] Joost, H. G. and Thorens, B. (2001) *Mol. Membr. Biol.* 18, 247-56.

[11] Mueckler, M. (1994) *Eur. J. Biochem.* 219, 713-25.

[12] Thorens, B. (2001) *Mol. Membr. Biol.* 18, 265-73.

[13] Shepherd, P. R., Gould, G. W., Colville, C. A., McCoid, S. C., Gibbs, E. M. and Kahn, B. B. (1992) *Biochem. Biophys. Res. Commun.* 188, 149-54.

[14] Haber, R. S., Weinstein, S. P., O'Boyle, E. and Morgello, S. (1993) *Endocrinology.* 132, 2538-43.

[15] Burant, C. F. and Davidson, N. O. (1994) *Am. J. Physiol.* 267, R1488-1495.

[16] Charron, M. J., Brosius, F. C., 3rd, Alper, S. L. and Lodish, H. F. (1989) *Proc. Natl. Acad. Sci. U S A.* 86, 2535-9.

[17] Uldry, M., Ibberson, M., Horisberger, J. D., Chatton, J. Y., Riederer, B. M. and Thorens, B. (2001) *Embo J.* 20, 4467-77.

[18] Wu, X. and Freeze, H. H. (2002) *Genomics.* 80, 553-557.

[19] Tomita, T. (2002) *Pathol. Int.* 52, 425-32.

[20] Vordermark, D. and Brown, J. M. (2003) *Strahlenther. Onkol.* 179, 801-811.

[21] Brown, R. S. and Wahl, R. L. (1993) *Cancer.* 72, 2979-85.

[22] Ravazoula, P., Batistatou, A., Aletra, C., Ladopoulos, J., Kourounis, G. and Tzigounis, B. (2003) *Eur. J. Gynaecol. Oncol.* 24, 544-6.

[23] Alo, P. L., Visca, P., Botti, C., Galati, G. M., Sebastiani, V., Andreano, T., Di Tondo, U. and Pizer, E. S. (2001) *Am. J. Clin. Pathol.* 116, 129-34.

[24] Younes, M., Brown, R. W., Mody, D. R., Fernandez, L. and Laucirica, R. (1995) *Anticancer Res.* 15, 2895-8.

[25] Zamora-Leon, S. P., Golde, D. W., Concha, II, Rivas, C. I., Delgado-Lopez, F., Baselga, J., Nualart, F. and Vera, J. C. (1996) *Proc. Natl. Acad. Sci. U S A.* 93, 1847-52.

[26] Rogers, S., Macheda, M. L., Docherty, S. E., Carty, M. D., Henderson, M. A., Soeller, W. C., Gibbs, E. M., James, D. E. and Best, J. D. (2002) *Am. J. Physiol. Endocrinol. Metab.* 282, E733-8.

[27] Haber, R. S., Rathan, A., Weiser, K. R., Pritsker, A., Itzkowitz, S. H., Bodian, C., Slater, G., Weiss, A. and Burstein, D. E. (1998) *Cancer.* 83, 34-40.

[28] Furudoi, A., Tanaka, S., Haruma, K., Yoshihara, M., Sumii, K., Kajiyama, G. and Shimamoto, F. (2001) *Oncology.* 60, 162-9.

[29] Cooper, R., Sarioglu, S., Sokmen, S., Fuzun, M., Kupelioglu, A., Valentine, H., Gorken, I. B., Airley, R. and West, C. (2003) *Br. J. Cancer.* 89, 870-6.

[30] Mellanen, P., Minn, H., Grenman, R. and Harkonen, P. (1994) *Int. J. Cancer.* 56, 622-9.

[31] Mineta, H., Miura, K., Takebayashi, S., Misawa, K., Araki, K., Misawa, Y. and Ueda, Y. (2002) *Anticancer Res.* 22, 3489-94.

[32] Kato, H., Takita, J., Miyazaki, T., Nakajima, M., Fukai, Y., Masuda, N., Fukuchi, M., Manda, R., Ojima, H., Tsukada, K. and Kuwano, H. (2002) *Anticancer Res.* 22, 2635-9.

[33] Kunkel, M., Reichert, T. E., Benz, P., Lehr, H. A., Jeong, J. H., Wieand, S., Bartenstein, P., Wagner, W. and Whiteside, T. L. (2003) *Cancer.* 97, 1015-24.

[34] Younes, M., Brown, R. W., Stephenson, M., Gondo, M. and Cagle, P. T. (1997) *Cancer.* 80, 1046-51.

[35] Minami, K., Saito, Y., Imamura, H. and Okamura, A. (2002) *Lung Cancer.* 38, 51-7.

[36] Younes, M., Juarez, D., Lechago, L. V. and Lerner, S. P. (2001) *Anticancer Res.* 21, 575-8.

[37] Kim, Y. W., Park, Y. K., Yoon, T. Y. and Lee, S. M. (2002) *Hepatogastroenterology.* 49, 907-11.

[38] Kawamura, T., Kusakabe, T., Sugino, T., Watanabe, K., Fukuda, T., Nashimoto, A., Honma, K. and Suzuki, T. (2001) *Cancer.* 92, 634-41.

[39] Airley, R., Loncaster, J., Davidson, S., Bromley, M., Roberts, S., Patterson, A., Hunter, R., Stratford, I. and West, C. (2001) *Clin. Cancer Res.* 7, 928-34.

[40] Schonberger, J., Ruschoff, J., Grimm, D., Marienhagen, J., Rummele, P., Meyringer, R., Kossmehl, P., Hofstaedter, F. and Eilles, C. (2002) *Thyroid.* 12, 747-54.

[41] Higashi, T., Tamaki, N., Honda, T., Torizuka, T., Kimura, T., Inokuma, T., Ohshio, G., Hosotani, R., Imamura, M. and Konishi, J. (1997) *J. Nucl. Med.* 38, 1337-44.

[42] Boado, R. J., Black, K. L. and Pardridge, W. M. (1994) *Brain Res. Mol. Brain Res.* 27, 51-7.

[43] Moriyama, N., Kurimoto, S., Kawabe, K., Takata, K. and Hirano, H. (1997) *Histochem. J.* 29, 273-8.

[44] Kalir, T., Wang, B. Y., Goldfischer, M., Haber, R. S., Reder, I., Demopoulos, R., Cohen, C. J. and Burstein, D. E. (2002) *Cancer.* 94, 1078-82.

[45] Cantuaria, G., Magalhaes, A., Penalver, M., Angioli, R., Braunschweiger, P., Gomez-Marin, O., Kanhoush, R., Gomez-Fernandez, C. and Nadji, M. (2000) *Gynecol. Oncol.* 79, 33-7.

[46] Cantuaria, G., Fagotti, A., Ferrandina, G., Magalhaes, A., Nadji, M., Angioli, R., Penalver, M., Mancuso, S. and Scambia, G. (2001) *Cancer.* 92, 1144-50.

[47] Yamamoto, T., Seino, Y., Fukumoto, H., Koh, G., Yano, H., Inagaki, N., Yamada, Y., Inoue, K., Manabe, T. and Imura, H. (1990) *Biochem. Biophys. Res. Commun.* 170, 223-30.

[48] Younes, M., Lechago, L. V., Somoano, J. R., Mosharaf, M. and Lechago, J. (1997) *Anticancer Res.* 17, 2747-50.

[49] Baer, S., Casaubon, L., Schwartz, M. R., Marcogliese, A. and Younes, M. (2002) *Laryngoscope.* 112, 393-6.

[50] Song, C. W., Lee, C. K., Rhee, J. G. and Levitt, S. H. (1982) *Int. J. Radiat. Oncol. Biol. Phys.* 8, 749-52.

[51] Tannock, I. F., Guttman, P. and Rauth, A. M. (1983) *Cancer Res.* 43, 980-3.

[52] Jain, V. K., Kalia, V. K., Sharma, R., Maharajan, V. and Menon, M. (1985) *Int. J. Radiat. Oncol. Biol. Phys.* 11, 943-50.

[53] Purohit, S. C. and Pohlit, W. (1982) *Int. J. Radiat. Oncol. Biol. Phys.* 8, 495-9.

[54] Jha, B. and Pohlit, W. (1992) *Int. J. Radiat. Biol.* 62, 409-15.

[55] Sharma, R. K. and Jain, V. (2002) *Indian J. Physiol. Pharmacol.* 46, 51-60.

[56] Cantuaria, G., Magalhaes, A., Angioli, R., Mendez, L., Mirhashemi, R., Wang, J., Wang, P., Penalver, M., Averette, H. and Braunschweiger, P. (2000) *Cancer.* 88, 381-8.

[57] Reinhard, J., Eichhorn, U., Wiessler, M. and Kaina, B. (2001) *Int. J. Cancer.* 93, 373-9.

[58] Paridaens, R., Uges, D. R., Barbet, N., Choi, L., Seeghers, M., van der Graaf, W. T., Groen, H. J., Dumez, H., Buuren, I. V., Muskiet, F., Capdeville, R., Oosterom, A. T. and de Vries, E. G. (2000) *Br. J. Cancer.* 83, 594-601.

[59] Styczynski, J., Wysocki, M., Debski, R., Balwierz, W., Rokicka-Milewska, R., Matysiak, M., Balcerska, A., Kowalczyk, J., Wachowiak, J., Sonta-Jakimczyk, D. and Chybicka, A. (2002) *Acta Biochim. Pol.* 49, 221-5.

[60] Mueckler, M., Caruso, C., Baldwin, S. A., Panico, M., Blench, I., Morris, H. R., Allard, W. J., Lienhard, G. E. and Lodish, H. F. (1985) *Scienc.e* 229, 941-5.

[61] Hockel, M., Schlenger, K., Aral, B., Mitze, M., Schaffer, U. and Vaupel, P. (1996) *Cancer Res.* 56, 4509-15.

[62] Hockel, M., Knoop, C., Schlenger, K., Vorndran, B., Baussmann, E., Mitze, M., Knapstein, P. G. and Vaupel, P. (1993) *Radiother. Oncol.* 26, 45-50.

[63] Harrison, L. B., Chadha, M., Hill, R. J., Hu, K. and Shasha, D. (2002) *Oncologist.* 7, 492-508.

[64] Fyles, A. W., Milosevic, M., Wong, R., Kavanagh, M. C., Pintilie, M., Sun, A., Chapman, W., Levin, W., Manchul, L., Keane, T. J. and Hill, R. P. (1998) *Radiother. Oncol.* 48, 149-56.

[65] Hall Eric, J. (2000) *Radiobiology for the radiologist.* (Lippincott Williams and Wilkins, Philadelphia ; London).

[66] Nias, A. H. W. (1998) *An introduction to radiobiology.* (Wiley, Chichester).

[67] Denekamp, J., Michael, B. D. and Harris, S. R. (1974) *Radiat. Res.* 60, 119-32.

[68] Murayama, C. and Mori, T. (1989) *Gan To Kagaku Ryoho.* 16, 2135-41.

[69] Aoki, M., Furusawa, Y., Shibamoto, Y., Kobayashi, A. and Tsujitani, M. (2002) *J. Radiat. Res. (Tokyo)* 43, 161-6.

[70] Nemoto, K., Shibamoto, Y., Ohmagari, J., Baba, Y., Ebe, K., Ariga, H., Takai, Y., Ouchi, A., Sasai, K., Shinozaki, M., Tsujitani, M., Sakaguchi, M., Yamada, S. and Sakamoto, K. (2001) *Anticancer Drugs.* 12, 1-6.

[71] Teicher, B. A. (1994) *Cancer Metastasis Rev.* 13, 139-68.

[72] Buettner, G. R. and Oberley, L. W. (1979) *FEBS Lett.* 101, 333-5.

[73] Hockel, M. and Vaupel, P. (2001) *J. Natl. Cancer Inst.* 93, 266-76.

[74] Vaupel, P., Kallinowski, F. and Okunieff, P. (1989) *Cancer Res.* 49, 6449-65.

[75] Vaupel, P., Kallinowski, F. and Okunieff, P. (1990) *Adv. Exp. Med. Biol.* 277, 895-905.

[76] Denekamp, J. and Dasu, A. (1999) *Acta Oncol.* 38, 903-18.

[77] Liu, X. D., Pan, G. Y., Xie, L., Hou, Y. Y., Lan, W., Su, Q. and Liu, G. Q. (2002) *Acta Pharmacol. Sin.* 23, 225-9.

[78] Brown, J. M. (1993) *Br. J. Cancer.* 67, 1163-70.

[79] Brown, J. M. (2000) *Drug Resist. Updat.* 3, 7-13.

[80] Patterson, L. H. and McKeown, S. R. (2000) *Br. J. Cancer.* 83, 1589-93.

[81] Ulhaq, S., Naylor, M. A., Chinje, E. C., Threadgill, M. D. and Stratford, I. J. (1997) *Anticancer Drug Des.* 12, 61-5.

[82] Wood, P. J., Horsman, M. R., Khalil, A. A., Steinberg, F., Streffer, C., Overgaard, J., Stratford, I. J. and Adams, G. E. (1996) *Acta Oncol.* 35, 989-94.

[83] Brown, J. M. and Siim, B. G. (1996) *Semin. Radiat. Oncol.* 6, 22-36.

[84] Stratford, I. J., Williams, K. J., Cowen, R. L. and Jaffar, M. (2003) *Semin. Radiat. Oncol.* 13, 42-52.

[85] Stratford, I. J. and Workman, P. (1998) *Anticancer Drug Des.* 13, 519-28.

[86] Brown, J. M. and Wang, L. H. (1998) *Anticancer Drug Des.* 13, 529-39.

[87] Bremner, J. C., Stratford, I. J., Bowler, J. and Adams, G. E. (1990) *Br. J. Cancer.* 61, 717-21.

[88] Patterson, A. V., Saunders, M. P., Chinje, E. C., Patterson, L. H. and Stratford, I. J. (1998) *Anticancer Drug Des.* 13, 541-73.

[89] Ema, M., Taya, S., Yokotani, N., Sogawa, K., Matsuda, Y. and Fujii-Kuriyama, Y. (1997) *Proc. Natl. Acad. Sci. U S A.* 94, 4273-8.

[90] Gu, Y. Z., Moran, S. M., Hogenesch, J. B., Wartman, L. and Bradfield, C. A. (1998) *Gene Expr.* 7, 205-13.

[91] Wenger, R. H. (2000) *J. Exp. Biol.* 203 Pt 8, 1253-63.

[92] Huang, L. E., Gu, J., Schau, M. and Bunn, H. F. (1998) *Proc. Natl. Acad. Sci. U S A.* 95, 7987-92.

[93] Huang, L. E., Arany, Z., Livingston, D. M. and Bunn, H. F. (1996) *J. Biol. Chem.* 271, 32253-9.

[94] Ratcliffe, P. J., O'Rourke, J. F., Maxwell, P. H. and Pugh, C. W. (1998) *J. Exp. Biol.* 201 ( Pt 8), 1153-62.

[95] Semenza, G. L., Roth, P. H., Fang, H. M. and Wang, G. L. (1994) *J. Biol. Chem.* 269, 23757-63.

[96] Semenza, G. L., Jiang, B. H., Leung, S. W., Passantino, R., Concordet, J. P., Maire, P. and Giallongo, A. (1996) *J. Biol. Chem.* 271, 32529-37.

[97] Wykoff, C. C., Beasley, N. J., Watson, P. H., Turner, K. J., Pastorek, J., Sibtain, A., Wilson, G. D., Turley, H., Talks, K. L., Maxwell, P. H., Pugh, C. W., Ratcliffe, P. J. and Harris, A. L. (2000) *Cancer Res.* 60, 7075-83.

[98] Maxwell, P. H., Dachs, G. U., Gleadle, J. M., Nicholls, L. G., Harris, A. L., Stratford, I. J., Hankinson, O., Pugh, C. W. and Ratcliffe, P. J. (1997) *Proc. Natl. Acad. Sci. U S A.* 94, 8104-9.

[99] Wiesener, M. S., Munchenhagen, P. M., Berger, I., Morgan, N. V., Roigas, J., Schwiertz, A., Jurgensen, J. S., Gruber, G., Maxwell, P. H., Loning, S. A., Frei, U., Maher, E. R., Grone, H. J. and Eckardt, K. U. (2001) *Cancer Res.* 61, 5215-22.

[100] Williams, K. J., Telfer, B. A., Airley, R. E., Peters, H. P., Sheridan, M. R., van der Kogel, A. J., Harris, A. L. and Stratford, I. J. (2002) *Oncogene.* 21, 282-90.

[101] Chen, J., Zhao, S., Nakada, K., Kuge, Y., Tamaki, N., Okada, F., Wang, J., Shindo, M., Higashino, F., Takeda, K., Asaka, M., Katoh, H., Sugiyama, T., Hosokawa, M. and Kobayashi, M. (2003) *Am. J. Pathol.* 162, 1283-91.

[102] Forsythe, J. A., Jiang, B. H., Iyer, N. V., Agani, F., Leung, S. W., Koos, R. D. and Semenza, G. L. (1996) *Mol. Cell Biol.* 16, 4604-13.

[103] Salceda, S., Beck, I. and Caro, J. (1996) *Arch. Biochem. Biophys.* 334, 389-94.

[104] Wood, S. M., Gleadle, J. M., Pugh, C. W., Hankinson, O. and Ratcliffe, P. J. (1996) *J. Biol. Chem.* 271, 15117-23.

[105] Jiang, B. H., Agani, F., Passaniti, A. and Semenza, G. L. (1997) *Cancer Res.* 57, 5328-5335.

[106] Greiner, E. F., Guppy, M. and Brand, K. (1994) *J. Biol. Chem.* 269, 31484-90.

[107] Hiraki, Y., Rosen, O. M. and Birnbaum, M. J. (1988) *J. Biol. Chem.* 263, 13655-62.

[108] Kitagawa, T., Tanaka, M. and Akamatsu, Y. (1989) *Biochim. Biophys. Acta.* 980, 100-8.

[109] Hatanaka, M. (1974) *Biochim. Biophys. Acta.* 355, 77-104.

[110] Dang, C. V., Lewis, B. C., Dolde, C., Dang, G. and Shim, H. (1997) *J. Bioenerg. Biomembr.* 29, 345-54.

[111] Osthus, R. C., Shim, H., Kim, S., Li, Q., Reddy, R., Mukherjee, M., Xu, Y., Wonsey, D., Lee, L. A. and Dang, C. V. (2000) *J. Biol. Chem.* 275, 21797-800.

[112] Baron-Delage, S., Mahraoui, L., Cadoret, A., Veissiere, D., Taillemite, J. L., Chastre, E., Gespach, C., Zweibaum, A., Capeau, J., Brot-Laroche, E. and Cherqui, G. (1996) *Am. J. Physiol.* 270, G314-23.

[113] Onetti, R., Baulida, J. and Bassols, A. (1997) *FEBS Lett.* 407, 267-70.

[114] Chen, C., Pore, N., Behrooz, A., Ismail-Beigi, F. and Maity, A. (2001) *J. Biol. Chem.* 276, 9519-25.

[115] Kallinowski, F., Brownell, A. L., Vaupel, P. and Brownell, G. L. (1991) *Br. J. Radiol.* 64, 350-9.

[116] Seagroves, T. N., Ryan, H. E., Lu, H., Wouters, B. G., Knapp, M., Thibault, P., Laderoute, K. and Johnson, R. S. (2001) *Mol. Cell Biol.* 21, 3436-44.

[117] Behrooz, A. and Ismail-Beigi, F. (1997) *J. Biol. Chem.* 272, 5555-62.

[118] Behrooz, A. and Ismail-Beigi, F. (1999) *News Physiol. Sci.* 14, 105-110.

[119] Zhang, J. Z., Behrooz, A. and Ismail-Beigi, F. (1999) *Am. J. Kidney Dis.* 34, 189-202.

[120] Diamond, D. L. and Carruthers, A. (1993) *J. Biol. Chem.* 268, 6437-44.

[121] Carruthers, A. and Helgerson, A. L. (1989) *Biochemistry.* 28, 8337-46.

[122] Cloherty, E. K., Diamond, D. L., Heard, K. S. and Carruthers, A. (1996) *Biochemistry.* 35, 13231-9.

[123] Wheeler, T. J. (1988) *J. Biol. Chem.* 263, 19447-54.

[124] Young, L. H., Renfu, Y., Russell, R., Hu, X., Caplan, M., Ren, J., Shulman, G. I. and Sinusas, A. J. (1997) *Circulation.* 95, 415-22.

[125] Shetty, M., Loeb, J. N. and Ismail-Beigi, F. (1992) *Am. J. Physiol.* 262, C527-32.

[126] Shetty, M., Ismail-Beigi, N., Loeb, J. N. and Ismail-Beigi, F. (1993) *Am. J. Physiol.* 265, C1224-9.

[127] Hamilton, B. J., Nichols, R. C., Tsukamoto, H., Boado, R. J., Pardridge, W. M. and Rigby, W. F. (1999) *Biochem. Biophys. Res. Commun.* 261, 646-51.

[128] Bos, R., van Der Hoeven, J. J., van Der Wall, E., van Der Groep, P., van Diest, P. J., Comans, E. F., Joshi, U., Semenza, G. L., Hoekstra, O. S., Lammertsma, A. A. and Molthoff, C. F. (2002) *J. Clin. Oncol.* 20, 379-87.

[129] Kietzmann, T., Krones-Herzig, A. and Jungermann, K. (2002) *Biochem. Pharmacol.* 64, 903-11.

[130] Krones, A., Jungermann, K. and Kietzmann, T. (2001) *Endocrinology.* 142, 2707-18.

[131] Patterson, A. V., Williams, K. J., Cowen, R. L., Jaffar, M., Telfer, B. A., Saunders, M., Airley, R., Honess, D., van der Kogel, A. J., Wolf, C. R. and Stratford, I. J. (2002) *Gene Ther.* 9, 946-54.

[132] Stratford, I. J. (1992) *BJR Suppl.* 24, 128-36.

[133] De Jaeger, K., Merlo, F. M., Kavanagh, M. C., Fyles, A. W., Hedley, D. and Hill, R. P. (1998) *Int. J. Radiat. Oncol. Biol. Phys.* 42, 717-21.

[134] Hodgkiss, R. J. and Wardman, P. (1992) *BJR. Suppl.* 24, 105-10.

[135] Brizel, D. M., Scully, S. P., Harrelson, J. M., Layfield, L. J., Bean, J. M., Prosnitz, L. R. and Dewhirst, M. W. (1996) *Cancer Res.* 56, 941-3.

[136] Nordsmark, M., Overgaard, M. and Overgaard, J. (1996) *Radiother Oncol* 41, 31-9.

[137] Nordsmark, M., Hoyer, M., Keller, J., Nielsen, O. S., Jensen, O. M. and Overgaard, J. (1996) *Int. J. Radiat. Oncol. Biol. Phys.* 35, 701-8.

[138] Siemann, D. W., Johansen, I. M. and Horsman, M. R. (1998) *Int. J. Radiat. Oncol. Biol. Phys.* 40, 1171-6.

[139] Cruickshank, G. S. and Rampling, R. (1994) *Acta Neurochir. Suppl. (Wien)* 60, 375-7.

[140] West, C. M., Cooper, R. A., Loncaster, J. A., Wilks, D. P. and Bromley, M. (2001) *Cancer Res.* 61, 2907-10.

[141] Cooper, R. A., West, C. M., Wilks, D. P., Logue, J. P., Davidson, S. E., Roberts, S. A. and Hunter, R. D. (1999) *Br. J. Cancer.* 81, 354-8.

[142] Cooper, R. A., Wilks, D. P., Logue, J. P., Davidson, S. E., Hunter, R. D., Roberts, S. A. and West, C. M. (1998) *Clin. Cancer Res.* 4, 2795-800.

[143] Rocchetti, R., Talevi, S., Margiotta, C., Calza, R., Corallini, A. and Possati, L. (2005) *Chemotherapy.* 51, 291-9.

[144] Hodgkiss, R. J. (1998) *Anticancer Drug Des.* 13, 687-702.

[145] Begg, A. C., Janssen, H., Sprong, D., Hofland, I., Blommestijn, G., Raleigh, J. A., Varia, M., Balm, A., Van Velthuyzen, L., Delaere, P., Sciot, R. and Haustermans, K. M. G. (2001) *Acta Oncol.* 40, 924-8.

[146] Varia, M. A., Calkins-Adams, D. P., Rinker, L. H., Kennedy, A. S., Novotny, D. B., Fowler, W. C., Jr. and Raleigh, J. A. (1998) *Gynecol. Oncol.* 71, 270-7.

[147] Kaanders, J. H., Wijffels, K. I., Marres, H. A., Ljungkvist, A. S., Pop, L. A., van den Hoogen, F. J., de Wilde, P. C., Bussink, J., Raleigh, J. A. and van der Kogel, A. J. (2002) *Cancer Res.* 62, 7066-74.

[148] Thrall, D. E., Rosner, G. L., Azuma, C., McEntee, M. C. and Raleigh, J. A. (1997) *Radiother. Oncol.* 44, 171-6.

[149] Raleigh, J. A., Chou, S. C., Arteel, G. E. and Horsman, M. R. (1999) *Radiat. Res.* 151, 580-9.

[150] Nordsmark, M., Loncaster, J., Aquino-Parsons, C., Chou, S. C., Ladekarl, M., Havsteen, H., Lindegaard, J. C., Davidson, S. E., Varia, M., West, C., Hunter, R., Overgaard, J. and Raleigh, J. A. (2003) *Radiother. Oncol.* 67, 35-44.

[151] Nordsmark, M., Loncaster, J., Chou, S. C., Havsteen, H., Lindegaard, J. C., Davidson, S. E., Varia, M., West, C., Hunter, R., Overgaard, J. and Raleigh, J. A. (2001) *Int. J. Radiat. Oncol. Biol. Phys.* 49, 581-6.

[152] Loncaster, J. A., Harris, A. L., Davidson, S. E., Logue, J. P., Hunter, R. D., Wycoff, C. C., Pastorek, J., Ratcliffe, P. J., Stratford, I. J. and West, C. M. (2001) *Cancer Res.* 61, 6394-9.

[153] Airley, R. E., Loncaster, J., Raleigh, J. A., Harris, A. L., Davidson, S. E., Hunter, R. D., West, C. M. and Stratford, I. J. (2003) *Int. J. Cancer.* 104, 85-91.

[154] Wouters, B. G. and Brown, J. M. (1997) *Radiat. Res.* 147, 541-50.

[155] Cairns, R. A., Kalliomaki, T. and Hill, R. P. (2001) *Cancer Res.* 61, 8903-8.

[156] Zavada, J., Zavadova, Z., Pastorek, J., Biesova, Z., Jezek, J. and Velek, J. (2000) *Br. J. Cancer.* 82, 1808-13.

[157] Yasuda, S., Fujii, H., Takahashi, W., Takagi, S., Ide, M. and Shohtsu, A. (1999) *Gan To Kagaku Ryoho.* 26, 756-61.

[158] Smith, T. A. (1998) *Nucl. Med. Commun.* 19, 97-105.

[159] Price, P. (2000) *Eur. J. Cancer.* 36, 691-3.

[160] Pauwels, E. K., Ribeiro, M. J., Stoot, J. H., McCready, V. R., Bourguignon, M. and Maziere, B. (1998) *Nucl. Med. Biol.* 25, 317-22.

[161] Brown, R. S., Leung, J. Y., Fisher, S. J., Frey, K. A., Ethier, S. P. and Wahl, R. L. (1996) *J. Nucl. Med.* 37, 1042-7.

[162] Brown, R. S., Goodman, T. M., Zasadny, K. R., Greenson, J. K. and Wahl, R. L. (2002) *Nucl. Med. Biol.* 29, 443-53.

[163] Brown, R. S., Leung, J. Y., Kison, P. V., Zasadny, K. R., Flint, A. and Wahl, R. L. (1999) *J. Nucl. Med.* 40, 556-65.

[164] Haberkorn, U., Ziegler, S. I., Oberdorfer, F., Trojan, H., Haag, D., Peschke, P., Berger, M. R., Altmann, A. and van Kaick, G. (1994) *Nucl. Med. Biol.* 21, 827-34.

[165] Zimny, M., Bares, R., Fass, J., Adam, G., Cremerius, U., Dohmen, B., Klever, P., Sabri, O., Schumpelick, V. and Buell, U. (1997) *Eur. J. Nucl. Med.* 24, 678-82.

[166] Reske, S. N., Grillenberger, K. G., Glatting, G., Port, M., Hildebrandt, M., Gansauge, F. and Beger, H. G. (1997) *J. Nucl. Med.* 38, 1344-8.

[167] Adams, S., Baum, R., Rink, T., Schumm-Drager, P. M., Usadel, K. H. and Hor, G. (1998) *Eur. J. Nucl. Med.* 25, 79-83.

[168] Lodge, M. A., Lucas, J. D., Marsden, P. K., Cronin, B. F., O'Doherty, M. J. and Smith, M. A. (1999) *Eur. J. Nucl. Med.* 26, 22-30.

[169] Gallowitsch, H. J., Kresnik, E., Gasser, J., Kumnig, G., Igerc, I., Mikosch, P. and Lind, P. (2003) *Invest. Radiol.* 38, 250-6.

[170] Wu, D. and Gambhir, S. S. (2003) *Clin. Breast Cancer.* 4 Suppl 1, S55-63.

[171] Lonneux, M., Borbath, I. I., Berliere, M., Kirkove, C. and Pauwels, S. (2000) *Clin. Positron. Imaging.* 3, 45-49.

[172] Baum, R. P. and Przetak, C. (2001) *Q. J. Nucl. Med.* 45, 257-68.

[173] Krak, N. C., Van Der Hoeven, J. J., Hoekstra, O. S., Twisk, J. W., Van Der Wall, E. and Lammertsma, A. A. (2003) *Eur. J. Nucl. Med. Mol. Imaging.* 30, 674-81.

[174] Ohta, M., Tokuda, Y., Suzuki, Y., Kubota, M., Makuuchi, H., Tajima, T., Nasu, S., Yasuda, S. and Shohtsu, A. (2001) *Nucl. Med. Commun.* 22, 875-9.

[175] Di Chiro, G. (1987) *Invest. Radiol.* 22, 360-71.

[176] Lapela, M., Eigtved, A., Jyrkkio, S., Grenman, R., Kurki, T., Lindholm, P., Nuutinen, J., Sutinen, E., Solin, O., Bjornskov, I., Bretlau, P., Friberg, L., Holm, S., Jensen, M., Sand Hansen, H. and Minn, H. (2000) *Eur. J. Cancer.* 36, 858-67.

[177] Minn, H., Lapela, M., Klemi, P. J., Grenman, R., Leskinen, S., Lindholm, P., Bergman, J., Eronen, E., Haaparanta, M. and Joensuu, H. (1997) *J. Nucl. Med.* 38, 1907-11.

[178] Burgman, P., Odonoghue, J. A., Humm, J. L. and Ling, C. C. (2001) *J. Nucl. Med.* 42, 170-5.

[179] Clavo, A. C. and Wahl, R. L. (1996) *J. Nucl. Med.* 37, 502-6.

[180] Clavo, A. C., Brown, R. S. and Wahl, R. L. (1995) *J. Nucl. Med* .36, 1625-32.

[181] Minn, H., Clavo, A. C. and Wahl, R. L. (1996) *Nucl. Med. Biol.* 23, 941-6.

[182] Kubota, R., Kubota, K., Yamada, S., Tada, M., Ido, T. and Tamahashi, N. (1994) *J. Nucl. Med.* 35, 1067-75.

[183] Lehtio, K., Oikonen, V., Gronroos, T., Eskola, O., Kalliokoski, K., Bergman, J., Solin, O., Grenman, R., Nuutila, P. and Minn, H. (2001) *J. Nucl. Med.* 42, 1643-52.

[184] Leenders, K. L. (1994) *J. Neurooncol.* 22, 269-73.

[185] Bentzen, L., Keiding, S., Horsman, M. R., Falborg, L., Hansen, S. B. and Overgaard, J. (2000) *Acta Oncol.* 39, 629-37.

[186] Dehdashti, F., Mintun, M. A., Lewis, J. S., Bradley, J., Govindan, R., Laforest, R., Welch, M. J. and Siegel, B. A. (2003) *Eur. J. Nucl. Med. Mol. Imaging.*

[187] Rajendran, J. G., Wilson, D. C., Conrad, E. U., Peterson, L. M., Bruckner, J. D., Rasey, J. S., Chin, L. K., Hofstrand, P. D., Grierson, J. R., Eary, J. F. and Krohn, K. A. (2003) *Eur. J. Nucl. Med. Mol. Imaging.* 30, 695-704.

[188] Patt, M., Sorger, D., Scheunemann, M. and Stocklin, G. (2002) *Appl. Radiat. Isot.* 57, 705-12.

[189] Bavetsias, V., Marriott, J. H., Melin, C., Kimbell, R., Matusiak, Z. S., Boyle, F. T. and Jackman, A. L. (2000) *J. Med. Chem.* 43, 1910-26.

[190] Fung, K. P., Ng, S. W., Ha, D. K. and Choy, Y. M. (1986) *Chemotherapy.* 32, 458-63.

[191] North, P. E., Waner, M., Mizeracki, A. and Mihm, M. C., Jr. (2000) *Hum. Pathol.* 31, 11-22.

[192] Simpson, I. A., Appel, N. M., Hokari, M., Oki, J., Holman, G. D., Maher, F., Koehler-Stec, E. M., Vannucci, S. J. and Smith, Q. R. (1999) *J. Neurochem.* 72, 238-47.

[193] Augustin, R., Carayannopoulos, M. O., Dowd, L. O., Phay, J. E., Moley, J. F. and Moley, K. H. (2004) *J. Biol. Chem.* 279, 16229-36.

In: Lung Cancer in Women
Editor: Varetta N. Torres, pp. 73-93

ISBN: 978-1-60021-659-6


*Chapter III*

# LUNG CANCER IN WOMEN

***Marcelo Blaya[1], Edgardo S. Santos[2], Eloy Roman[1], Melissa Karr and Luis E. Raez*[1]***

[1] Division of Hematology-Oncology, Sylvester Comprehensive Cancer Center, University of Miami Miller's School of Medicine, Miami, FL., USA

[2] Tulane Cancer Center, Tulane University School of Medicine, New Orleans, LA., USA

## ABSTRACT

Although breast cancer is the most common malignant disease diagnosed in women, lung cancer has become the most common cancer-related death in women. Noteworthy, lung cancer mortality in women is superior to mortality rate seen from breast, ovarian, and uterine cancers combined. Cigarette smoking is one of the causes directly responsible for this malignancy; however, the disease appears to be different in women, as can be demonstrated by variations in histologic types in men and women. There are also differences in terms of survival where women have shown to have better survival rates after surgical resection in earlier stage or even in the metastatic setting. Recently, genetic variation among men and women and its possible role in oncogenesis has become evident, including those of CYP1A1 gene or gastrin-releasing peptide receptor. Furthermore, studies have shown that estrogens may be involved in lung tumorigenesis at many different levels, as they may act as estrogen-receptor ligands, activating cellular proliferation or may be activated into reactive intermediates that can cause oxidative damage. The possible role of estrogen in lung tumorigenesis has been shown in case control studies where factors such as early menopause, association between tobacco use and estrogen, and hormonal replacement therapy have been associated with an increased

* Corresponding Author: Luis E. Raez, M.D., FACP; Assistant Professor of Medicine; Director of Hematology-Oncology Clinics; Co-Leader of the Thoracic Oncology Group; University of Miami, Miller School of Medicine; Division of Hematology-Medical Oncology; Sylvester Comprehensive Cancer Center; 1475 N.W. 12$^{th}$ Avenue, Miami, FL 33136; Phone: 305-243-6644; Facsimile: 305-243-5326; Email: lraez@med.miami.edu

risk of lung cancer. Nevertheless, the role and impact of genetic and hormonal variations in lung carcinogenesis in women is still under study.

Interestingly, younger women with lung cancer seem to have better responses with tyrosine kinase inhibitors like gefinitib and erlotinib. In fact, the identification of mutations in the ATP-binding domain of the epidermal growth factor receptor has been shown to predict dramatic responses and introduced the possibility of more individualized therapy. It is already known that factors such as Asian descendant, never-smoker, and female gender confer a better response to epidermal growth factor receptor inhibitors mainly because mutations on that domain appear to be more prevalent in these patients. Thus, it is expected that a better understanding of tumor biology and genetic profile differences among both gender may lead to a more precisely targeted therapy in lung cancer, and consequently, better outcomes.

**Keywords:** lung cancer, non-small cell lung cancer (NSCLC), risk factors, small cell lung cancer (SCLC), smoking, women.

## Introduction

Carcinoma of the lung is the leading cause of cancer death in both men and women not only in the United States, but also throughout the world [1]. It was long thought that this was a disease which primarily affected men. However, this perception has recently started to change when lung cancer incidence in women began to rise and ultimately, surpassed breast cancer in 1987 as the leading cause of cancer deaths in females. In 2001, a report of the Surgeon General titled *"Women and Smoking"* noted that the 600% increase in death rate from lung cancer in women was a "full-blown epidemic" [2]. Women started smoking in significant numbers during and following World War II. The lung cancer death rate for women rose slowly from about 2.5 cases per 100,000 women in 1930 to about 5 cases per 100,000 in 1960. Since 1960, the lung cancer death rate has increased rapidly and steadily, and in 1990 it was over 30 per 100,000 women [3].

The prevalence of cigarette smoking in women, although decreased, it did not do so as much as that of men. Some beliefs such as smoking help control weight have motivated many young women to smoke [5]. Over 20 million American women smoke and nowadays there are a large proportion of teenage girls who use tobacco products.

## Lung Cancer and Smoking in Women

"You've come a long way, baby" at least that is what the 1960 Virginia Slim ad depicting a beautiful young woman wearing stylish fashionable clothes wanted us to believe. They are absolutely right; women have come a long way. Before 1960, it was rare for a woman to smoke. The gender gap between men and women was immense. Today, about 22 million American women are smokers. This is a 600% increase compared to half a century ago [4]. In 2003, 44% of the 157,200 lung cancer deaths were reported to be women. This gives a new meaning to that old 1960 Philip Morris magazine ad. At present, women and society are much more aware and focused on breast cancer because it is ranked as the *"# 1"* most common cancer in women but let us step back and take a look at the big picture. Lung cancer, ranked *"# 2"* in women, is the leading cause of cancer deaths and is primarily due to an increase in tobacco use [4]. There are actually more women dying from lung cancer than the combined total of breast, ovarian and uterine cancer [5].

Many things come into consideration when we talk about women and smoking such as smoking patterns and trends, risk factors, and interventions for prevention. We can also see how the tobacco industry has historically created marketing specifically targeted at women and teenage girls. A number of things need to be acted on to end this preventable epidemic of smoking and smoking-related deaths among women in the United States and throughout the world. The highest frequency of smoking can be seen among American Indian and Alaska Native women, an intermediate occurrence is seen in Caucasian and African American women, and the lowest incidence is among Hispanic, Asian or Pacific Islander women [2].

Smoking prevalence is nearly three times higher among women with 9 to 11 years of education than among women with 16 or more years of education [2]. According to the United States Centers for Disease Control and Prevention (CDC), at least 500,000 teenage girls use tobacco products. Some of the reasons why girls and women may be attracted to smoking are: belief that smoking makes you liberated sexually attractive, athletic, fun loving and slim. Yet, it is quite the contrary with smokers being nicotine dependant, physically unhealthy, and socio-economically disadvantaged and depressed. A 2005 study in the journal "*Tobacco Control*" found that cigarette advertisements for younger women focused on the themes of friendship with other women, self-confidence, freedom, and independence [4].

Despite increased knowledge of the adverse health and teratogenic effects of smoking, its incidence during pregnancy has slightly decreased. Of the 4 million women who deliver babies each year, approximately one million of them smoke during pregnancy. Moreover, we have also noticed that there is a predilection pattern with certain types of cancers related to women smokers. Women appear to have a greater risk of developing small cell lung cancer (SCLC) than men who smoke, and they are more prone to develop adenocarcinoma of the lung than men smokers, and evidence which suggests a possible role of exogenous and endogenous estrogens [6].

## Risk Factors for Women Smokers

- The risk for lung cancer increases with quantity, duration, and intensity of smoking [7]
- The risk for dying of lung cancer is 20 times higher among women who smoke two or more packs of cigarettes per day than among women who do not smoke [7].
- Women smokers face some unique additional risks:
  - menstrual irregularities and earlier menopause
  - infertility
  - bone-thinning osteoporosis
  - arthritis
  - cervical cancer

    - dangerous blood clots if using birth control pills
    - if pregnant: low-birth weight, stillbirths, miscarriages and sudden infant death syndrome

- Findings suggest that having two gene mutations, XPD and cyclin D1, increase lung cancer risks in smokers [8, 9].
    - XPD is involved in repairing everyday damage that occurs naturally when cells divide. Damage to this gene causes genetic damage which accumulates in the cell.
    - Cyclin D1 plays a role in regulating the life cycle of the cell. Damage to this gene allows cells to divide and proliferate abnormally.
- Dr. Curtis Harris from the National Cancer Institute (NCI) states that there is a genetic difference in the lung of women which may contribute to a greater lung cancer risk among women smokers. A gene called the gastrin-releasing peptide receptor (GRPR) is linked with abnormal cell growth and is much more active in females than males. Because the gene is found on the X chromosome, it may explain why female smokers are more than twice more likely to develop lung cancer than male smokers. This gene prompts cells to link up with the GPR hormone and that link in turn causes abnormal cell growth that can lead to lung cancer [10].
- More and more, we are seeing an increase risk of lung cancer in women who smoke than in men who smoke [11]. Sharon Shriver, a biologist from Pennsylvania State University, stated that *"women are much more likely to develop lung cancer after less smoking exposure than are men"* [10]. This is a very common idea whatever the evidence needs to be presented. We will mention later genetic or hormonal differences that might explain this, however stronger evidence remains to be obtained and validated.

## Reducing Prevalence of Smoking among Women

Prevention is critical to reduce the millions of premature deaths caused by smoking. The first step should be geared toward keeping tobacco out of the hands of our teenage girls. We need to educate parents, teachers and community leaders on antismoking strategies. Currently, less than 20% of the states in the United States of America require schools to offer tobacco prevention services [12]. If tobacco prevention programs are properly developed and put into place in our school systems, we can inevitably succeed in preventing adolescents from smoking at all. The Secretary of Health and Human Services, Tommy Thomson, put it best when he said, *"what starts as a single puff is turning into a death sentence"*. David Sacher, the 16$^{th}$ Surgeon General from 1998-2002, urged the American states to establish a course of action to effectively fight against female smoking. A few states did just that. In the state of California, a combination of higher cigarette taxes and massive education caused lung cancer to drop almost 5% among Californian women in the last decade even as it rose by 13% elsewhere. Powerful ads in the state of Massachusetts showed a cigarette pack with a real smoker's photograph saying: "*WARNING: Pam Laffin died from smoking at 31. How old will you be?*" And lastly, a Florida campaign by teenagers educating other teens reduced smoking by middle-school girls from 18.1% in 1998 to 10.9% last year. Smoking-related lung cancer deaths kill more women every year than any other cancer, and yet many people know very little about it. How many more mothers, sisters and daughters have to die prematurely for our voice to be heard?

## Other Factors Linked to Women with Lung Cancer

### Family History

It is well known that patients with lung cancer have a higher number of relatives with lung cancer than control subjects according to some publications [13-15]. There are several potential factors that can explain this situation; however, the simplest explanation for this problem is the clustering of cigarette smokers within families. Perhaps, it is also true that there is an increased risk of lung cancer regardless of family smoking history. In term of the increased risk associated with smoking in women [16, 17], Horwitz et al. showed odd ratios (ORs) for developing lung cancer in women non-smokers with family history of lung cancer, in women smokers, and in women smokers with family history of lung cancer of 2.8, 11.3, and 30, respectively [17]. A history of prior lung disease, another known risk factor for men, was associated with a relative risk (RR) of developing lung cancer of 1.2 and 1.56 in two case-control studies limited to women [18, 19].

We still need to have more evidence that both genetic and perhaps environmental factors may be present in these cases [20]. An American case-control study done in non-smokers tried to estimate the familial risk for lung cancer [21]. Cases were significantly more likely than controls to have a family history of aerodigestive cancers (OR = 2.78) and a trend toward an excess of lung cancer (OR = 4.14; $P = 0.07$). Previous studies done in non-smokers also demonstrated an increased risk in nonsmoking women, and this risk was found to be greater for adenocarcinoma of the lung [13, 22]. Schwartz et al. demonstrated a similar trend in nonsmokers in general; in particular, the risk was found to be greater in women than in men (OR: 1.7 vs 0.5, respectively), and again adenocarcinoma was the predominant tissue type [13].

### Diet

Several investigators have postulated that diet is considered a potential risk factor for the development of lung cancer. Several publications have mentioned that greater dietary intake of fruit and vegetables were associated with a reduced risk of lung cancer [23, 24]. According to the authors, there were considerable dietary differences among the ethnic and racial populations in these studies; however, adjustment for mean daily fruit and vegetable intake among these groups could not explain the strong differences in risk among the populations. A study was conducted to examine the relationship between smoking, dietary antioxidants, and lung cancer risk found that women who consumed five or more carrots per week had a RR of

0.4 (95% CI, 0.2 to 0.8) compared with the risk for women who had not consumed carrots [25]. This is something that was also verified by two prospective studies done in the United States [26]. A 10-year follow-up of a cohort of men in the Health Professionals Follow-up Study and a 12-year follow-up period of a cohort of women in the Nurses Health Study found that new lung cancers were diagnosed in 275 of 46,924 men and 519 of 77,283 women. The risk of lung cancer was significantly reduced in those who had consumed a variety of carotenoids for a maximum protective period of 4 to 8 years even after adjusting for residual confounding from smoking (RR, 0.68; 95% CI, 0.49 to 0.94 for the highest compared with the lowest total carotenoid intake). Of note, the association was stronger in women than in men. Among female never smokers, a significant 63% lower risk was noted [26]. Another hospital-based, case-control study demonstrated that fruit intake and the use of soy in Chinese women provided a protective effect against lung cancer [27]. The same protective effect was observed with the consumption of green tea in a population-based, case-control study [28]. Due to the lack of consistent, reproducible, and strong evidence, many researchers believe that the relationship between diet and vitamins with lung carcinogenesis is unsolved [29-32].

## Ethnic and Racial Differences

The age-adjusted lung cancer incidence in the African American women population was 10% to 20% higher than in White women. Since 1975, the increase has been 120% in African American and 89% in White women, respectively. The incidence rates have continued to increase at an average annual rate of 2.4% for African American and 2.2% for White women, respectively, since 1985.

The Multiethnic Cohort Study consisted in more than 215,000 men and women in the states of California and Hawaii and comprises mainly five self-reported racial and ethnic populations: African Americans, Japanese Americans, Hispanic, Native Hawaiians, and Whites living in Hawaii and California. Between 1993 and 1996, adults between the ages of 45 to 75 were enrolled into the study by completing a 26-page mailed questionnaire asking detailed information about dietary habits, demographic factors, level of education, occupation, personal behavior, prior medical conditions, and family history of common cancers [33]. This study showed that among cigarette smokers, African Americans and Native Hawaiians are more susceptible to lung cancer than Whites, Japanese Americans, and Hispanic. In this study, the level of education was related to risk, with the highest risk among those with less than 8 years of schooling. Education is very likely a surrogate variable for other important exposures, but what these are and whether they are disproportionately distributed in the observed high-risk groups of African Americans and Native Hawaiians are not clear. These findings are unlikely to be explained by differences in socioeconomic status, since over 50% of the African Americans in the Multiethnic Cohort Study had some college education, as compared with only 20% to 30% of Hispanic in this study [33].

### Human Papilloma Virus (HPV) Infection

Human papilloma virus (HPV) types 6 and 11 infections are well-recognized events in the pathogenesis of cervical cancer. These HPVs are associated with cervical intraepithelial neoplasia (CIN), and HPV types 16 and 18 are associated with invasive cervical carcinoma. HPV DNA utilizing polymerase chain reaction (PCR) and *in situ hybridization* was detected in the tumors of 49% of women with lung cancer who also had a history of high-grade CIN grade 3 [34]. A Taiwanese study revealed the presence of HPV DNA (types 16 and 18) in the cancer cells of nonsmoking women with lung cancer [35]. Interestingly, HPV infection seems to be more associated with squamous cell carcinoma of the lung. Yousem et al. demonstrated the occurrence of HPV 6 and 11, 16 and 18, and 31, 33, and 35 serotypes in squamous metaplasia of the bronchus, but no association was found in adenocarcinoma or SCLC [36]. Japanese studies have detected HPV DNA (serotypes 6, 11, 16, and 18) in well-differentiated squamous cell carcinoma and adenocarcinoma cells that were adjacent to squamous cell carcinoma [37, 38]. There is far from universal agreement that HPV is an etiologic agent in lung cancer [39, 40]. An analysis of paraffin-embedded tissue from 32 squamous bronchial carcinomas and 15 cervical cancers utilizing both *in situ* hybridization and PCR techniques was negative for HPV in the lung cancer cases, while 12 of the 15 cervical cases were positive [41]. It is also quite possible that an association of HPV in lung cancer reflects the coexistence of increased and earlier smoking behavior and sexual intercourses.

## Epidermal Growth Factor Receptor (EGFR) and Lung Cancer

Currently, combination chemotherapy is the standard of care for patients with advanced non-small cell lung cancer (NSCLC), but little progress towards improving the efficacy has been made in the past 20 years [42-44]. More recently, EGFR inhibitors have emerged as effective therapies for selected patients with previously treated NSCLC. EGFR is a member of a closely related family of receptors, including EGFR (ErbB1), HER-2/neu (ErbB2), HER-3 (ErbB3) and HER-4 (ErbB4). Ligand binding to EGFR leads to tyrosine kinase activation and a series of events that mediate increases in cellular proliferation, invasion, blocking of apoptosis and resistance to chemotherapy [45]. This led to the development of tyrosine kinase inhibitors (TKIs), initially with gefitinib, and later, erlotinib. Gefitinib achieved encouraging response rates and symptomatic relief, which lead to its approval by the United States Food and Drug Administration (FDA) for use in patients who had progressed after platinum- and docetaxel-containing regimens. Erlotinib has been the only TKI studied in a phase III randomized study that showed a survival benefit. Patients with treatment failure after one or two prior chemotherapy regimens were randomized to either erlotinib or placebo. The erlotinib group had a statistically significant increase in median and 1-year survival rates compared to placebo. Based on this, the US FDA approved erlotinib for patients with NSCLC who had progressed after one or two systemic chemotherapy regimens.

Early in the development of TKIs several phase II studies showed that female sex, adenocarcinoma, Asian origin and never having smoked are all associated with responsiveness of NSCLC to erlotinib or gefitinib [46-48]. It became a very popular idea that if you are a young, non-smoker female you should have the chance to be treated with a TKI. These findings were further confirmed by another study which looked at tumor-biopsy samples from participants of the phase III erlotinib trial and investigated whether responsiveness to erlotinib and its impact on survival were associated with expression by the tumor of EGFR and EGFR gene amplification and mutations [49]. In this study, the authors concluded that the presence of an EGFR mutation among patients with NSCLC who received erlotinib had an increased responsiveness to the agent, but this did not translate into a survival benefit.

Why are these EGFR mutations more prevalent in women and in people with Asian heritage? Paez et al. found EGFR mutations in 16 out of 119 tumors, with predominance of mutations in 15 (28%) of 58 specimens from Japan as compared to one (2%) of 61 from the United States [50]. The mutations were much more common in women (9/45; 20%) than in men (seven of 74; 9%). The highest fraction of EGFR mutations was observed in Japanese women with adenocarcinoma (8/14; 57%) [50]. In another recent study, Huang et al. performed mutational analysis of the EGFR coding sequence on 101 fresh-frozen lung tumor tissues [51]. Among the 101 patients, 39% carried EGFR mutations within the tumor. Of the 69 patients with adenocarcinoma, 56% had at least one mutation in exons 18 to 21 of the EGFR gene. In this study, there was no significant difference in the EGFR mutation rate between male (18/33; 54.5%) and female (20/36; 55.5%) patients with adenocarcinoma, and the mutation patterns were also similar between the two groups [51]. It remains to be determined whether sex might play a role in gefinitib or erlotinib responses in patients with EGFR mutations.

## Hormonal Influences in Women with Lung Cancer

Recent studies have demonstrated how lung cancer therapy may be tailored in the near future in part by the different response rates seen among men and women. Due to these observed differences it is then reasonable to postulate that testosterone and estrogen levels may play an important role in cancer evolution. Estrogen has long been linked to the development of breast and endometrial cancer. Because of this observations as well as the negative impact seen on the cardiovascular system the use of exogenous estrogens has been abandoned as a means of hormone replacement therapy (HRT) [52]. Decreasing circulating estrogen levels by either chemical or medical castration or the use of partial estrogen agonists is now standard of care in the treatment of breast cancer. With further studies we may exploit these treatments in women with other solid tumors including lung cancer.

The classic estrogen receptor (ER) is a ligand-activated transcription factor that influences several bodily functions by its effects on the steroid hormone 17β- estradiol in both men and women. Estrogen functions include female differentiation, fertility, bone stability and cardiovascular health as well as endometrial proliferation. It was long believed that there was only one ER. The exciting discovery of a second ER, ERβ, was later discovered in 1996 and localized to chromosome 14 [53]. The first ER to be cloned was vital for maintenance of the above-mentioned functions. However, studies of ER knockout mice show that the gene deletion has little or no effect on bone stability or on the cardiovascular system. The function of this second ER was then put in question. Both receptors hold several distinct functional domains which include a central DNA binding domain that is highly conserved between the classical ER (ER α) and ER β [54]. The C-terminus encodes the ligand-dependent transcription activation function of the protein. Located at the N-terminus is a second transcription activation function, which is ligand independent and is activated by growth factor mediated phosphorylation. These two ERs possess different biological roles and are found within different tissue through out the body. The ER β is required for differentiation of estrogen dependent tissue and is found in high frequency within human endothelial cells, the ovaries, and the lungs [53]. Tissue that expresses both ERs α and β may possess extremely complex gene regulation via hetero-dimer formation. Interestingly enough, alternatively spliced variants of both types of ERs have been identified in lung tissue [55]. Estrogen can bind to its receptor elements or AP-1 enhancer elements in the promoter region of a variety of target genes and activate transcription by recruiting co-activator proteins. Both ERs have been shown to signal in opposite directions when complexed with estradiol from an AP-1 site. The ER α when bound by estrogen has been found to activate transcription whereas the ER β inhibits it [56]. Moreover, the estrogen antagonists (tamoxifen and raloxifene) were found to be potent transcriptional activators with ERs at an AP1 site. Thus, the two receptors signal in different ways depending on ligand and response element. This suggests that these receptors may play different roles in gene regulation.

It has been observed that lung cancer specimens from women are more likely to express ERs than that of male specimens. These differences may thus partly contribute to observed differences with disease progression and response to therapy among women and men. The most striking difference being the recently noted response to TKIs among Asian women (whom never smoked) containing broncho-alveolar cell carcinoma [57]. As mention before, several reports have linked lung cancer to estrogen by finding its receptor in tumor specimens at high numbers and almost null in normal pulmonary tissue. Immunohistochemistry detects expression of the ER in 7%-97% of cases. However, results from these investigators are thus far inconsistent and clinically irrelevant [58-61]. ERs have also been found in the different histological subtypes of NSCLC [59]. Investigators have also shown that ER mRNA and protein are expressed at extremely low levels in the lung, and that splice variants with uncertain functionality represent the majority of the ER transcripts in the lung [62]. Researchers have shown that β-estradiol produced a proliferative response in vitro in both normal lung fibroblasts and cultured NSCLC tumor cells. *In vitro* and *in vivo studies* have shown that β-estradiol stimulated growth of the NSCLC tumor line, H23, grown as tumor xenografts in SCID mice [63].

Other evidence presented shows that in paraffin sections of NSCLC cells the ER β immunoreactivity was localized to the nucleus, whereas ER α immunoreactivity was localized to the cytoplasm, suggesting that both nuclear and cytoplasmic signaling is involved in estrogenic responses in the lung. They demonstrated that β-estradiol stimulated transcription of an estrogen response element-luciferase construct transfected in NSCLC tumor cell lines. Antiestrogens blocked this effect. Stimulation of lung fibroblasts with β-estradiol also increased production of hepatocyte growth factor by 2-fold. These results suggest that estrogen signaling plays an important biological role in lung tissue and that estrogen could possibly promote lung cancer. Additionally, it is intuitive to postulate that anti-estrogen therapy may have therapeutic value in treating or preventing lung cancer. The caveat to these above observations is that under normal physiologic conditions the ER β has also been found to serve biological functions [64]. This same receptor has been found to regulate surfactant homeostasis and alveolar formation in mouse models [65].

A strong correlation with carcinogen-metabolizing enzymes such as CYP1B1 has been noticed in studies of patients with lung cancer and ER expression. These may possibly translate into differences in lung cancer behavior and response to therapy [66]. In the next section we will explore genetic differences in lung carcinogenesis between male and female patients.

Besides the classic estrogenic effects seen by its interaction with nuclear proteins, it is now more obvious that signaling pathways via the cell plasma membrane may be taking place. In this interaction, several growth factors may come into play including insulin like growth factor (IGF) and epidermal growth factor (EGF) among others [67]. These cytoplasmic ERs may in fact activate the EGFR and the phosphor-inositol (PI)-3 kinase family of receptors there by stimulating cell proliferation and growth. It is also believed that interactions with these growth factors and the ER may be taking place and causing estrogen independent receptor activation.

Exogenous estrogens have also been linked as a possible culprit in lung cancer development. Taioli and Wynder published data that both endogenous and exogenous estrogens may be involved in lung cancer development in women [68]. In their work using case control data they demonstrated how menopause prior to age 40 was associated with a reduction in lung cancer (OR = 0.3). The use of exogenous estrogens was also associated with modest increase risk for lung cancer (OR = 1.7). Smoking was also found to have a possible interaction with estrogen replacement and the development of adenocarcinoma of the lung (OR = 32).

Another trial using a similar method of analysis among women whom used estrogen replacement therapy for a minimum of three months had an OR of 1.0 for the development of lung cancer [69]. Schabath et al., again using a case-control design, evaluated the association between HRT and the risk of lung cancer in almost 500 women with lung cancer and 519 age-matched controls [70]. They found that the use of HRT was associated with a 34% overall reduction in lung cancer risk after controlling for age, menopausal status, ethnicity, body mass index and tobacco exposure. This study however did not thoroughly assess the dose or the duration of estrogen therapy thereby leaving much doubt.

Hormonal disparities among men and women continue to be an area of debate with many questions still unanswered. With the availability of effective estrogen and testosterone blocking agents and their ease of administration it is of some disappointment that more research is not aimed at identifying this potential advantage. A full understanding of the effects estrogens posses at the cellular level is required to begin understanding its role in tumorigenesis.

## THE ROLE OF GENETICS

Definitely, lung cancer seems to be different in women. Histological subtype, etiologies, aberrant enzymatic pathways, biological behavior and disease course have shown important differences between both males and females [35, 71-74]. Sometimes, these observations have been consistently confirmed, and in other instances, the data is conflicting.

Perhaps, the most striking factor between male and female is their hormonal differences as we discussed previously. The role of sex steroid hormones in women has been postulated as a factor for lung carcinogenesis due to increased incidence in women with lung cancer as well as different susceptibility to tobacco effect when compared with matched males. In fact, the ability of estrogen to induce differentiation and maturation in the lung has been demonstrated [58, 75]. ER is expressed not only in normal lung but also in the malignant transformed lung tissue [76]. In lung cancer, an ER variant is the most common ER found in malignant lung tissue, and it differs from the classic ER $\alpha$ expressed in hormonal sensitive breast cancer patients [77]. Moreover, the $\beta$-estradiol has shown *in vitro* proliferative effect on normal lung fibroblasts and lung cancer cell lines [53, 64]. However, the proliferation is 17-fold increased on the lung cancer-derived cells, suggesting a responsive predisposition of the malignant clone to estrogen. To date, the exact role of estrogens in lung cancer formation is still under investigation. However, it has been found that both ERs ($\alpha$ and $\beta$) act on gene regulation and may modulate the expression of polycyclic aryl hydrocarbon enzymatic pathways as well as other signal transduction pathways. In this sense, a case-control study showed that early age at menopause (40 years or younger) is associated with a decreased risk for the development of adenocarcinoma of the lung while estrogen replacement therapy was associated with an increased risk for adenocarcinoma [68]. The study also observed a synergistic effect between estrogen replacement, smoking, and lung adenocarcinoma. More intriguing findings were provided by Stabile et al. who showed that estradiol causes NSCLC cell proliferation and antiestrogen induces growth inhibition [77]. Estrogens may also act as direct carcinogens affecting DNA configuration [78, 79]. Other possible roles include activation of growth factor genes such as IGF-1, EGF, and others [80].

In recent years, genetic aberrations, epigenetic changes, and putative carcinogens have been described in lung carcinogenesis. One of them, the p53 mutation is induced by smoking via the formation of DNA adducts, and thus, mutations in the p53 gene commonly reflect exposure to environmental carcinogens [81]. It is believed that DNA adducts are important in lung tumorigenesis because the extent of DNA adduct formation depends on the balance between the rates of oxidation of the carcinogenic compounds in tobacco smoke, DNA repair capacity, and the rates of detoxification of the reactive products via conjugation [82]. Moreover, the level of DNA adduct in the lung could be an exposure marker to carcinogens as well as a useful factor to be considered for lung cancer susceptibility. These DNA adducts have been found in higher levels in women than in male smokers when compared by pack-year of tobacco smoking [83]. Furthermore, DNA adducts have been found in higher levels in a series of nonsmoking Taiwanese women than nonsmoking men, and it may reflect the environmental exposure to carcinogens in Asian population [84]. A higher frequency of a specific mutation (G:C—T:A) in the p53 gene and higher average of DNA adduct level were found by Kure et al. in lung tumors from both men and women. However, the exposure to cigarette carcinogens was lower in women (23 pack-years vs. 39 pack-years) [74]. Interestingly, this specific mutation in p53 gene was found to be significantly higher in women smokers than in non-smokers [85]. Thus, the study concluded that lung tumors from women smokers have more tobacco-related mutations than women non-smokers and men smokers.

*K-ras*, a proto-oncogene of the *Ras* family, has been found in lung cancer, and its incidence is 3-fold higher in women than men [86, 87]. In women smokers, *K-ras* mutations have been found more frequently in NSCLC than male smokers [86]. The prognostic role of *K-ras* in lung cancer is still controversial. The *Ras* proteins are pivotal regulators of cellular proliferation, differentiation, motility, and apoptosis. Mutations on this gene have been found in 20%-30% of NSCLC and are believed to play a key role in this malignancy. Although *K-ras* mutation was initially found to be a negative prognostic marker, more recent studies have failed to reproduce those findings. Also, there are differences in *K-ras* mutation incidence based on ethnicity. *K-ras* oncogene activation by point mutation occurs in about 30% of lung adenocarcinoma in Caucasians. However, *K-ras* gene mutation was found in 13-19% of lung adenocarcinomas in Asian men and it was not present in female patients [88, 89]. An explanation for these findings is the fact that point mutation in the *K-ras* is secondary to the mutagenic effect of tobacco, and most of Chinese women are non-smokers [81].

Another important gene which encodes an enzyme for the metabolism of carcinogenic polycyclic aromatic hydrocarbons, *CYP1A1* gene, has shown to be overexpressed in lung tumors from women smokers compared with men smokers [83, 90]. *CYP1A1* overexpression leads to the activation of polycyclic aromatic hydrocarbons, inducing DNA binding by highly reactive substances, and hence, forming adducts [91]. The metabolic pathway regulated by *CYP1A1* gene takes a more crucial role when phase 2 enzymes such as glutathione S-transferase M1 (*GSTM1*) is deleted, and cannot compete with the phase 1 carcinogen-activating enzymes (like *CYP1A1*). The *GSTM1* null genotype is the most common polymorphism observed, and it is found in 40-60% of the general population due to a gene deletion [92]. *GSTM1* inhibits the formation of free radicals and also catalyzes the conversion of reactive intermediates to inactivate conjugates which are more water soluble and easier to be excreted [93]. Tang et al. conducted a molecular epidemiologic case-control study of lung cancer in which 3 biomarkers: *GSTM1* null genotype, polycyclic aromatic hydrocarbon-DNA adducts (PAH-DNA), and sister chromatid exchanges (SCE) were analyzed in 136 NSCLC surgical patients and 115 control subjects [94]. *GSTM1* null genotype was significantly associated with lung cancer (OR = 2.04). Interestingly, ORs for *GSTM1* and lung cancer were significant in females (OR: 2.50) and smokers (OR: 2.25), and not significant in males and non-smokers. When males were compared against females and smokers versus non-smokers, no significant differences were found. However, OR for *GSTM1* and lung cancer in women smokers was 3.03 compared with 1.42 in men smokers. No difference was found between cases and controls in terms of PAH-DNA and SCE. When elevated PAH-DNA is combined with *GSTM1* null genotype, it appeared to be multiplicative on case-control status (OR: 16.19) [94]. The study concluded that *GSTM1* null genotype effect is higher in female smokers, which is consistent with other reports in which females are at increased risk for lung tumorigenesis than males at equal tobacco exposure, especially when both *CYP1A1* and *GSTM1* gene polymorphism are combined [95].

Moreover, other prognostic markers in lung cancer such as ERCC1, Her-2 neu, and RXRβ appeared to be sex specific [96]. In a study conducted by Dannenberg et al., high levels of these receptors predicted for a better survival in women, but not in men. Conversely, high ornithine decarboxylase expression and low level of cyclooxygenase-2 predicted for better survival in men, but not in women [96]. Although the study included a small number of patients, it emphasized important differences between both gender when we analyze risk factor and predictive and prognostic markers.

## Prognosis of Women with Lung Cancer

In general, women with lung cancer respond better to therapy than male patients regardless of histology, stage, and modality of treatment. Because the incidence of lung cancer is higher in women and it has steadily increased in the last years, lung cancer in women has gained the attention from researchers. The Surveillance, Epidemiology and End Results (SEER) database of 31,226 lung cancer patients analyzed several variables in terms of prognosis. Female sex was identified as a favorable prognostic factor [97]. Another epidemiologic study from Poland revealed that female patients had better prognosis than males with lung cancer regarding the treatment modality used, were younger, adenocarcinoma and SCLC were the most common histological subtypes, and more women were non-smokers than male patients [98]. In a multivariate analysis of this population-based study of 20,561 cases of lung cancer, the RR of death was significantly higher in men (1.15; $P < 0.001$).

The available data in terms of outcome based on gender is also conflicting. Some reports have suggested that women had better outcome when surgery, concurrent chemoradiation or triple modality (surgery, chemotherapy, and radiation) are used [99-101]. Nevertheless, other surgical studies have shown better outcome in males affected by lung cancer [102-104]. In SCLC series, a multivariate analysis from Cancer and Leukemia Group B (CALGB) showed a significantly better response and survival rates for women when compared with their male counterparts [105]. Some studies have found female gender to be a favorable prognostic factor in terms of SCLC survival; however, these observations have not been uniformly confirmed [106-111].

Although female gender has been associated with longer survival in lung cancer, it has not been correlated with radiographic response to chemotherapy. Nonetheless, a clinical trial using an EGFR inhibitor, gefitinib, showed a better radiographic response in female patients as well as adenocarcinoma histological type [46, 47]. Clearly, this observation of survival improvement in lung cancer women may have implication in future clinical trial design and interpretation.

## References


[1] Patel J, Bach P, Kris M. Lung cancer in US women: a contemporary epidemic. *JAMA.* 2004; 291(14):1763-1768.

[2] U.S. Department of Health and Human Services. Women and Smoking: A Report of the Surgeon General. U.S. Department of Health and Human Services, Centers for Disease Control and Prevention, National Center for Chronic Disease Prevention and Health Promotion, Office on Smoking and Health, 2001.of Health and Human Services, Public Health Service, Office of Surgeon General; 2001.

[3] Parker SL, Tong T, Bolden S, Wingo PA. Cancer statistics, 1997. *CA Cancer J. Clin.* 1997; 47(1):5-27.

[4] Patel J. Lung cancer in women. *J. Clin. Oncol.* 2005; 23(14):3212-3218.

[5] Fu JB, Kau TY, Severson RK, Kalemkerian GP. Lung cancer in women: analysis of the national Surveillance, Epidemiology, and End Results database. *Chest.* 2005; 127(3): 768-777.

[6] Baldini EH, Strauss GM. Women and Lung Cancer: waiting to exhale. *Chest.* 1997; 112(4Suppl):229s-234s.

[7] American Cancer Society. Cancer Facts and Figures 2004. Atlanta, GA: American Cancer Society: www.cancer.org accessed january 6th 2007.

[8] Buch S, Zhu B, Davis AG, et al. Association of polymorphisms in the cyclin D1 and XPD genes and susceptibility to cancers of the upper aero-digestive tract. *Mol. Carcinog.* 2005 Apr; 42(4):222-8.

[9] Friend, Tim. "Gene mutations May Raise Lung Cancer Risk in Smokers", *USA Today,* July 2003.

[10] Shriver SP, Bourdeau HA, Gubish CT, et al. Sex-specific expression of gastrin-releasing peptide receptor: relationship to smoking history and lung cancer. *J. Natl. Cancer Inst.* 2000; 92(1):24-33.

[11] Pope M, Ashley MJ, Ferrence R. The Carcinogenic and Toxic Effects of tobacco smoke: are women particularly susceptible? *J. Gend. Specif. Med.* 1999; 2(6):45-51.

[12] Wyman J, Price JH, Jordan T, Dake JA, Telljohann SK. Parents perception of the role of schools in tobacco use prevention and cessation for youths. *J. Community Health.* 2006; 31(3):225-248.

[13] Schwartz AG, Yang P, Swanson GM. Familial risk of lung cancer among nonsmokers and their relatives. *Am. J. Epidemiol.* 1996; 144(6):554–562.

[14] Ooi WL, Elston RC, Chen VW, Bailey-Wilson JE, Rotschild H. Increased familial risk for lung cancer. *J. Natl. Cancer Inst.* 1986; 76(2):217–222.

[15] Wu AH, Yu MC, Thomas DC, Pike MC, Henderson DE.. Personal and family history of lung disease as risk factors for adenocarcinoma of the lung. *Cancer Res.* 1988; 48:7279–7284.

[16] Osann KE. Lung cancer in women: the importance of smoking, family history of cancer, and medical history of respiratory disease. *Cancer Res.* 1991; 51:4893-97

[17] Horwitz RI, Smaldone LF, Viscoli CM. An ecogenetic hypothesis for lung cancer in women. *Arch. Intern. Med.* 1988; 148:2609-12

[18] Wu AH, Fontham ET, Reynolds P, et al. Previous lung disease and risk of lung cancer among lifetime nonsmoking women in the United States. *Am. J. Epidemiol.* 1995; 141 (11):1023-32

[19] Alavanja MC, Brownson RC, Boice JD Jr Hock E. Preexisting lung disease and lung cancer among nonsmoking women. *Am. J. Epidemiol.* 1992; 136:623-32

[20] Tokuhata GK, Lilienfeld AM. Familial aggregation of lung cancer in humans. *J. Natl. Cancer Inst.* 1963; 30:289–312.

[21] Mayne ST, Buenconsejo J, Janerich DT. Familial cancer history and lung cancer risk in United States nonsmoking men and women. *Cancer Epidemiol. Biomarkers Prev.* 1999; 8(12)1065–1069.

[22] Wu AH, Fontham ET, Reynolds P, et al. Family history of cancer and risk of lung cancer among lifetime nonsmoking women in the United States. *Am. J. Epidemiol.* 1996; 143:535–542.

[23] Ziegler RG, Mayne ST, Swanson CA. Nutritionand lung cancer. *Cancer Causes Control.* 1996; 7(1):157-177.

[24] Smith-Warner SA, Spiegelman D, Yaun SS, et al. Fruits, vegetables and lung cancer: a pooled analysis of cohort studies. *Int. J. Cancer.* 2003; 107 (6):1001-1011.

[25] Speizer FE, Colditz GA, Hunter DJ, et al. Prospective study of smoking, antioxidant intake and lung cancer in middle aged women (USA). *Cancer Causes Control.* 1999; 10:475–482.

[26] Michaud DS, Feskanich D, Rimm EB, et al. Intake of specific carotenoids and risk of lung cancer in 2 prospective US Cohorts. *Am. J. Clin. Nutr.* 2000; 72:990–997.

[27] Seow A, Poh WT, Teh M, et al. Diet, reproductive factors and lung cancer risk among Chinese women in Singapore: evidence for a protective effect of soy in nonsmokers. *Int. J. Cancer.* 2002; 97:365–371.

[28] Zhong L, Goldberg MS, Gao YT, et al. A population based case-control study of lung cancer and green tea consumption among women living in Shanghai China. *Epidemiology.* 2001; 12(6):695–700

[29] The Alpha-Tocopherol, Beta-Carotene Cancer Prevention Study Group. The effect of vitamin E and beta-carotene on the incidence of lung cancer and other cancer in male smokers. *N. Engl. J. Med.* 1994; 330:1029-1035

[30] Menkes MS, Comstock GW, Vuilleumier JP, et al. Serum beta-carotene, vitamins A and E, selenium, and the risk of lung cancer. *N. Engl. J. Med.* 1986; 315:1250-54

[31] Steinmetz KA, Potter JD, Folsom AR. Vegetables, fruit, and lung cancer in the Iowa Women's Health Study. *Cancer Res.* 1993; 53:536-43

[32] Wu AH, Henderson BE, Pike MC, et al. Smoking and other risk factors for lung cancer in women. *J. Natl. Cancer Inst.* 1985; 74:747-51

[33] Haiman CA, Stram DO, Wilkens LR, et al. Ethnic and Racial Differences in the Smoking-Related Risk of Lung Cancer. *N. Engl. J. Med.* 2006; 354(4): 4:333-342.

[34] Hennig EM, Suo Z, Karlsen F, et al. HPV positive bronchopulmonary carcinomas in women with previous high-grade cervical intraepithelial neoplasia (CIN III). *Acta Oncol.* 1999; 38:639–647

[35] Cheng Y-W, Chiou H-L, Sheu G-T, et al. The association of human papillomavirus 16/18 infection with lung cancer among nonsmoking Taiwanese women. *Cancer Res.* 2001; 61:2799-2803.

[36] Yousem SA, Ohori, Sonmez-Alpan E. Occurrence of human papillomavirus DNA in primary lung neoplasms. *Cancer.* 1992; 69:693–697.

[37] Hirayasu T, Iwamasa T, Kamada Y, et al. Human papillomavirus DNA in squamous cell carcinoma of the lung. *J. Clin. Pathol.* 1996; 49:810-817.

[38] Tsuhako K, Nakazato I, Hirayasu T, et al. Human papillomavirus DNA in adenosquamous cell carcinoma of the lung. *J. Clin. Pathol.* 1998; 51:741-749.

[39] Kaya H, Kotiloglu E, Inanli S, et al. Prevalence of human papillomavirus in laryngeal and lung cancer. *Pathologica.* 2001; 93:531-534.

[40] Gorgoulis VG, Zachartous P, Kotsinas A, et al. Human papillomavirus (HPV) is possibly involved in laryngeal but not in lung carcinogenesis. *Hum. Pathol.* 1999; 30:274-283.

[41] Welt A, Hummel M, Niedobitek G, et al. Human papillomavirus infection is not associated with bronchial carcinoma: evaluation by in situ hybridization and the polymerase chain reaction. *J. Pathol.* 1997; 181:276-280.

[42] Schiller JH, Harrington D, Belani CP et al: Comparison of four chemotherapy regimens for advanced non small cell lung cancer. *N. Engl. J. Med.* 2002; 346:92-98.

[43] Kelly K, Crowley J, Bunn PA Jr et al: Randomized phase III trial of paclitaxel plus carboplatin versus vinorelbine plus Cisplatin in the treatment of patients with advanced non small cell lung cancer: A Southwest Oncology Group trial. *J. Clin. Oncol.* 2001; 19:3210-3218.

[44] Breathnach OS, Freidlin B, Conley B et al: Twenty-two years of phase III trials for patients with advanced non small cell lung cancer: Sobering results. *J. Clin. Oncol.* 2001; 19:1734-1742.

[45] Janne PA, Engelman JA, Johnson BE. Epidermal growth factor receptor mutations in non-small-cell lung cancer: implications for treatment and tumor biology. *J. Clin. Oncol.* 2005; 23(14):3227-3234.

[46] Fukuoka M, Yano S, Giaccone G, et al. Multi-institutional randomized phase II trial of gefitinib for previously treated patients with advanced non-small cell lung cancer. *J. Clin. Oncol.* 2003; 21(12):2237-2246.

[47] Kris MG, Natale RB, Herbst RS, et al. Efficacy of gefitinib, an inhibitor of the epidermal growth factor receptor tyrosine kinase, in symptomatic patients with non-small cell lung cancer: a randomized trial. *JAMA.* 2003; 290:2149-2158.

[48] Perez-Soler R, Chachoua A, Hammond LA et al. determinants of tumor response and survival with erlotinib in patients with non-small cell lung cancer. *J. Clin. Oncol.* 2004; 22:3238-3247.

[49] Tsao MS, Sakurada A, Cutz JC, et al: Erlotinib in Lung Cancer – molecular and clinical predictors of outcome. *N. Engl. J. Med.* 2005; 353:133-144.

[50] Paez J, Janne P, Lee J, et al. EGFR mutations in lung cancer: Correlation with clinical response to gefitinib therapy. *Science.* 2004; 304:1497-1500.

[51] Huang S, Liu H, Ling-Hui L, et al. High frequency of epidermal growth factor receptor mutations with complex patterns in non-small cell lung cancers related to gefitinib responsiveness in Taiwan. *Clin. Cancer Res.* 2004; 10:8195-8203.

[52] Hulley S, Grady D, Bush T, et al. Randomized trial of estrogen plus progestin for secondary prevention of coronary heart disease in postmenopausal women. Heart and Estrogen/progestin Replacement Study (HERS) Research Group. *JAMA.* 1998; 280(7) 605-13.

[53] Enmark E, Pelto-Huikko M, Grandien K, et al: Human estrogen receptor beta-gene structure, chromosomal localization, and expression pattern. *J. Clin. Endocrinol. Metab.* 1997; 82:4258-4265.

[54] Pettersson K, Gustafsson J. Role of estrogen receptor beta in estrogen action. *Annu. Rev. Physiol.* 2001; 63:165-192.

[55] Fasco M, Hurteau G, Spivack S. Gender-dependent expression of alpha and beta estrogen receptors in human nontumor and tumor lung tissue. *Mol. Cell Endocrinol.* 2002; 188:125-140.

[56] Paech K, Webb P, Kuiper GG, et al. Differential ligand activation of estrogen receptors ERalpha and ERbeta at AP1 sites. *Science.* 1997; 277:1508-1510.

[57] Pao W, Miller VA. Epidermal growth factor receptor mutations, small-molecule kinase inhibitors, and non-small-cell lung cancer: current knowledge and future directions. *J. Clin. Oncol.* 2005; 23(11):2556-2568.

[58] Canver CC, Memoli VA, Vanderveer PL, et al. Sex hormone receptors in non-small-cell lung cancer in human beings. *J. Thorac Cardiovasc. Surg.* 1994; 108:153-157.

[59] Cagle PT, Mody DR, Schwartz MR. Estrogen and progesterone receptors in bronchogenic carcinoma. *Cancer Res.* 1990; 50:6632-6635.

[60] Ollayos CW, Riordan GP, Rushin JM. Estrogen receptor detection in paraffin sections of adenocarcinoma of the colon, pancreas, and lung. *Arch. Pathol. Lab. Med.* 1994; 118:630-632.

[61] Beattie CW, Hansen NW, Thomas PA. Steroid receptors in human lung cancer. *Cancer Res.* 1985; 45:4206-4214.

[62] Matsuda S, Kadowaki Y, Ichino M, et al: 17 beta-estradiol mimics ligand activity of the c-erbB2 protooncogene product. *Proc. Natl. Acad. Sci. U S A.* 1993; 90:10803-10807.

[63] Stabile LP, Davis AL, Gubish CT, et al. Human non-small cell lung tumors and cells derived from normal lung express both estrogen receptor alpha and beta and show biological responses to estrogen. *Cancer Res.* 2002; 62:2141-2150.

[64] Omoto Y, Kobayashi Y, Nishida K, et al. Expression, function, and clinical implications of the estrogen receptor beta in human lung cancers. *Biochem. Biophys. Res. Commun.* 2001; 285(2):340-347..

[65] Patrone C, Caseel T, Pettersson K, et al. Regulation of postnatal lung development and homeostasis by estrogen receptor beta. *Mol. Cell Biol.* 2003; 23:8542-8552.

[66] Spivack S, Hurteau G, Fasco M, et al. Phase I and II carcinogen metabolism gene expression in human lung tissue and tumors. *Clin. Cancer Res.* 2003; 9:6002-6011.

[67] Levin ER. Bidirectional signaling between the estrogen receptor and the epidermal growth factor receptor. *Mol. Endocrinol.* 2003; 17(3):309-317.

[68] Taioli E, Wynder EL: Re: Endocrine factors and adenocarcinoma of the lung in women. *J. Natl. Cancer Inst.* 1994; 86:869-870.

[69] Blackman J, Coogan P, Rosenberg L, et al. Estrogen replacement therapy and risk of lung cancer. *Pharmacoepidemiol. Drug Saf.* 2002; 11(7):561-567.

[70] Schabath M, Wu X, Vassilopoulou-Sellin R, et al. Hormone replacement therapy and lung cancer risk: A case-control analysis. *Clin. Cancer Res.* 2004; 10:113-123.

[71] Osann KE, Anton-Culver H, Kurosaki T, Taylor T. Sex differences in lung-cancer risk associated with cigarette smoking. *Int. J. Cancer.* 1993; 54:44-48.

[72] Thun MJ, Lally CA, Flannery JT, Calle EE, Flanders WD, Heath CW Jr. Cigarette smoking and changes in the histopathology of lung cancer. *J. Natl. Cancer Inst.* 1997; 89:1580-1586.

[73] Wong MP, Fung LF, Wang E, et al. Chromosomal aberrations of primary lung adenocarcinomas in nonsmokers. *Cancer.* 2003; 97:1263-1270.

[74] Kure EH, Ryberg D, Hewer A, et al. p53 Mutations in lung tumours: relationship to gender and lung DNA adduct levels. *Carcinogenesis.* 1996; 17:2201-2205.

[75] Khosia S, Brehler A, Eisenfeld A, Ingelson L, Parks P, Rooney S. Influence of sex hormones on maturation in the fetal rabbit. *Biochem. Biophys. Acta.* 1983; 250:112-126.

[76] Mollerup S, Jorgensen K, Berge G, Haugen A. Expression of estrogen receptors in human lung tissue and cell lines. *Lung Cancer.* 2002; 37(2):153-159.

[77] Stabile LP, Davis AL, Gubish CT, et al. Human non-small cell lung tumors and cells derived from normal lung express both estrogen receptor alpha and beta and show biological responses to estrogen. *Cancer Res.* 2002; 62(7):2141-2150.

[78] Yager JD, Liehr JG. Molecular mechanisms of estrogen carcinogenesis. *Annu. Rev. Pharmacol. Toxicol.* 1996; 36:203-232.

[79] Fishman J. Biological action of catechol estrogens. *J. Endocrinol.* 1981; 85:59-65.

[80] Ignar-Trowbridge DM, Pimentel M, Parker MG, et al. Peptide growth factor cross-talk with the estrogen receptor requires the A/B domain and occurs independently of protein kinas C or estradiol. *Endocrinology.* 1996; 137:1735-1744.

[81] Lam WK. Lung cancer in Asian women-the environment and genes. *Respirology.* 2005; 10(4):408-17.

[82] Haugen A. Women who smoke: are women more susceptible to tobacco-induced lung cancer? *Carcinogenesis.* 2002; 23:227-229.

[83] Mollerup S, Ryberg D, Hewer A. Sex differences in lung CYP1A1 expression and DNA adduct levels among lung cancer patients. *Cancer Res.* 1999; 59:3317–3320.

[84] Cheng YW, Hsieh LL, Lin PP, et al. Gender difference in DNA adduct levels among nonsmoking lung cancer patients. *Environ. Mol. Mutagen.* 2001; 37:304-310.

[85] Toyooka S, Shimizu N, Gazdar A. The TP53 gene, tobacco exposure, and lung cancer. *Hum. Mutat.* 2003; 21:229-239.

[86] Nelson HH, Christiani DC, Mark EJ, Wiencke JK, Wain JC, Kelsey KT. Implications and prognostic value of K-ras mutation for early-stage lung cancer in women. *J. Natl. Cancer Inst.* 1999; 91:2032-2038.

[87] Ahrendt SA, Decker PA, Alawi EA, et al. Cigarette smoking is strongly associated with mutation of the K-ras gene in patients with primary adenocarcinoma of the lung. *Cancer.* 2001; 92:1525-1530.

[88] Lung M, Wong M, Lam WK et al. Incidence of ras oncogene activation in lung carcinoma in Hong Kong. *Cancer.* 1992; 70:760-763.

[89] Wang YC, Lee HS, Chen SK, Yang SC, Chen CY. Analysis of K-ras gene mutations in lung carcinomas: correlation with gender, histological subtypes and clinical outcome. *J. Cancer Res. Clin. Oncol.* 1998; 124(9): 517-522.

[90] McLemore TL, Adelberg S, Liu MC, et al. Expression of CYP1A1 gene in patients with lung cancer: evidence for cigarette smoke-induced gene expression in normal lung tissue and for altered gene regulation in primary pulmonary carcinomas. *J. Natl. Cancer Inst.* 1990; 82:1333-1339.

[91] Guengerich FP, Shimada T. Oxidation of toxic and carcinogenic chemicals by human cytochrome P-450 enzymes. *Chem. Res. Toxicol.* 1991; 4:391-407.

[92] Bell D, Taylor J, Paulson D, Robertson C, Mohler J, Lucier G. Genetic risk and carcinogen exposure: a common inherited defect of the carcinogenmetabolism gene glutathione S-transferase M1 (GSTM1) that increases susceptibility to bladder cancer. *J. Natl. Cancer Inst.* 1993; 85:1159-1164.

[93] Daniel V. Glutathione S-transferases: gene structure and regulation of expression. *Crit. Rev. Biochem. Mol. Biol.* 1993; 28:173-207.

[94] Tang D, Rundle A, Warburton D, et al. Associations between both genetic and environmentals biomarkers and lung cancer: evidence of a greater risk of lung cancer in women smokers. *Carcinogenesis.* 1998; 19:1949-1953.

[95] Dresler C, Fratelli C, Babb J, Everley L, Evans A, Clapper M. Gender differences in genetic susceptibility for lung cancer. *Lung Cancer.* 2000; 30:153-160.

[96] Dannenberg K, Brabender J, Schneider S. et al. Gender differences in the predictive power of prognostic factors in NSCLC. *Proc. Am. Soc. Clin. Oncol.* 2004; 22(14S):619s (abstr 7008).

[97] Ramalingam S, Pawlish K, Gadgeel S. Lung cancer in young patients: analysis of a Surveillance, Epidemiology, and End Results Database. *Am. J. Clin. Oncol.* 1998; 6:651-657.

[98] Radzikowska E, Glaz P, Roszkowski K. Lung cancer in women: age, smoking, histology, performance status, stage, initial treatment and survival: population-based study of 20,561 cases. *Ann. Oncol.* 2002; 13:1087–1093.

[99] Mitsudomi T, Tateishi M, Oka T, et al. Longer survival after resection of non-small cell lung cancer in Japanese women. *Ann. Thorac. Surg.* 1989; 48:639-642.

[100] Albain KS, Rusch VW, Crowley JJ, et al. Concurrent cisplatin/etoposide plus chest radiotherapy followed by surgery for stages IIIA(N2) and IIIB non-small cell lung cancer: mature results of Southwest Oncology Group phase II study 8805. *J. Clin. Oncol.* 1995; 13:1880-1992.

[101] Graham MV, Purdy JA, Emami B, et al. Preliminary results of a prospective trial using three dimensional radiotherapy for lung cancer. *Int. J. Radiat. Oncol. Biol. Phys*. 1995; 33:993-1000.

[102] Kirsh MM, Tashian J, Sloan H. Carcinoma of the lung in women. *Ann. Thorac. Surg.* 1982; 34:34-39.

[103] Bignall JR, Martin M. Survival experience of women with bronchial carcinoma. *Lancet.* 1972; 2:60-62.

[104] Harley HRS. Cancer of the lung in women. *Thorax.* 1976; 31:254-264.

[105] Spiegelman D, Maurer LH, Ware JH, et al. Prognostic factors in small-cell carcinoma of the lung: an analysis of 1,521 patients. *J. Clin. Oncol.* 1989; 7:344-354.

[106] Osterlind K, Andersen PK. Prognostic factors in small cell lung cancer: multivariate model based on 778 patients treated with chemotherapy with or without irradiation. *Cancer Res.* 1986; 46(8):4189-4194.

[107] Skarin AT. Analysis of long-term survivors with small-cell lung cancer. *Chest.* 1993; 103:440S-444S.

[108] Sagman U, Maki E, Evans WK, et al. Small-cell carcinoma of the lung: derivation of a prognostic staging system. *J. Clin. Oncol.* 1991; 9:1639-1649.

[109] Feld R, Sagman U. Prognostic Factors in Small Cell Lung Cancer. *Semin. Radiat. Oncol.* 1995; 5(1):27-32.

[110] Albain KS, Crowley JJ, Le Blanc M, et al. Determinants of improved outcome in small-cell lung cancer: an analysis of the 2,580-patient Southwest Oncology Group data base. *J. Clin. Oncol.* 1990; 8:1563-1574.

[111] Lassen U, Osterlind K, Hansen M, Dombernowsky P, Bergman B, Hansen HH. Long-term survival in small-cell lung cancer: posttreatment characteristics in patients surviving 5 to 18+ years--an analysis of 1,714 consecutive patients. *J. Clin. Oncol.* 1995; 13(5):1215-1220.

In: Lung Cancer in Women
Editor: Varetta N. Torres, pp. 95-113
ISBN: 978-1-60021-659-6


*Chapter IV*

# WOMEN'S SUSCEPTIBILITY TO RISK AND SURVIVAL FROM LUNG CANCER

***Jong Y. Park*[*], *Tatyana Zhukov and Melvyn S. Tockman***
Division of Cancer Prevention and Control, H. Lee Moffitt Cancer Center,
Department of Interdisciplinary Oncology, School of Medicine,
University of South Florida, Tampa, FL.,USA

## ABSTRACT

Lung cancer had been considered a disease of men. However, incidence and morality rates of lung cancer among women have risen rapidly in the past few decades. The increase in lung cancer among women parallels their cigarette consumption as had been earlier demonstrated in men. Currently, lung cancer is the leading cause of cancer mortality in women, exceeding the second and third causes (breast and colon cancers) combined. 73,020 deaths from lung cancer in women are estimated in 2006 in the US, slightly fewer than the estimated men's lung cancer mortality. There is controversy whether women have a higher relative risk of developing lung cancer than men. Previous studies reported that women do not have a greater susceptibility to lung cancer than men, given equal smoking exposure. However, this hypothesis has not received universal support. The purpose of this chapter is to review the literature addressing: 1) whether women have a higher susceptibility to tobacco carcinogens than men, 2) whether women have better survival after the diagnosis of lung cancer, and 3) the potential biological mechanisms for a gender difference in lung cancer risk and survival. This information may change strategies for cancer prevention, such as smoking cessation efforts toward women, and has implications for targeted lung cancer therapy.

[*] Corresponding author: Jong Park, Ph.D., H. Lee Moffitt Cancer Center, University of South Florida, MRC3047A, 12902 Magnolia Drive, Tampa, FL 33612; Tel: (813) 745-1703; Fax: (813) 745-1720; Email: Jong.Park@moffitt.org

# 1. Introduction

Compared to men, the relative susceptibility of women for developing lung cancer remains controversial. The published reports of gender-specific risk effects remain inconsistent. Many confounding factors, such as amount and depth of smoking, second hand smoking, diet, occupation, indoor exposure, different life span, hormonal pattern, and genetic profiles have affected the differences in lung cancer risk between men and women.

Until 1950, lung cancer was a disease of men. However since 1950, female lung cancer incidence and mortality rates increased in developed counties, including the U.S. From the late 1980s, lung cancer has become the leading cause of cancer mortality among women in the U.S. Although mortality rates have continued to decrease across all major cancer sites in men and in women, mortality rates of female lung cancer continued to increase by 0.3% per year from 1995 to 2002 [1]. Due in large measure to smoking cessation over the past 3 decades, fewer people developed lung cancer and mortality in most age groups declined during the 1990s, except lung cancer mortality rates for women age 65 to 74 which continue to rise [2]. The increased mortality rates among this age group are due to the lag in the temporal trend of cigarette smoking between men and women. [1]

# 2. Gender Difference in Lung Cancer Risk

Several studies have reported that women receive diagnoses at a younger age, suggesting a higher susceptibility to the development of lung cancer [3, 4]. A study of lung cancer detected by baseline computed tomography (CT) screening provided evidence that for a given level of smoking, lung cancer was found more often in women than men [5]. However, other studies have contradicted these findings, and the effect of gender on lung cancer risk associated with tobacco use remains controversial [6]. Although not definitive, some studies have shown that female smokers appear to be at higher risk of developing small cell lung cancer than squamous cell lung cancer, whereas male smokers have a similar risk for the two lung cancer histological cell types [7, 8]. Furthermore, female smokers are more likely to develop adenocarcinoma of the lung at a younger age, and estrogens may play a causative role in this phenomenon [9, 10]. Zang and Wynder (1996) reported that women had ~1.5 fold higher risk of developing lung cancer than men, given the same level of smoking exposure [4]. They observed that the gender differences in lung cancer risk were statistically significant for all histological types, showing a dose-response pattern of higher risk with heavier smoking exposure.

## 2.A. Different Smoking Pattern between Men and Women

Previous studies have shown that ~90 percent of the gender difference in lung cancer incidence was attributable to differences in smoking habits [4, 11]. Several important smoking related factors are often ignored in most epidemiological studies. The risk for lung cancer is associated with level and duration of smoking in both genders. However, this association was suggested to be stronger for women than for men. In general, female lung cancer patients had less exposure to smoking than male patients. Among lung cancer patients, roughly 98% of men, and 70-90% of women, reported a history of smoking. Therefore, the association between smoking levels and the risk for lung cancer may increase faster for women than for men [12].

Women smoke for different reasons than men. Women reported smoking more in emotional and social situations; men reported smoking more in situations requiring close attention to a task [13]. The age at initiation of smoking conveys a different independent risk for lung cancer between genders. In men, the relative risk is higher for those who began to smoke before age 20 (OR = 12.7; 95% CI = 6.4 - 25.2) compared with men who began smoking at age 20 or older (OR = 6.0, 95% CI = 2.8 -12.9). For women, many of whom start smoking at an older age, the risk increase continues until age 25 (OR = 10.0; 95% CI = 4.7 - 21.2) compared with women who began smoking at age 26 or older (OR = 2.6; 95% CI = 0.5 - 12.4) [14]. Female lung cancer patients aged >55 years were more likely to have never smoked than men.

Men usually inhale more deeply than women and smoke more than 75% of each cigarette [4]. In addition, men smoked cigarettes with higher tar content than those smoked by women. The roles of these factors in smoking-related lung cancer risk is interrelated and complicated.

## 2.B. Histological Subtypes of Lung Cancer

The distribution of histological subtypes differs significantly between men and women with lung cancer in US [6]. In women, adenocarcinoma (45%) was the most common histological subtype, followed by small cell cancer (23%) and squamous cell carcinomas (21%). In men, squamous cell carcinoma (36%) was the most common subtype, followed closely by adenocarcinoma (33%) and remotely by small cell carcinoma (18%) (table 1). This difference in histological distribution may be related to cigarette smoke exposure. 10-20% of female lung adenocarcinoma cancer patients are never-smokers while small-cell carcinoma had the lowest frequency of never smokers (2%) [4]. Conversely, adenocarcinoma accounted for the majority (49-65%) of female non-smokers with lung cancer [15, 16]. Changes in the design of the cigarette filter and smoking patterns also may contribute to the recent changes in the distribution of lung cancer histological subtypes. Different distribution of histological types of lung cancer were observed in different countries [17] (table 1) possibly related to smoking frequency. In Asia, the prevalence of smoking for women over 18 years of age (3-15%) was significantly lower that that for men (40-60%).

**Table 1. Histological distribution of lung cancer patients**

| Population | AD[1] | SCC[2] | Large cell | Small cell | First author, year (Ref) |
|---|---|---|---|---|---|
| US.Men<br>US Women | 48,772 (33)[3]<br>36,561 (45) | 53,178 (36)<br>17,493 (21) | 17,786 (12)<br>92,61 (11) | 26,973 (18)<br>18,528 (23) | Fu 2005 [6] |
| Polish Men<br>Polish Women | 1,376 (10)<br>505 (22) | 7,946 (55)<br>759 (33) | 2,204 (15)<br>450 (19) | 2,859 (20)<br>620 (27) | Radzikowska, 2002 [17] |

[1] Adenocarcinoma
[2] Squamous cell carcinoma
[3] Numbers in bracket denote percentages

## 2.C. Comparisons of Gender-Specific Lung Cancer Susceptibility

Several studies reported that women may have a higher susceptibility to the development of lung cancer [3, 4, 12, 17-23]. Most of the studies that found a significant risk increase among women were retrospective in design, reporting excess lung cancer odds ratios of 0.7-2.9 fold (table 2). A large case-control study conducted in Ontario, Canada showed an odds ratio (OR) of lung cancer for female smokers of 27.9 (95% CI = 14.9 - 52.0) compared with 9.6 (95% CI = 5.6 - 16.3) for male smokers [12]. Another case-control study reported that female smokers were 1.7-1.8 times more likely to develop lung cancer than male smokers [22]. Zang and Wynder (1996) showed that women had a ~1.5 fold higher estimated odds of developing lung cancer than men, given the same smoking exposure [4]. An earlier study from 1977 showed a lung cancer OR for female smokers of 16 vs. a OR for male smokers of 10 [18] (table 2).

More recently using prospective data, Bain, *et al* (2004) have drawn a direct comparison of lung cancer incidence rates from Caucasian female and male cohorts (the Nurses' Health Study and the Health Professional's Follow-up Study, respectively) with common age ranges and follow-up periods. Cigarette smoking status and intensity were ascertained on biennial questionnaires over 7 questionnaire follow-up cycles [24]. From 1986 through 2000, 60,296 Nurses' Health Study women contributed 994 lung cancer diagnoses over 738,000 person-years, while 25,397 Health Professionals Follow-up Study men contributed 319 lung cancers over 297,000 person-years. Sex- and age-specific incidence rates were compared by smoking status and intensity. Adjusted hazard ratios were also calculated, conditioned on age and follow-up cycle. Bain, *et al.* (2004) found no statistical gender differences in standardized age- and dose-specific incidence rate ratios, either by direct comparison or by hazard ratios calculated from models adjusted for smoking characteristics (OR = 1.1, 95%CI = 0.95 - 1.3) [24]. At most, these investigators found a small (10%), non-significant excess female risk. This female excess seemed more pronounced over age 65, although even these older age rate differences were not statistically significant. Further, in their literature review of six prospective studies that examined lung cancer incidence or mortality by gender, Bain, *et al.* (2004) report that no excess risk was identified among women. Prescott *et al.* (1998) reported identical incidence rates of lung cancer for male and female never smokers, and this similar rate held across current and former smokers [25]. Thun *et al.* (1995) reported the data gathered by ACS volunteers from the 1,051,038 participants in the Cancer Prevention Study I

(CPS I) and the 1,185,106 participants in CPS II, showing that the male lung cancer mortality rates exceeded the comparable female rates [26] (table 2). This substantial body of prospective evidence shows no gender-specific difference in smoking-related lung cancer susceptibility.

**Table 2. Retrospective and prospective lung cancer studies reporting comparisons of lung cancer rates for women and men**

| Population | Cases # Women/Men | OR or RR (95%CI) | Study design | First author, year (Ref) |
|---|---|---|---|---|
| Third National Cancer Survey | | 1.6 | Retro[1] | Williams, 1977 [18] |
| New Jersey | 994/763 | 0.7 | Retro | Schoenberg, 1989 [19] Schoenberg, 1987 [87] |
| Missouri | | 1.4 | Retro | Brownson, 1992 [20] |
| CSPOC[2] | 833/1153 | 1.3 | Retro | Osann, 1993 [21] |
| Ontario, Canada | 442/403 | 2.9 | Retro | Risch, 1993 [12] |
| AHF[3] | | 1.7-1.8 | Retro | Harris, 1993 [22] |
| AHF | 781/1108 | 1.2 – 1.5 | Retro | Zang and Wynder, 1996 [4] |
| Taiwanese | 291/236 | 1.7 | Retro | Le, 2001 [23] |
| NTLDRIR[4] | 2875/17686 | 0.9 | Retro | Radzikowska, 2002 [17] |
| ACS[5] | 1871/1905 | 0.6 | Pros[6] | Thun, 1995 [26] |
| Kaiser-Permanente | 50/51<br>14/26 | 0.8 (0.6-1.2)<br>0.6 (0.3-1.0) | Pros | Friedman, 1997 [88] |
| Danish | 188/619 | 0.8 (0.3-2.1) | Pros | Prescott, 1998 [25] |
| Swedish | 199/243 | NS[7] | Pros | Nilsson, 2001[89] |
| Scottish | 217/446 | <1.0 | Pros | Marang-vande Mheen, 2001 [90] |
| CARET[8] | 338/732 | 0.9 (0.9-1.1) | Pros | Bach, 2003 [91] |
| Nurses' Health study<br>Health professional follow-up | 955/311 | 1.1 (0.95-1.3) | Pros | Bain, 2004 [24] |

[1] Retrospcetive
[2] Cancer Surveillance Program of Orange County
[3] American Health Foundation
[4] The National Tuberculosis and Lung Diseases Research Institute
[5] American Cancer Society
[6] Prospcetive
[7] Non significant
[8] Carotene and Retinol Efficacy Trial

In addition to common limitations associated with retrospective studies (selection bias, recall bias, confounding), the earlier case-control studies may have been influenced by baseline rates and control selection that occurred when the smoking epidemic was less "mature", when fewer women smoked, when female smoking began at an older age, women smoked fewer cigarettes per day, and inhaled less deeply [27]. While the prospective studies are incomplete and lack precision, they are less likely to mislead, and support the observed convergence of lung cancer risks among men and women that correspond to their smoking habits [28].

# 3. Genetic and Biologic Factors

## 3.A. Hormonal Factors

Any gender differences in lung cancer presentation and susceptibility could be explained by different hormonal factors between men and women. There is evidence supporting the hypothesis that early menopause decreases risk of adenocarcinoma of the lung, whereas hormone replacement therapy is associated with higher risk of lung cancer [29]. Cigarette smoking may alter the estrogen metabolism pathway in female smokers leading to changes in estrogen level [30]. Previous study suggested that estrogen receptor signaling pathways might play important roles both in normal lung biology and in controlling the growth of lung cancer [29]. Stabile *et al.* (2004) reported that estrogen can directly stimulate the transcription of estrogen-responsive genes in lung cells, and it can also transactivate growth factor signaling pathways. Therefore, estrogen may promote lung cancer through direct actions on pre-cancer or cancer cells, or through indirect action on lung fibroblasts [31]. Estrogen levels are often elevated in female lung cancer patients compared with control women [32]; local synthesis of estrogen might be increased within lung cancer cells [31]. Estrogen receptors (ERs), mainly ER-β, are expressed and functional in normal lung and tumor cell lines and tissues. However, clinical analyses of ER expression in lung cancer has been contradictory [33, 34].

### *3.A.1. Estrogen Receptors*

Although the importance of ERs in breast tumor carcinogenesis has been recognized, only limited data describe the roles of ER pathways in lung cancer [31]. Two ERs, ER-α and ER-β, are encoded by separate genes, and function as ligand-activated transcription factors [35]. Whether ERs mediate the ligand-dependent transcriptional response of non-small cell lung cancer (NSCLC) cells to estrogen, remains controversial. Kawai *et al.* (2005) reported that the absence of ER-β expression is associated with a poorer prognosis among NSCLC patients. ER-β immunostaining was found more often in adenocarcinomas, compared to squamous cell carcinomas of the lung [36]. In contrast, Pietras *et al.* (2005) investigated roles of ERs in growth-promoting pathways in NSCLC cells. They found that estrogen-induced growth of NIH-H23 lung cancer cells *in vitro* correlated closely with acute hormonal activation of mitogen-activated protein kinase signaling and was significantly reduced by treatment with Faslodex, a pure anti-estrogen [34].

Estrogen can also directly stimulate the transcription of estrogen-responsive genes along the EGF pathway in lung cancer cells [37]. ER-β is expressed in the lung tissue and estrogen could stimulate lung tumor growth, while ER-β inhibits the carcinogenesis of other tissues, such as mammary and prostate [38]. The mechanisms of these observations are unknown and may occur through the function of ER-α. These diverse effects of the ER were mediated by interacting with other transcription factors. Lai *et al.* (2005) reported that the expression of the ER is more commonly detected in female than in male lung cancer, because less hypermethylation of the ER promoter is seen in female patients. ER was also shown to be involved in the attenuation of antioxidant response element (ARE)-driven gene regulation [39]. Therefore, an alternative ER mechanism may involve the regulation of tobacco carcinogen inactivation enzymes, such as dihydrodiol dehydrogenase (DDH) transcription [40].

The tumor suppressor protein p53 can play a role as a negative regulator of estrogen receptor signaling pathways in a tissue-specific manner, as was found in endometrial and breast cancer cells. Wild-type p53 physically interacts with the ER and represses estrogen-activated transcriptional activity. However, p53 mutants had no or reduced repression effect, depending on the sites of mutation [41]. Liu *et al.* (2006) reported that ER-α binds p53 directly and represses its function by affecting transcription of downstream p53 targets (p21, PCNA) [42]. Together these findings indicate that p53 may play dual roles, and can cross-talk with the ER in hormone-activated signaling pathways. Balanced in normal cells, and likely unbalanced in cancer cells, this cross-talk may favor the direct binding of p53 directly to ER, repressing the transcriptional activity of ER-responsive genes, leading to an anti-proliferative role. Conversely, this may allow for ER to directly bind p53 and inhibit its role as a tumor suppressor by enhancing transcription of p53- responsive genes.

It is intriguing to speculate that blocking ER function might be an important therapeutic strategy against lung cancer in female patients. There are experimental data that ER-α functioning might be critically affected through requirement of cofactors, i.e. ATP-dependent chromatin remodeling proteins, such as the SWI/SNF complex that control estrogen-responsive transcriptional activity of genes involved in cell proliferation [43]. In support of involvement of SWI/SNF core subunits in lung cancer progression, there is a report that loss of expression of BRM/BRG1 in tumor cells is associated with poor prognosis in NSCLC [44]. The ER role in modulation of p53 regulation of DNA damage checkpoints may reveal novel data on gender-based risk and prognosis in lung cancer, and lead in a future to ER-specific drug intervention in the treatment of early stages NSCLC.

## 3.B. Metabolism

### *3.B.1. Nicotine*

Nicotine, the active reinforcing substance in tobacco, changes the level of several neuroregulators and provides improvement in specific neural performance. There is speculation of gender differences in nicotine effects. Lower nicotine metabolism by women is supported by several animal studies [45, 46]. Kyerematen *et al.* (1988) investigated sex differences in nicotine metabolism and disposition in animals. They observed that female rats had lower plasma cotinine concentrations than did male rats; urinary recoveries of nicotine were higher in female than in male rats; and total urinary output of nicotine metabolites was higher in male than female rats. Therefore, the reduced rate of nicotine metabolism, as well as a larger volume of distribution of nicotine was observed in female rats [45]. Men and women are thought to regulate their smoking differently and to differ in their susceptibility to nicotine addiction. Zeman *et al.* (2002) observed that women had significantly lower nicotine levels than men even though there is no significant difference in the number of cigarettes per day between the genders. Therefore, they suggested that gender differences exist in smoking behaviors, nicotine sensitivity, and nicotine requirements.[47].

Previous studies indicated that female smokers tend to be less dependent on nicotine and more dependent on the environmental cues associated with smoking [47]. Gender differences in nicotine addiction may modulate the metabolism and clearance of nicotine. Benowitz and Jacob (1984) estimated the metabolic clearances of nicotine in men and women. They observed that men metabolized nicotine faster than did women [48]. Hecht and Hoffman demonstrated that nicotine can be a precursor for tobacco-specific lung carcinogens (N-nitrosamines) [49]. The most carcinogenic tobacco-specific nitrosamines in laboratory animals are 4-(methylnitrosamino)-1-(3-pyridyl)-1-butanone (NNK), 4-(methylnitrosamino)-1-(3-pyridyl)-1-butanol (NNAL), and N'-nitrosonornicotine (NNN). NNK and NNN form DNA adducts after metabolic activation by cytochromes P450. The resulting adducts have been detected in cells and tissues susceptible to NNK carcinogenesis in rodents. NNK also induces single strand breaks and increases levels of 8-oxodeoxyguanosine in DNA of treated animals [50].

More than the addictive component of tobacco and a carcinogenic precursor, nicotine modulates cellular proteins responsible for proliferation and survival of transformed (neoplastic) cells. This may have clinical implications since continued smoking after a diagnosis of lung cancer is associated with poorer responses to chemotherapy and/or radiation and with decreased survival [51-53]. Tsurutani et al. (2005) identify Akt and NFκB as the key cellular targets of nicotine in established lung cancer cells [54]. Jin et al (2004) show that through activation of Akt, ERK 1/2 and PKA, nicotine induces multi-site phosphorylation of Bad which is then sequestered from mitochondria by the scaffold protein 14-3-3, inhibiting the proapoptotic function of Bad resulting in neoplastic cell survival [55]. Describing that propranolol inhibits nicotine-induced Bad phosphorylation and restores apoptosis, Jin et al (2004) suggest that the β-adrenergic receptor may be the nicotine target in human cancer cells, a potential focus for targeted therapy development [55].

The observation that nicotine stimulates Akt-dependent proliferation and NFκB-dependent survival of lung cancer cells underscores the importance of smoking cessation even after a lung cancer diagnosis. It is never 'too late' to quit smoking. These observations also raise the question whether enhanced female survival after a diagnosis of lung cancer is due to more frequent smoking cessation among female lung cancer patients, or to other biological causes.

### *3.B.2. Other Tobacco Carcinogens*

Benzo[a]pyrene (BaP) is a polycyclic aromatic hydrocarbon (PAH) that is produced from incomplete combustion and is found in cigarette smoke. BaP is initially oxidized to BaP-epoxide then eventually converted to BaP 7,8-dihydrodiol-9,10-epoxide (BPDE) by CYP1A1, which is a central enzyme in the metabolic activation of PAHs. BPDE can bind to DNA creating DNA adducts. DNA adduct levels have been shown to correlate with the level of CYP1A1 mRNA and activity [56]. Reyberg *et al.* (1994) have reported that a higher level of lung hydrophobic DNA adducts in the lung tumors of smoking female lung cancer patients, which supports higher risk of developing smoke-induced lung cancer among women [57]. Mollerup *et al.* (1999) have found that female smokers had a significantly higher level of

DNA adducts in their non-tumor lung tissues than male smokers. Females also had significantly higher levels of adducts/pack-year. Further, Mollerup et al. found that female smokers exhibited a significantly higher expression level of lung *CYP1A1* compared with males [56]. However, BaP metabolites are also metabolized by several detoxifying enzymes, such as dihydrodiol dehydrogenase (DDH), Gluththione S transferases (GSTs), and UDP-glucuronosyl transferases (UGTs), to hydrophilic, inactivated forms. Chen *et al.* (2001) reported that female lung tumor tissues expressed significantly lower DDH than those of male lung tumors. These data suggested that lower DDH expression in women may lead to higher levels of BaP metabolites and result in higher levels of DNA adducts [58]. Recently they expanded their study to investigate a possible role for DHH in lung tumor tissues. They observed that DDH expression was inversely related to BaP-DNA adduct levels in lung tumor. Furthermore, the absence of DDH expression in lung cancer patients was more common for women that for men [40].

## 3.C. DNA Damage/Repair Signaling

Hofer *et al.* (2002) analyzed background levels of DNA damage in non-smoking individuals and the relationship between damage and gender. The authors found that men had higher ($p < 0.001$) levels of DNA single strand breaks than women. These data suggested that gender can affect DNA damage and/or damage repair [59].

It has been shown that phosphorylation of histone H2AX is linearly correlated to the number of double strand breaks [60]. H2AX, a member of the histone H2A family, is rapidly phosphorylated in response to ionizing radiation. This phosphorylation, at an evolutionary conserved C-terminal phosphatidylinositol 3-OH-kinase-related kinase (PI3KK) motif, is thought to be critical for recognition and repair of DNA double strand breaks (DSB). Immunofluorescence studies have shown that several proteins involved in DNA repair including BRCA1, BRCA2, Rad51 and MRE11 are recruited to sites of γ-H2AX (phosphorylated H2AX) [61].

γ-H2AX seems to localize specifically at sites of DNA damage and has been recognized as one of the earliest markers of damaged DNA [62, 63]. Recent data suggest that H2AX is a tumor suppressor gene, raising the possibility that mutations or changes in levels of H2AX may be causally involved in cancer development [64]. ATR/ATM-regulated DNA damage checkpoints (phosphorylated kinases ATM and Chk2; γ-H2AX and p53) might become activated in the early stages of human tumorigenesis that delay or prevent cancer [65, 66]. As a central indicator of DNA damage signaling, dephosphorylation of γ-H2AX is necessary for the termination of checkpoint signaling after DNA repair is complete, but is not necessary for the completion of the repair process [67, 68]. Addressing the fundamental question of how chromatin structure is changed in response to DSB. Yano *et al.* (2005) report that chromatin remodeling not only takes place at the DSB site, but also controls the accessibility of DNA repair factors [69]. The evolutionary conserved INO80 chromatin remodeling complex directly participates in the DSB repair through specific interaction with γ-H2AX, suggesting that an ATP-dependent chromatin remodeling complex can read post-translational histone code in the repair of DNA damage [70]. How damaged DNA activates DNA-damaged response proteins, and whether there are specific gender differences in these mechanisms related to cancer development and progression are still questions to be addressed.

Our data suggested that estrogen binding to estrogen receptors activates ER signaling pathways that modulate the DNA damage/repair response, and may be responsible for the gender bias in lung cancer risk and progression. We observed that expression of estrogen receptors and a marker of the DNA damage/repair signaling pathway (γ-H2AX) are correlated with gender-specific lung cancer frequency and patient survival [71]. Using a novel marker labeling strategy, we quantitatively assessed their sub-cellular localization by applying our computer assisted pathology diagnosis (CAPD) imaging. Immunohistochemisty (IHC) with image analysis was performed on a teaching set of clinical lung tumor and adjacent normal tissue specimens. Similar analyses of marker expression were performed on lung cancer and non-neoplastic cultured cell lines. We observed significant increases in expression of ER-α, ER-β (nuclear) and γ-H2AX in malignant tumors compared to normal adjacent lung tissues. The NSCLC lung tumor specimens from women were observed to be at earlier TNM stage than the male specimens. Our preliminary observations that half of the female lung cancer patients were non-smokers compared to male patients who were all smokers led us to investigate the existence of additional factors contributing to the different prognosis of female NSCLC patients, beyond smoking status and tumor stage. The association of gender-specific overexpression of ER-α, ER-β and γ-H2AX in lung cancer patients with different prognosis must now be confirmed in an independent set of lung tumor specimens. If these analyses are validated, future study will seek clinical validation to demonstrate that markers of ER activation and DNA damage/repair pathway may serve as prognostic biomarkers identifying high- risk patients, specifically in women diagnosed with early stage lung cancer.

### 3.D. Genetic Profile

There is evidence of genetic predisposition to lung cancer, especially in women [10]. A family history for lung cancer was identified as a risk factor in 1963 by Tokuhata and Lilienfeld [72]. Horwitz *et al.* (1988) assessed the possible role of family history and its interrelationship with smoking as risk factors for lung cancer in women. A significant risk increase for lung cancer was identified in female never smoker patients with family history of lung cancer as compared to female never smoker patients with no family history (OR = 5.7). Furthermore, they observed that smoker patients without a family history had an odds ratio of 15.1; and smoker patients with a family history had an odds ratio of almost 30 [73]. These data suggested that family history may be an important risk factor for lung cancer in women.

Numerous studies demonstrated that tobacco carcinogen metabolizing enzymes, such as CYP1A1 and GSTM1 are involved in the activation and detoxification of genotoxic components in cigarette smoke. Early studies reported that the gender difference in the activation of drugs is due to the higher activity of p450 enzymes of male rats [74] [75, 76]. Therefore, differences in the activity of these enzymes could also influence the lung cancer susceptibility in men and women. Gender variation has been studied in enzymes that are involved in the metabolism of tobacco-related carcinogens [75, 76]. It is conceivable that genetically determined variations in the activity of carcinogen metabolizing enzymes modify individual susceptibility to lung cancer [77, 78].

Among lung cancer patients, female smokers have been found to have higher levels of PAH-related DNA adducts and *CYP1A1* gene expression in their normal lung tissue compared to male smokers [56]. Steroid hormones might differentially interact with aryl hydrocarbon receptor- and estrogen receptor-mediated cellular effects. However, current data do not support any role of estrogen in regulating the metabolic activation of polycyclic aromatic hydrocarbons in lung [79].

Nicotine is primarily metabolized to cotinine through the P450 enzymes, especially CYP2A6. Cotinine is then further converted to 3-hydroxycotinine again through CYP2A6 [80]. Genetic variations in CYP2A6, such as gene deletion and gene duplication, have been reported. These genetic variations caused the formation of low-activity or loss of CYP2A6 enzymes [81]. These genotype polymorphisms may lead to low rates of nicotine conversion. Therefore, smokers with *CYP2A6* variant alleles have been reported to smoke different amounts compared with those with wild-type in an effort to maintain nicotine levels in their system [82]. Thus, smokers with slow nicotine metabolizer genotypes smoke fewer cigarettes than those with normal metabolizer genotypes.

Men and women are thought to regulate their smoking differently and to differ in their susceptibility to nicotine addiction. Although difference was not found in the number of cigarettes per day between the sexes, females had significantly lower nicotine levels than males [47]. Nakajima et al. (2006) reported that the capability for nicotine metabolism was higher in women than in men based upon phenotype studies [83]. This suggests that men and women smoke differently to regulate and obtain comparable nicotine levels.

# 4. Survival Rates

Numerous studies report that women have better survival rates than men regardless of the stage of lung cancer at diagnosis [17, 32, 84]. Once cancer is detected, the overall 5-year relative survival rates from the NCI-Surveillance Epidemiology and End Results (SEER) data were significantly higher in women than in men ($p < 0.0001$) (table 3). During the course of the period from 1975-1999, overall survival rates increased in both men and women, with a slightly greater increase noted in men, resulting in a modest narrowing of the gender gap. For the time period from 1975 to 1987, the 5-year relative survival rates were 4.2% greater in women, while for the time period from 1988 to 1999, they were 3.5% higher in women [6].

Survival from lung cancer is directly related to stage at diagnosis. However, women have been reported to have higher survival rates at all stages of lung cancer [17, 32, 84]. This trend has continued in more recent studies from the Mayo clinic [85] and the University of Alabama at Birmingham [86]. Once diagnosed with lung cancer, women have a significantly better 5-year survival at Stage I, Stage II, Stage III and over all stages [86]. However, the favorable prognostic effect of female gender was restricted to patients aged less than 60 years (average survival 13.3 mo *vs.* 10.1 mo; 2ys survival 26% vs. 5%), whereas for older women no advantage over men's results were reported (average survival 9.3 mo vs. 9.1 mo; 2ys survival 8% vs. 7%) [6].

Female patients with ages less than 60 years achieved a 32% 3-year survival rate. It was concluded (a) that sex constitutes a major prognostic factor in small cell lung cancer (SCLC) and is especially useful as a predictor for long-term survival, and (b) that the favorable prognostic value of the female is restricted to younger patients [22]. We observed poorer prognoses for women older than 60 years diagnosed with early stages of the disease, compared to men.

**Table 3. Temporal comparison of relative 5-Year survival between genders**

| 1975–1987 | | | 1988–1999 | | |
|---|---|---|---|---|---|
| Men | Women | p-value | Men | Women | p-value |
| 0.13 | 0.17 | $< 0.0001$ | 0.14 | 0.17 | $< 0.0001$ |

## 5. Conclusion

Smoking is the leading cause for lung cancer in both genders. While the prevalence of smoking has declined in both sexes, the decline in smoking is slower in women than men. Seven prospective studies of lung cancer incidence rates and mortality form a substantial body of evidence that shows no significant gender-specific difference in smoking-related lung cancer susceptibility. Males and females with similar cigarette smoke exposure develop lung cancer at similar rates. While male/female differences exist in estrogen level, estrogen receptor expression, nicotine response, DNA damage/repair signaling, and genetic profile, it is unlikely that these factors contribute more than 10% excess to female lung cancer susceptibility.

Once lung cancer has been diagnosed however, females experience a 3-4% more favorable 5-year survival. The favorable prognosis for female lung cancer patients was observed for each stage, but seemed limited to those less that 60 years of age. The observation that nicotine stimulates Akt-dependent cancer cell proliferation and NFκB-dependent lung cancer cell survival underscores the importance of smoking cessation even after a lung cancer diagnosis. It is never ‘too late’ to quit smoking. These observations also raise the question whether enhanced female survival after a diagnosis of lung cancer is due to more frequent smoking cessation among female lung cancer patients, or to other biological causes.

## References

[1] Jemal, A., R. Siegel, E. Ward, T. Murray, J. Xu, C. Smigal, and M.J. Thun, Cancer statistics, 2006. *CA Cancer J. Clin,* 2006. 56(2): p. 106-30.

[2] Clegg, L.X., F.P. Li, B.F. Hankey, K. Chu, and B.K. Edwards, Cancer survival among US whites and minorities: a SEER (Surveillance, Epidemiology, and End

Results) Program population-based study. *Arch. Intern. Med,* 2002. 162(17): p. 1985-93.

[3] Payne, S., 'Smoke like a man, die like a man'?: a review of the relationship between gender, sex and lung cancer. *Soc. Sci. Med,* 2001. 53(8): p. 1067-80.

[4] Zang, E.A. and E.L. Wynder, Differences in lung cancer risk between men and women: examination of the evidence. *J. Natl. Cancer Inst,* 1996. 88(3-4): p. 183-92.

[5] Henschke, C.I. and O.S. Miettinen, Women's susceptibility to tobacco carcinogens. *Lung Cancer,* 2004. 43(1): p. 1-5.

[6] Fu, J.B., T.Y. Kau, R.K. Severson, and G.P. Kalemkerian, Lung cancer in women: analysis of the national Surveillance, Epidemiology, and End Results database. *Chest,* 2005. 127(3): p. 768-77.

[7] Kazerouni, N., C.J. Alverson, S.C. Redd, J.A. Mott, and D.M. Mannino, Sex differences in COPD and lung cancer mortality trends--United States, 1968-1999. *J. Womens Health.* (Larchmt), 2004. 13(1): p. 17-23.

[8] de Perrot, M., M. Licker, C. Bouchardy, M. Usel, J. Robert, and A. Spiliopoulos, Sex differences in presentation, management, and prognosis of patients with non-small cell lung carcinoma. *J. Thorac. Cardiovasc. Surg,* 2000. 119(1): p. 21-6.

[9] Baldini, E.H. and G.M. Strauss, Women and lung cancer: waiting to exhale. *Chest,* 1997. 112(4 Suppl): p. 229S-234S.

[10] Sellers, T.A., J.D. Potter, J.E. Bailey-Wilson, S.S. Rich, H. Rothschild, and R.C. Elston, Lung cancer detection and prevention: evidence for an interaction between smoking and genetic predisposition. *Cancer Res,* 1992. 52(9 Suppl): p. 2694s-2697s.

[11] Tong, L., M.R. Spitz, J.J. Fueger, and C.A. Amos, Lung carcinoma in former smokers. *Cancer,* 1996. 78(5): p. 1004-10.

[12] Risch, H.A., G.R. Howe, M. Jain, J.D. Burch, E.J. Holowaty, and A.B. Miller, Are female smokers at higher risk for lung cancer than male smokers? A case-control analysis by histologic type. *Am. J. Epidemiol,* 1993. 138(5): p. 281-93.

[13] Zuckerman, M., S. Ball, and J. Black, Influences of sensation seeking, gender, risk appraisal, and situational motivation on smoking. *Addict. Behav,* 1990. 15(3): p. 209-20.

[14] Hegmann, K.T., A.M. Fraser, R.P. Keaney, S.E. Moser, D.S. Nilasena, M. Sedlars, L. Higham-Gren, and J.L. Lyon, The effect of age at smoking initiation on lung cancer risk. *Epidemiology,* 1993. 4(5): p. 444-8.

[15] Koo, L.C. and J.H. Ho, Worldwide epidemiological patterns of lung cancer in nonsmokers. *Int. J. Epidemiol,* 1990. 19 Suppl 1: p. S14-23.

[16] Pauk, N., A. Kubik, P. Zatloukal, and E. Krepela, Lung cancer in women. *Lung Cancer,* 2005. 48(1): p. 1-9.

[17] Radzikowska, E., P. Glaz, and K. Roszkowski, Lung cancer in women: age, smoking, histology, performance status, stage, initial treatment and survival. Population-based study of 20 561 cases. *Ann. Oncol,* 2002. 13(7): p. 1087-93.

[18] Williams, R.R. and J.W. Horm, Association of cancer sites with tobacco and alcohol consumption and socioeconomic status of patients: interview study from the Third National Cancer Survey. *J. Natl. Cancer Inst,* 1977. 58(3): p. 525-47.

[19] Schoenberg, J.B., H.B. Wilcox, T.J. Mason, J. Bill, and A. Stemhagen, Variation in smoking-related lung cancer risk among New Jersey women. *Am. J. Epidemiol,* 1989. 130(4): p. 688-95.

[20] Brownson, R.C., J.C. Chang, and J.R. Davis, Gender and histologic type variations in smoking-related risk of lung cancer. *Epidemiology,* 1992. 3(1): p. 61-4.

[21] Osann, K.E., H. Anton-Culver, T. Kurosaki, and T. Taylor, Sex differences in lung-cancer risk associated with cigarette smoking. *Int. J. Cancer,* 1993. 54(1): p. 44-8.

[22] Harris, R.E., E.A. Zang, J.I. Anderson, and E.L. Wynder, Race and sex differences in lung cancer risk associated with cigarette smoking. *Int. J. Epidemiol,* 1993. 22(4): p. 592-9.

[23] Le, C.H., Y.C. Ko, L.S. Cheng, Y.C. Lin, H.J. Lin, M.S. Huang, J.J. Huang, E.L. Kao, and H.Z. Wang, The heterogeneity in risk factors of lung cancer and the difference of histologic distribution between genders in Taiwan. *Cancer Causes Control,* 2001. 12(4): p. 289-300.

[24] Bain, C., D. Feskanich, F.E. Speizer, M. Thun, E. Hertzmark, B.A. Rosner, and G.A. Colditz, Lung cancer rates in men and women with comparable histories of smoking. *J. Natl. Cancer Inst,* 2004. 96(11): p. 826-34.

[25] Prescott, E., M. Osler, H.O. Hein, K. Borch-Johnsen, P. Lange, P. Schnohr, and J. Vestbo, Gender and smoking-related risk of lung cancer. The Copenhagen Center for Prospective Population Studies. *Epidemiology,* 1998. 9(1): p. 79-83.

[26] Thun, M.J., C.A. Day-Lally, E.E. Calle, W.D. Flanders, and C.W. Heath, Jr., Excess mortality among cigarette smokers: changes in a 20-year interval. *Am. J. Public Health,* 1995. 85(9): p. 1223-30.

[27] Ezzati, M. and A.D. Lopez, Measuring the accumulated hazards of smoking: global and regional estimates for 2000. *Tob. Control,* 2003. 12(1): p. 79-85.

[28] Jemal, A., W.D. Travis, R.E. Tarone, L. Travis, and S.S. Devesa, Lung cancer rates convergence in young men and women in the United States: analysis by birth cohort and histologic type. *Int. J. Cancer,* 2003. 105(1): p. 101-7.

[29] Taioli, E. and E.L. Wynder, Re: Endocrine factors and adenocarcinoma of the lung in women. *J. Natl. Cancer Inst,* 1994. 86(11): p. 869-70.

[30] Baron, J.A., C. La Vecchia, and F. Levi, The antiestrogenic effect of cigarette smoking in women. *Am. J. Obstet Gynecol,* 1990. 162(2): p. 502-14.

[31] Stabile, L.P. and J.M. Siegfried, Estrogen receptor pathways in lung cancer. *Curr. Oncol. Rep,* 2004. 6(4): p. 259-67.

[32] Tiutiunova, A.M., E.D. Chirvina, T.V. Mironenko, S.Z. Kartashov, and V.A. Luntovskaia, [Hormonal balance in women with lung cancer and its changes after combined treatment]. *Vopr. Onkol,* 1986. 32(4): p. 26-30.

[33] Kawai, H., A. Ishii, K. Washiya, T. Konno, H. Kon, C. Yamaya, I. Ono, Y. Minamiya, and J. Ogawa, Estrogen receptor alpha and beta are prognostic factors in non-small cell lung cancer. *Clin. Cancer Res,* 2005. 11(14): p. 5084-9.

[34] Pietras, R.J., D.C. Marquez, H.W. Chen, E. Tsai, O. Weinberg, and M. Fishbein, Estrogen and growth factor receptor interactions in human breast and non-small cell lung cancer cells. *Steroids,* 2005. 70(5-7): p. 372-81.

[35] Pettersson, K. and J.A. Gustafsson, Role of estrogen receptor beta in estrogen action. *Annu. Rev. Physiol,* 2001. 63: p. 165-92.

[36] Omoto, Y., Y. Kobayashi, K. Nishida, E. Tsuchiya, H. Eguchi, K. Nakagawa, Y. Ishikawa, T. Yamori, H. Iwase, Y. Fujii, M. Warner, J.A. Gustafsson, and S.I. Hayashi, Expression, function, and clinical implications of the estrogen receptor beta in human lung cancers. *Biochem. Biophys. Res. Commun,* 2001. 285(2): p. 340-7.

[37] Stabile, L.P., J.S. Lyker, C.T. Gubish, W. Zhang, J.R. Grandis, and J.M. Siegfried, Combined targeting of the estrogen receptor and the epidermal growth factor receptor in non-small cell lung cancer shows enhanced antiproliferative effects. *Cancer Res,* 2005. 65(4): p. 1459-70.

[38] Roger, P., M.E. Sahla, S. Makela, J.A. Gustafsson, P. Baldet, and H. Rochefort, Decreased expression of estrogen receptor beta protein in proliferative preinvasive mammary tumors. *Cancer Res,* 2001. 61(6): p. 2537-41.

[39] Lai, J.C., Y.W. Cheng, H.L. Chiou, M.F. Wu, C.Y. Chen, and H. Lee, Gender difference in estrogen receptor alpha promoter hypermethylation and its prognostic value in non-small cell lung cancer. *Int. J. Cancer,* 2005. 117(6): p. 974-80.

[40] Cheng, Y.W., H.J. Tsai, J.Y. Wu, Y.F. Hsu, C.Y. Chen, N.J. Hao, and H. Lee, A possible role for dihydrodiol dehydrogenase in the formation of benzo[a]pyrene-DNA adducts in lung cancer cells and tumor tissues. *Environ. Mol. Mutagen,* 2006.

[41] Yu, C.L., P. Driggers, G. Barrera-Hernandez, S.B. Nunez, J.H. Segars, and S. Cheng, The tumor suppressor p53 is a negative regulator of estrogen receptor signaling pathways. *Biochem. Biophys. Res. Commun,* 1997. 239(2): p. 617-20.

[42] Liu, W., S.D. Konduri, S. Bansal, B.K. Nayak, S.A. Rajasekaran, S.M. Karuppayil, A.K. Rajasekaran, and G.M. Das, Estrogen receptor-alpha binds p53 tumor suppressor protein directly and represses its function. *J. Biol. Chem,* 2006. 281(15): p. 9837-40.

[43] Osborne, C.K. and R. Schiff, Estrogen-receptor biology: continuing progress and therapeutic implications. *J. Clin. Oncol,* 2005. 23(8): p. 1616-22.

[44] Fukuoka, J., T. Fujii, J.H. Shih, T. Dracheva, D. Meerzaman, A. Player, K. Hong, S. Settnek, A. Gupta, K. Buetow, S. Hewitt, W.D. Travis, and J. Jen, Chromatin remodeling factors and BRM/BRG1 expression as prognostic indicators in non-small cell lung cancer. *Clin. Cancer Res,* 2004. 10(13): p. 4314-24.

[45] Kyerematen, G.A., G.F. Owens, B. Chattopadhyay, J.D. deBethizy, and E.S. Vesell, Sexual dimorphism of nicotine metabolism and distribution in the rat. Studies in vivo and in vitro. *Drug Metab. Dispos,* 1988. 16(6): p. 823-8.

[46] Seaton, M., G.A. Kyerematen, M. Morgan, E.V. Jeszenka, and E.S. Vesell, Nicotine metabolism in stumptailed macaques, Macaca arctoides. *Drug Metab. Dispos,* 1991. 19(5): p. 946-54.

[47] Zeman, M.V., L. Hiraki, and E.M. Sellers, Gender differences in tobacco smoking: higher relative exposure to smoke than nicotine in women. *J. Womens Health Gend. Based Med,* 2002. 11(2): p. 147-53.

[48] Benowitz, N.L. and P. Jacob, 3rd, Daily intake of nicotine during cigarette smoking. *Clin. Pharmacol. Ther,* 1984. 35(4): p. 499-504.

[49] Hecht, S.S. and D. Hoffmann, The relevance of tobacco-specific nitrosamines to human cancer. *Cancer Surv,* 1989. 8(2): p. 273-94.

[50] Hecht, S.S., DNA adduct formation from tobacco-specific N-nitrosamines. *Mutat. Res,* 1999. 424(1-2): p. 127-42.

[51] Browman, G.P., G. Wong, I. Hodson, J. Sathya, R. Russell, L. McAlpine, P. Skingley, and M.N. Levine, Influence of cigarette smoking on the efficacy of radiation therapy in head and neck cancer. *N. Engl. J. Med,* 1993. 328(3): p. 159-63.

[52] Videtic, G.M., L.W. Stitt, A.R. Dar, W.I. Kocha, A.T. Tomiak, P.T. Truong, M.D. Vincent, and E.W. Yu, Continued cigarette smoking by patients receiving concurrent chemoradiotherapy for limited-stage small-cell lung cancer is associated with decreased survival. *J. Clin. Oncol,* 2003. 21(8): p. 1544-9.

[53] Johnston-Early, A., M.H. Cohen, J.D. Minna, L.M. Paxton, B.E. Fossieck, Jr., D.C. Ihde, P.A. Bunn, Jr., M.J. Matthews, and R. Makuch, Smoking abstinence and small cell lung cancer survival. *An association. Jama,* 1980. 244(19): p. 2175-9.

[54] Tsurutani, J., S.S. Castillo, J. Brognard, C.A. Granville, C. Zhang, J.J. Gills, J. Sayyah, and P.A. Dennis, Tobacco components stimulate Akt-dependent proliferation and NFkappaB-dependent survival in lung cancer cells. *Carcinogenesis,* 2005. 26(7): p. 1182-95.

[55] Jin, Z., F. Gao, T. Flagg, and X. Deng, Nicotine induces multi-site phosphorylation of Bad in association with suppression of apoptosis. *J. Biol. Chem,* 2004. 279(22): p. 23837-44.

[56] Mollerup, S., D. Ryberg, A. Hewer, D.H. Phillips, and A. Haugen, Sex differences in lung CYP1A1 expression and DNA adduct levels among lung cancer patients. *Cancer Res,* 1999. 59(14): p. 3317-20.

[57] Ryberg, D., A. Hewer, D.H. Phillips, and A. Haugen, Different susceptibility to smoking-induced DNA damage among male and female lung cancer patients. *Cancer Res,* 1994. 54(22): p. 5801-3.

[58] Cheng, Y.W., L.L. Hsieh, P.P. Lin, C.P. Chen, C.Y. Chen, T.S. Lin, J.M. Su, and H. Lee, Gender difference in DNA adduct levels among nonsmoking lung cancer patients. *Environ. Mol. Mutagen,* 2001. 37(4): p. 304-10.

[59] Hofer, T., H.L. Karlsson, and L. Moller, DNA oxidative damage and strand breaks in young healthy individuals: a gender difference and the role of life style factors. *Free Radic. Res,* 2006. 40(7): p. 707-14.

[60] Hatch, C.L., W.M. Bonner, and E.N. Moudrianakis, Minor histone 2A variants and ubiquinated forms in the native H2A:H2B dimer. *Science,* 1983. 221(4609): p. 468-70.

[61] Ward, I.M. and J. Chen, Histone H2AX is phosphorylated in an ATR-dependent manner in response to replicational stress. *J. Biol. Chem,* 2001. 276(51): p. 47759-62.

[62] Rogakou, E.P., C. Boon, C. Redon, and W.M. Bonner, Megabase chromatin domains involved in DNA double-strand breaks in vivo. *J. Cell Biol,* 1999. 146(5): p. 905-16.

[63] Monteiro, A.N., S. Zhang, C.M. Phelan, and S.A. Narod, Absence of constitutional H2AX gene mutations in 101 hereditary breast cancer families. *J. Med. Genet,* 2003. 40(4): p. e51.

[64] Burma, S., B.P. Chen, M. Murphy, A. Kurimasa, and D.J. Chen, ATM phosphorylates histone H2AX in response to DNA double-strand breaks. *J. Biol. Chem,* 2001. 276(45): p. 42462-7.

[65] Bartkova, J., Z. Horejsi, K. Koed, A. Kramer, F. Tort, K. Zieger, P. Guldberg, M. Sehested, J.M. Nesland, C. Lukas, T. Orntoft, J. Lukas, and J. Bartek, DNA damage response as a candidate anti-cancer barrier in early human tumorigenesis. *Nature,* 2005. 434(7035): p. 864-70.

[66] Bassing, C.H. and F.W. Alt, The cellular response to general and programmed DNA double strand breaks. *DNA Repair.* (Amst), 2004. 3(8-9): p. 781-96.

[67] Rios-Doria, J., A. Fay, A. Velkova, and A.N. Monteiro, DNA damage response: determining the fate of phosphorylated histone H2AX. *Cancer Biol. Ther,* 2006. 5(2): p. 142-4.

[68] Keogh, M.C., J.A. Kim, M. Downey, J. Fillingham, D. Chowdhury, J.C. Harrison, M. Onishi, N. Datta, S. Galicia, A. Emili, J. Lieberman, X. Shen, S. Buratowski, J.E. Haber, D. Durocher, J.F. Greenblatt, and N.J. Krogan, A phosphatase complex that dephosphorylates gammaH2AX regulates DNA damage checkpoint recovery. *Nature,* 2006. 439(7075): p. 497-501.

[69] Yano, M., S. Toyooka, K. Tsukuda, H. Dote, M. Ouchida, T. Hanabata, M. Aoe, H. Date, A.F. Gazdar, and N. Shimizu, Aberrant promoter methylation of human DAB2 interactive protein (hDAB2IP) gene in lung cancers. *Int. J. Cancer,* 2005. 113(1): p. 59-66.

[70] Dai, Z., A.P. Popkie, W.G. Zhu, C.D. Timmers, A. Raval, S. Tannehill-Gregg, C.D. Morrison, H. Auer, R.A. Kratzke, G. Niehans, S. Amatschek, W. Sommergruber,

G.W. Leone, T. Rosol, G.A. Otterson, and C. Plass, Bone morphogenetic protein 3B silencing in non-small-cell lung cancer. *Oncogene,* 2004. 23(20): p. 3521-9.

[71] Zhukov TA, P.S., Monteiro A, Martino M, Lancaster J, Qian W, Song DS, Cantor AB, Sellers TA, Tockman MS. . Novel Lung Cancer Biomarker g-H2AX (Marker of DNA Damage Response) and Estrogen Receptors Pathways: Do They Crosstalk? . in AACR Frontiers in Cancer Prevention Research meeting. 2005. Baltimore, MD.

[72] Tokuhata, G.K. and A.M. Lilienfeld, Familial aggregation of lung cancer in humans. *J. Natl. Cancer Inst,* 1963. 30: p. 289-312.

[73] Horwitz, R.I., L.F. Smaldone, and C.M. Viscoli, An ecogenetic hypothesis for lung cancer in women. *Arch. Intern. Med,* 1988. 148(12): p. 2609-12.

[74] Kato, R., Sex-related differences in drug metabolism. *Drug Metab. Rev,* 1974. 3(1): p. 1-32.

[75] Park, J.Y., J.E. Muscat, Q. Ren, S.P. Schantz, R.D. Harwick, J.C. Stern, V. Pike, J.P. Richie, Jr., and P. Lazarus, CYP1A1 and GSTM1 polymorphisms and oral cancer risk. *Cancer Epidemiol. Biomarkers Prev,* 1997. 6(10): p. 791-7.

[76] Dresler, C.M., C. Fratelli, J. Babb, L. Everley, A.A. Evans, and M.L. Clapper, Gender differences in genetic susceptibility for lung cancer. *Lung Cancer,* 2000. 30(3): p. 153-60.

[77] Berge, G., S. Mollerup, O.V. S, A. Hewer, D.H. Phillips, E. Eilertsen, and A. Haugen, Role of estrogen receptor in regulation of polycyclic aromatic hydrocarbon metabolic activation in lung. *Lung Cancer,* 2004. 45(3): p. 289-97.

[78] Vineis, P., F. Veglia, S. Benhamou, D. Butkiewicz, I. Cascorbi, M.L. Clapper, V. Dolzan, A. Haugen, A. Hirvonen, M. Ingelman-Sundberg, M. Kihara, C. Kiyohara, P. Kremers, L. Le Marchand, S. Ohshima, R. Pastorelli, A. Rannug, M. Romkes, B. Schoket, P. Shields, R.C. Strange, I. Stucker, H. Sugimura, S. Garte, L. Gaspari, and E. Taioli, CYP1A1 T3801 C polymorphism and lung cancer: a pooled analysis of 2451 cases and 3358 controls. *Int. J. Cancer,* 2003. 104(5): p. 650-7.

[79] Shriver, S.P., H.A. Bourdeau, C.T. Gubish, D.L. Tirpak, A.L. Davis, J.D. Luketich, and J.M. Siegfried, Sex-specific expression of gastrin-releasing peptide receptor: relationship to smoking history and risk of lung cancer. *J. Natl. Cancer Inst,* 2000. 92(1): p. 24-33.

[80] Benowitz, N.L., G.E. Swan, P. Jacob, 3rd, C.N. Lessov-Schlaggar, and R.F. Tyndale, CYP2A6 genotype and the metabolism and disposition kinetics of nicotine. *Clin. Pharmacol. Ther,* 2006. 80(5): p. 457-67.

[81] Xu, C., S. Goodz, E.M. Sellers, and R.F. Tyndale, CYP2A6 genetic variation and potential consequences. *Adv. Drug Deliv. Rev,* 2002. 54(10): p. 1245-56.

[82] Malaiyandi, V., E.M. Sellers, and R.F. Tyndale, Implications of CYP2A6 genetic variation for smoking behaviors and nicotine dependence. *Clin. Pharmacol. Ther,* 2005. 77(3): p. 145-58.

[83] Nakajima, M., T. Fukami, H. Yamanaka, E. Higashi, H. Sakai, R. Yoshida, J.T. Kwon, H.L. McLeod, and T. Yokoi, Comprehensive evaluation of variability in nicotine metabolism and CYP2A6 polymorphic alleles in four ethnic populations. *Clin. Pharmacol. Ther,* 2006. 80(3): p. 282-97.

[84] Chatkin, J.M., C.M. Abreu, C.C. Fritscher, M.B. Wagner, and J.A. Pinto, Is there a gender difference in non-small cell lung cancer survival? *Gend Med,* 2004. 1(1): p. 41-7.

[85] Visbal, A.L., B.A. Williams, F.C. Nichols, 3rd, R.S. Marks, J.R. Jett, M.C. Aubry, E.S. Edell, J.A. Wampfler, J.R. Molina, and P. Yang, Gender differences in non-small-cell lung cancer survival: an analysis of 4,618 patients diagnosed between 1997 and 2002. *Ann Thorac Surg*, 2004. **78**(1): p. 209-15; discussion 215..

[86] Cerfolio, R.J., A.S. Bryant, E. Scott, M. Sharma, F. Robert, S.A. Spencer, and R.I. Garver, Women with pathologic stage I, II, and III non-small cell lung cancer have better survival than men. *Chest*, 2006. **130**(6): p. 1796-802.

[87] Schoenberg, J.B., A. Stemhagen, T.J. Mason, J. Patterson, J. Bill, and R. Altman, Occupation and lung cancer risk among New Jersey white males. *J Natl Cancer Inst,* 1987. **79**(1): p. 13-21.

[88] Friedman, G., Tekawa, I, and Sadler, M, Smoking and mortality:the Kaiser-Permanente experience. smoking and tobacco control monograph, ed. D. Burns, Garfinkel, l and Smet, *J. Vol.* 8. 1997. 477-499.

[89] Nilsson, S., J.M. Carstensen, and G. Pershagen, Mortality among male and female smokers in Sweden: a 33 year follow up. *J. Epidemiol. Community Health,* 2001. 55(11): p. 825-30.

[90] Marang-van de Mheen, P.J., G.D. Smith, C.L. Hart, and D.J. Hole, Are women more sensitive to smoking than men? Findings from the Renfrew and Paisley study. *Int. J. Epidemiol,* 2001. 30(4): p. 787-92.

[91] Bach, P.B., M.W. Kattan, M.D. Thornquist, M.G. Kris, R.C. Tate, M.J. Barnett, L.J. Hsieh, and C.B. Begg, Variations in Lung Cancer Risk Among Smokers. *J. Natl. Cancer Inst,* 2003. 95(6): p. 470-478.

In: Lung Cancer in Women
Editor: Varetta N. Torres, pp. 115-130
ISBN: 978-1-60021-659-6


*Chapter V*

# EPIDEMIOLOGY OF LUNG CANCER IN WOMEN

***Amit W. Panwalkar**[*1] **and Apar Kishor Ganti**[2]*

[1] Section of Oncology/Hematology, Department of Internal Medicine,
University of Nebraska Medical Center, Omaha, NE., USA
[2] Department of Internal Medicine,
Omaha VA Medical Center, Omaha, NE., USA

## INTRODUCTION

Lung cancer was a rare condition in the early twentieth century. It was only after World War I that this disease assumed epidemic proportions.[1] Unfortunately, a century later, it is estimated that lung cancer will cause 72,130 deaths in women and a much higher estimated 90,330, in men.[2] This is despite the publication of the U.S. Surgeon General's report, in 1964, that cigarette smoking was injurious to health and that the tobacco habit needed to be curbed.[3] Statistics related to smoking and lung cancer mortality have reflected male dominion, since reporting began a few decades ago.[2] However, in the post World War II era, women increasingly picked up the tobacco habit and their lung cancer incidence has risen since then. Lung cancer is now the foremost killer of women amongst all cancers, and kills more women than breast and colon cancer combined. Lung cancer incidence in women has increased fourfold over the last three decades, and is expected to increase further.[4] There are several differences between lung cancer in men and women of growing import. Women may be at increased risk of developing lung cancer as compared to men for any given rate of smoking.[5] Women who have never smoked have a 30% increased risk of lung cancer if they lived with spouses who smoked than if they lived with non-smokers.[6] It is possible that genetic mutations leading to lung cancer may be more frequently found in

* Address for Correspondence: Amit W. Panwalkar, MD; 987680 Nebraska Medical Center; Omaha, NE 68198-7680; Tel: (402) 559 5520; Fax: (402) 559 6520; Email: apanwalkar@unmc.edu

women.[7] The inability of women to repair DNA damage related to smoking vis-à-vis their male counterparts may lead to increased susceptibility to cancer.[8] Moreover, disease manifestations in pre-menopausal women may be different from post-menopausal women.[9] However, intriguingly, survival in women with lung cancer seems to be better than men with the same disease. Lung cancer in women apparently tends to be detected at an earlier stage, is of different histology and appears to be less aggressive.[10] It is now known that there are important differences in the biology of the tumors in the two sexes.[11] These differences are the focus of the following discussion.

## Incidence, Prevalence and Mortality

The fact that lung cancer is the most common cancer in the world is old news. However, the tremendous increase in the incidence of lung cancer in females over the last decade is not as well advertised. This upsurge began in the United States of America (USA) several years ago, and of late has been observed in Europe as well. The rise in tobacco-smoking rates post World War II appears to be the main cause of this increase. However, smoking habits in females are quite different to males, and other risk factors specific to females probably play a role as well.

Incidence rates of lung cancer in females are lower globally, (12.1 per 100,000 women compared with 35.5 per 100,000 in men). The highest rates are observed in North America and Northern Europe (figure 1). Of note, the incidence in China is rather high (19.0 per 100,000), similar to that in other developed countries. Sex ratios for lung cancer are also different depending on the country from which the data are taken and reflects differences in smoking habits. The lowest sex ratio (male/female) is 1.7 in Denmark and the highest is 13.4 in Spain. The sex ratio is 2.4 in Northern Europe, whereas it is 7.4 for Southern Europe and 5.0 for Western Europe. For the year 2000, an estimated 85% of lung cancer in men and 47% of lung cancer in women was the consequence of tobacco smoking. In the lowest incidence areas of East and West Africa and South-central Asia there are no cases attributable to smoking in women, while the highest fractions are seen in North America (85%), northern Europe (74%), and Australia/New Zealand (72%), where women have been smoking the longest. The estimated numbers of lung cancer cases worldwide has increased by 51% since 1985 (+44% in men and +76% in women). In men, this increase appears to be solely due to population growth and aging; with a small (–3.3%) decrease in the actual age-standardized incidence. In contrast, the age-standardized incidence has increased by 22% in women.

In men, several developed nations are now past the peak of the lung cancer epidemic, with declining incidence rates (e.g., United States[2] and the countries of Northern and Western Europe[12]). However, in women, the epidemic is still in its early stages and most Western countries currently show a rising trend in incidence and mortality. The incidence rates in men decreased by 2.3% per year in the early 1990s. In contrast, a sharp increase in the incidence of lung cancer, from 6/100,000 in 1960 to more than 40/100,000 in 1990, has occurred in women. However, more recent figures suggest that the incidence rates of lung cancer among women may have attained a plateau and the peak of the epidemic may have been reached in the USA, Spain and UK[2, 13] (table 1).

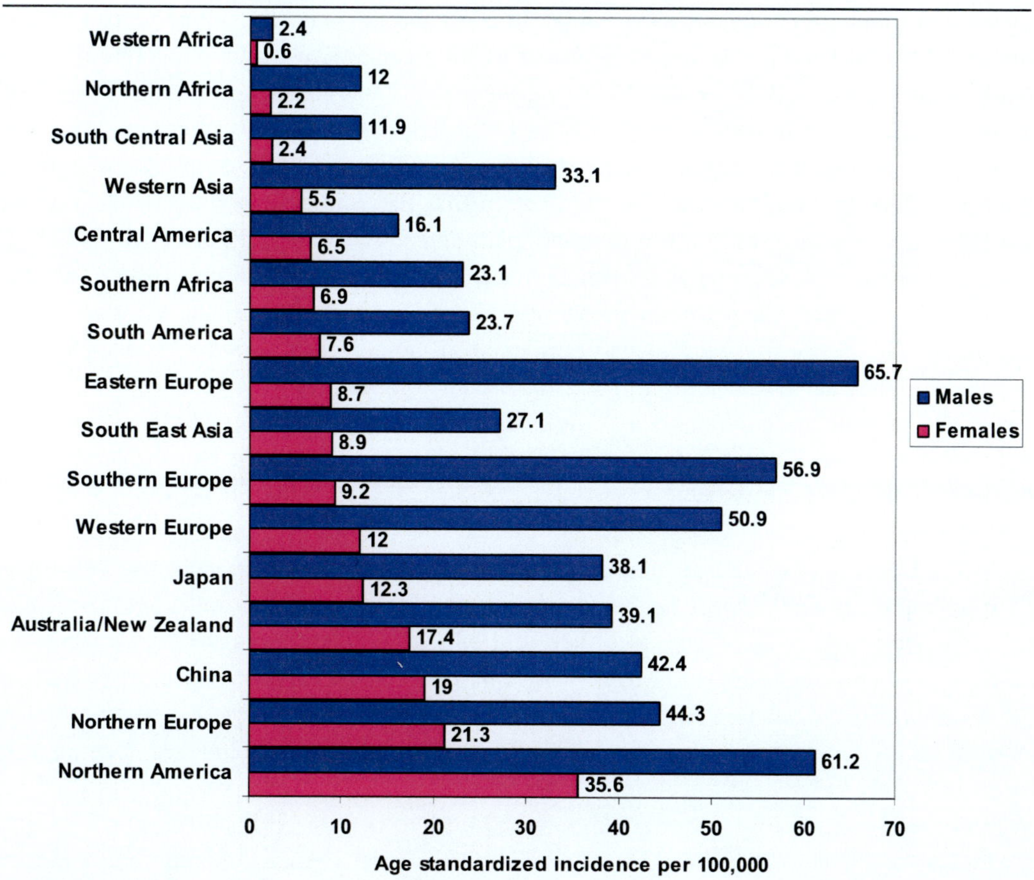


*Adapted from Parkin, D.M., et al., Global cancer statistics, 2002. CA Cancer J Clin, 2005. 55(2): p. 74-108.

Figure 1. Worldwide incidence of Lung Cancer*.

**Table 1. Comparative trend in lung cancer incidence and mortality by sex in the US***

| | Epoch | APC[@] | Epoch | APC | Epoch | APC |
|---|---|---|---|---|---|---|
| Incidence | | | | | | |
| Males | 1975-1982 | +1.5 | 1982-1991 | -0.4 | 1991-2002 | -1.8 |
| Females | 1990-1998 | +1.0 | 1998-2002 | -0.5 | 2002-2010 | ? |
| Mortality | | | | | | |
| Males | 1978-1984 | +1.2 | 1984-1991 | +0.3 | 1991-2002 | -1.9 |
| Females | 1990-1995 | +1.7 | 1995-2002 | +0.3 | 2002-2010 | ? |

[@]APC = annual percentage change.
**Adapted from Jemal, A., et al., Cancer statistics, 2006. CA Cancer J Clin, 2006. 56(2): p. 106-30.*

Lung cancer is one of the most lethal cancers due to its high incidence and high case fatality rate. In 2005, lung cancer killed 1.3 million people worldwide, representing 17.1% of cancer deaths. The 5-year survival in patients with lung cancer is about 15% in the USA, 10% in Western Europe and 9.8% in developing countries. In the US alone, it is estimated that 81,770 women will develop lung cancer in 2006 and the majority, about 72,130, of these will die of this disease.[2] While the number of lung cancers in males is declining in most countries in Europe, mortality due to lung cancer continues to rise in females [14] with a 600% increase in the mortality rate between 1990 and 1997.[15] In women, there are clear upsurges in death rates seen in younger and older women in almost all west European countries in recent decades with little indication that the epidemic will soon reach a peak, except the UK and Ireland. In these two nations lung cancer death rates are now declining in younger women and stabilizing in older women, reflecting a declining risk in younger women. It is too early to predict whether the observed plateau/decline in rates in women, born after 1950, in several countries is likely to be sustained. Evaluation of trends in cigarette consumption may provide insight into this uncertainty. Where national data are available, the proportion of adult male smokers has fallen steadily in the last five decades. In women, recent smoking trends are downwards in Belgium, Denmark, Sweden and the Netherlands, although in the USA, Austria and Spain, large increases in smoking prevalence amongst adults are emerging.

In the USA, lung cancer accounts for 13% of all cancers that are diagnosed each year, but it accounts for 28% of all cancer deaths annually (31% in men and 25% in women). However, women may have improved survival and responses to treatment. A recent large prospective cohort study analyzed data from 1,085 patients with lung cancer (671 men and 414 women), matched for race, pulmonary function, smoking history, co-morbidities, neoadjuvant therapy, histology, and resection rates. Women were younger at diagnosis and were more likely to have adenocarcinoma, but were found to have better stage-specific 5-year survival rates (stage I 69% versus 64%; $p = 0.034$; stage II 60% versus 50%; $p = 0.042$; and stage III 46% versus 37%; $p = 0.024$). Women receiving neoadjuvant chemotherapy alone ($n = 76$) were more likely to respond completely or partially as compared with men ($p = 0.025$).[16]

## Risk Factors Influencing Lung Cancer in Females

Approximately 85% to 90% of all patients who develop lung cancer have a history of cigarette smoking. Lung cancer develops only in 20% of cigarette smokers; suggesting that the causes of lung cancer are multi-factorial.[17] There is evidence to believe that some of these factors may be of particular significance in women (table 2).

**Table 2. Differences in risk factors by Sex**

| Variable | Difference (compared with men) |
|---|---|
| Smoking | Increased risk overall (?) |
| ETS | Increased risk overall |
| DNA repair capacity | Decreased, thereby increasing risk |
| GRPR overexpression | Increased risk in smokers or non-smokers |
| GSTM1 polymorphism | Increased risk with lower activity |
| K-ras mutation | Increased risk |
| HRT | Increased risk of incidence and mortality |
| Dietary antioxidants | Decreased risk |
| Family history | Increased risk of incidence |
| Response to treatment | Favorable |
| Overall survival | Superior |

## Implications of Lifestyle

Human behavior patterns are adapted by their biological, psychological, and social needs. These patterns may include certain ways of preparing and consuming food, physical inactivity, and the development of dependence on tobacco products. Many of these patterns have an impact on cancer.

### *Smoking*

Cigarette smoking is by far the major cause of lung cancer. Smokers are 22 times more likely to die from lung cancer than nonsmokers.[4] Initial studies of lung cancer and smoking emphasized men, who began smoking earlier and consumed greater quantities of tobacco than did women. The percentage of men who are current smokers has been declining since the Surgeon General's report in 1964, linking cigarette smoke to lung cancer. Conversely, since 1980, the prevalence of smoking among women has risen significantly in many countries, including the US. Smoking rates among women in the US now surpass those among men. Although the acceptance of smoking by women was initiated by "freedom" for women in the early days of tobacco use, an active campaign to encourage smoking amongst women was undertaken by the tobacco industry. As a result, the tobacco industry has marketed aggressively to women and teenage girls, portraying smoking as sophisticated, seductive, a weight loss tool, in addition to equality with men.

However, the rate of increase in the incidence of lung cancer among women in the United States is more rapid than would be expected based on changing smoking rates alone. A case-control study of 14,596 patients who had lung cancer found that the relative odds ratio (OR) for developing lung cancer was higher in women than in men — 12.7 and 9.1 respectively.[18] A hospital-based, case-control study of 1889 subjects (1108 men and 781 women) with lung cancer and 2070 control subjects (1122 men and 948 women) with diseases unrelated to smoking,[5] revealed that women who had lung cancer had less exposure to cigarette smoke than men who had lung cancer. Moreover, women were more likely to be never-smokers, started smoking at a later age, smoked fewer cigarettes, smoked brands that contained less tar, and inhaled less deeply than men. Despite this, women had a 1.2-fold to 1.7-fold higher odds ratio of developing lung cancer than men, at every level of tobacco exposure. The differences were more pronounced for small cell carcinoma and adenocarcinoma. A Canadian case-control study of 442 female and 362 male patients who had lung cancer also found a higher odds ratio for lung cancer for female smokers — 27.9 compared with 9.6 for male smokers.[19] Notably, one large study found no difference in susceptibility between males and females, despite a correction for the amount of cigarette exposure.[20] To lend credence to this a recent multicenter, case-control study from Germany and Italy indicated that the relative risk estimates of lung cancer due to smoking did not differ substantially between men and women with similar levels of tobacco exposure.[21]

### *Environmental Tobacco Smoke (ETS)*

ETS accounts for around 3,000 lung cancer deaths each year in the USA among nonsmokers, primarily women. Urinary levels of nicotine, cotinine, 4-(methylnitrosamino)-1-(3-pyridyl)-butanol, a tobacco-specific carcinogen, and its glucuronide were elevated in nonsmoking women exposed to ETS compared to the unexposed.[22] In another multi-center case-control study, non-smoking women with spouses who used tobacco had a 30% increased risk of lung cancer, with a higher risk in those women with increased levels of exposure, which was statistically significant.[6] However other studies have reported contrary results and currently there is no agreement with the concept of higher risk in females.[20, 21] Several biases such as the absolute risk being higher in non-smoking females compared to non-smoking males and the reluctance of females to express their true smoking habits may need to be accounted for while evaluating these studies. Factors specific to females also include exposure to smoke unrelated to tobacco. In developing countries, exposure to fossil fuel smoke and cooking fumes has been shown to be associated with an increased risk of developing lung cancer.[23]

### *Diet*

Dietary ingredients or a lack thereof, may pose a potential risk for the development of lung cancer. Two prospective cohort studies lend credence to this observation. A prospective study examined the relationship between smoking, dietary antioxidants, and lung cancer risk.[24] Women who consumed five or more carrots per week had a relative risk of 0.4 (95% CI, 0.2 to 0.8) compared with the risk for women who had not consumed carrots. A 10-year follow-up the cohort of men in the Health Professionals Follow-up Study and a 12-year follow-up period of the cohort of women in the Nurses Health Study showed that new lung cancers were diagnosed in 275 of 46,924 men and 519 of 77,283 women. The risk of lung cancer was significantly reduced in those who had consumed a variety of carotenoids for a maximum protective period of 4 to 8 years after adjustment for confounding factors like smoking (RR 0.68) for the highest compared with the lowest total carotenoid intake. Notably, the association was stronger in women than in men. Among female never-smokers, a significant 63% lower risk was noted.[25] A hospital-based, case-control study demonstrated that fruit intake and the use of soy in Chinese women provided a protective effect against lung cancer.[26] The same protective effect was observed with the consumption of green tea in another population-based, case-control study.[27]

## Socio-Economic Factors

Cancer and other chronic diseases are profoundly associated with social and economic status. Tobacco use and alcohol abuse are highest in groups with the least education.[28] In a study of females in Mumbai, India, a lower educational level was associated with a higher usage of tobacco. One of the reasons for this is that lower socio-economic groups are often explicitly targeted in the marketing of unhealthy products, and are also the least likely to be reached by preventive and other healthcare services.[29]

## Genetic Factors

### *Deoxyribonucleic Acid (DNA) Repair Capacity*

Carcinogens, such as polycyclic aromatic hydrocarbons (PAH) and nitrosamines, are present in tobacco smoke and exert their biologic effects after biotransformation through the formation of DNA adducts in target tissues and mutations in transforming genes.[30] Emerging literature implicates differences in DNA repair capacity in both the pathogenesis of lung cancer and response to therapy. A complex family of proteins effectively removes damaged DNA segments and repairs mismatched nucleotides. Deficiencies in these processes are unequivocally mutagenic and/or carcinogenic. Two classes of enzymes play a crucial role in the metabolism of tobacco-related carcinogens: the phase I and II detoxifying enzymes. While phase I enzymes (*e.g.* cytochrome P450, monooxygenases) activate carcinogens to reactive intermediates, their action is balanced by phase II enzymes, which serve to convert these same reactive intermediates (*e.g.* reactive oxygen species) to inactive conjugates that are more water soluble and hence excreted more readily. Polymorphisms have been found to alter the metabolic activity of detoxification enzymes. Those active metabolites that are not detoxified bind to DNA forming DNA adducts. Women have higher levels of these DNA adducts when compared to men.[31, 32] In a study of 632 subjects, evaluating the repair of tobacco carcinogen-induced DNA adducts and lung cancer risk, lymphocytes were obtained from newly diagnosed lung cancer patients and from control subjects matched for age, sex, and smoking status. These cells were cultured and transfected with a plasmid containing a reporter gene that would not be expressed if the plasmid DNA was damaged. The lymphocytes were then exposed to a known tobacco-derived carcinogen. Patients <60 years old, those with a family history of lung cancer, and female patients had a lower DNA repair capacity and thereby, a higher lung cancer risk.[33] These results were confirmed in a larger case-control study with 764 lung cancer patients and 677 control subjects.[8] The higher DNA adduct levels were also found to be associated with the expression of the cytochrome P4501A1 (*CYP1A1*) gene, an aryl hydrocarbon hydroxylase enzyme. This enhanced enzyme inducibility causes bioactivation of benzopyrene, a polycyclic aromatic hydrocarbon that is found in cigarette smoke.[34] Significantly higher levels of expression of *CYP1A1* were found in normal lung tissue of current female smokers with lung cancer, compared with male subjects with lung cancer.[32] The increase in *CYP1A1* expression correlated with increased levels of DNA adducts.[32] Ryberg et al found that DNA adduct levels were higher in female patients who had lung cancer than in male patients who had lung cancer after adjusting for smoking dose.[31] In addition, the subjects with higher DNA adduct levels generally had a shorter duration of smoking before the clinical onset of lung cancer. This led them to conclude that susceptibility to DNA damage caused by PAH-like compounds may be higher among women than in men. Interestingly, this deficiency in repair capacity may also be related to the observation that women respond better to treatment with platinum-based chemotherapy. Platinum agents act through the formation of DNA adducts resulting in cycle arrest and apoptosis. Repair of these adducts is a mechanism of resistance to platinum drugs. Recent studies have demonstrated that diminished repair capacity is associated with improved outcome in stage IV non-small cell lung cancer (NSCLC) treated with cisplatin-based chemotherapy and early stage lung cancer treated with adjuvant platinum-based therapy.[35, 36]

### *Glutathione-S-Transferase M1 (GSTM1)*

Genetic polymorphisms may explain some individual variations in risk due to smoking habits. The role of glutathion *S*-transferase M1 (*GSTM1*) has been demonstrated in lung cancer. A lack of activity is associated with an increased risk of lung cancer in smokers; deletion of the gene results in a greater increase in risk of lung cancer in female smokers than in male smokers[37]; and the combination of the null genotype of *GSTM1* with a mutation of *CYP1A1* also results in an increase in lung cancer risk for females as compared with males (odds ratio 6.54 versus 2.36).[34] The null genotype of *GSTM1* also seems to result in an increase in lung cancer risk (odds ratio 2.6) due to ETS exposure in females.[38]

### *Gastrin-Releasing Peptide Receptor (GRPR)*

GRPR, a receptor for the autocrine growth factor, has been identified in lung cancer.[39] The GRPR gene is on the X chromosome and escapes X-inactivation. It is expressed more frequently in female nonsmokers than male, and is activated earlier in response to tobacco exposure.[40] In a study evaluating GRPR mRNA expression in lung tissues and cultured cells from 78 individuals (40 men and 48 women), mRNA expression was detected more frequently in female nonsmokers than in male nonsmokers (55% versus 0%). Among smokers with lower levels of tobacco exposure (<25 pack years), a higher rate of expression of GRPR mRNA was observed for women (75%) compared with men (20%).[40] The investigators also found that female subjects developed lung cancer with significantly less tobacco exposure than did the males (41 versus 59.9 pack-years, $P = 0.032$). Additionally, almost all of the nonsmokers diagnosed with lung cancer were female (6 of 29 women versus 1 of 29 men). Of these six nonsmoking females, five demonstrated GRPR expression. The investigators concluded that the presence of two expressed copies of the GRPR gene in women may be a factor in their increased susceptibility to tobacco-induced lung cancer and that the ability to express the GRPR gene in the adult airway, irrespective of tobacco exposure, may predispose the individual to develop lung cancer.[40]

### *HER-2/neu*

Certain growth factors have been shown to stimulate the growth of both normal and neoplastic cells in the lung. ERBB2 (HER-2/neu) is one of four receptor-type tyrosine kinases that form a heterodimer with other members of the ERB-B class and mediates cell growth and survival. HER-2/neu has been found to be overexpressed in 25 to 30% of invasive breast cancers and is associated with a more aggressive clinical course. Its incidence in NSCLC varies from 27 to 63%. One study found inferior survival for patients with high serum levels of HER-2/neu compared to patients with lower levels (7.1 months versus 10.9 months; p=0.004), in advanced NSCLC.[41, 42] Previous series have found that overexpression of HER-2/neu is associated with a poorer prognosis and survival. HER-2/neu is most commonly expressed in adenocarcinoma, the most common subtype in women.[43] However, improved outcomes have not been seen with trastuzumab therapy in addition to standard chemotherapy.

### *TP53*

The p53 pathway has long been recognized as playing a key role in cell cycle regulation by causing arrest in both the G1 and G2 phases in cell division in response to DNA damage. This arrest allows for DNA repair or apoptosis. Mutations of the p53 gene lead to abrogation of this arrest and perpetuation of DNA damage and consequent inhibition of the normal apoptotic mechanism. The most frequent genetic alterations found are in p53 (in 90% of small cell lung cancers [SCLCs] 40 to 70% of [NSCLCs]).[7] Smoking has been found to induce p53 mutation via the formation of DNA adducts. As discussed above women have been found to have higher levels of pulmonary DNA adducts per pack-year than men.[32] Other studies have shown an association between mutations in the p53 tumor suppressor gene and smoking in lung cancer cases. The dominant mutation in the p53 gene is G:C to T:A transversions. The frequency of G:C to T:A transversions in p53 were greater in lung cancers from female smokers compared with male smokers and female never smokers (37% versus 12%).[17, 44]

### *K-ras Oncogene*

The K-ras oncogene encodes a protein that is known to be oncogenic when mutated or overexpressed. In a study to define patient characteristics associated with K-ras gene mutation and to determine whether the mutation is a biomarker of prognosis, lung cancer specimens resected from 365 patients were analyzed. Mutations in codon 12 of the K-ras oncogene occurring predominantly in adenocarcinomas, were found only in patients with a history of smoking, and were more common in women compared with men (26.2% versus 17.4%, p<0.05). The study also showed a significant association between the presence of K-ras gene mutation and inferior survival. The investigators concluded that cigarette smoking induces K-ras mutations and the resultant clones are further expanded by a second event that may involve the growth-promoting effects of hormones that may be specific for adenocarcinomas.[7] Women are three times more likely to carry the K-ras mutation than men.[7] Ras mutations seem to be predominantly associated with the adenocarcinoma histology.[7, 45] However, a recent study has yielded conflicting data regarding K-ras is an adverse prognostic variable.[46]

## Hormonal Factors

The most obvious biological differences between men and women are hormonal. With the increasing rates of lung cancer in women and their increased susceptibility to the detrimental effects of tobacco smoke compared to men, the role of female steroid sex hormones has been hypothesized to be a factor in lung carcinogenesis. It is well established that estrogens may act as direct carcinogens by means of chromosomal alterations and genetic mutations in breast and other female cancers. The role of hormone replacement therapy (HRT) and oral contraception in the development of lung cancer is controversial.[47] Estrogens receptors (ER-α) and (ER-β) have also been found in bronchial tumor cells and NSCLC, with a more frequent expression in females.[48, 49] Thus, estrogens could play an additional role in carcinogenesis through these receptors. In a recent study, mRNA for ER-α and ER-β was detected in cultured human NSCLC cells, cultured normal lung fibroblast cell lines, and normal bronchial epithelial cells. This study also demonstrated that treatment of lung fibroblasts with β-estradiol resulted in a two-fold increased secretion of hepatocyte growth factor, and induced mitogenesis and motility in normal and neoplastic cells.[49] Estrogens may be involved in lung carcinogenesis by acting as estrogen receptor ligands and activating cell proliferation through indirect actions on lung fibroblasts, or by metabolic activation to reactive intermediates that can produce DNA adducts or cause oxidative damage.[49] An increased risk of lung cancer in women who received hormone replacement therapy was noted in a large-scale epidemiologic cohort study; however, no adjustment was made for the amount of smoking.[50] In a case-control study, 180 women who had lung cancer were evaluated for the history of smoking and hormone replacement therapy. For women who had never smoked, hormone replacement therapy posed no additional risk.[47] There was, however, a statistically significant synergy between smoking and HRT; women who smoked but did not take hormone replacement therapy had an odds ratio of 13 for developing lung cancer compared with 32.4 for women who smoked and took hormone replacement therapy. In addition, the investigators reported an increased risk of adenocarcinoma associated with hormone replacement therapy (odds ratio 1.7). No comparable age-related difference in smoking was found among males with lung cancer or female control subjects. Adami et al also have shown an increased risk (RR 1.26) of lung cancer in women receiving HRT in their study.[50] It appears that the higher circulating levels of estrogen in women when compared to men, coupled with their lower rate of DNA repair, make women particularly susceptible to the carcinogenic influence of tobacco smoke. There are data that HRT may actually exert a protective effect, however these are of poor quality.[51] Moore et al analyzed the Surveillance, Epidemiology, and End Results Database to evaluate the influence of menopausal status on outcomes in lung cancer. Utilizing an average menopausal age of 51 years, they classified 14,676 women entered in the database into premenopausal and postmenopausal groups. In addition to comparisons between the two groups, there were also comparisons against men from similar age groups. Several intriguing differences emerged between the groups.[9] Premenopausal women tended to present with more extensive disease and adenocarcinoma as compared to postmenopausal women. They underwent more extensive surgical procedures (pneumonectomy vs. lobectomy) at every stage of disease ($p < 0.0001$) and were more likely to receive radiotherapy (58% vs. 48%, $p <$

0.0001). While premenopausal women and younger men had similar mortality (after adjustments for covariates), postmenopausal women had fewer lung cancer-related deaths compared with older men. A major limitation of this study was the potentially confounding effects of age. However the use of HRT in postmenopausal women was not examined. A more recent study examined the effects of HRT on survival. Evaluation of 429 subjects showed that overall survival was significantly higher in women with no HRT compared with patients who received HRT (79 versus 39 months, HR 1.97). The effect seemed to be more pronounced in women with a smoking history.[52]

## Family History

Patients with lung cancer have a higher number of relatives with lung cancer than control subjects.[53] The simplest explanation of this finding is the clustering of cigarette smokers within families. While this may be true, there is also an increased risk of lung cancer regardless of family smoking history. This finding suggests that other genetic and perhaps environmental factors that may be affect this population. A population-based, case-control study estimated the familial risk for lung cancer by restricting the analysis to nonsmokers.[54] Cases were significantly more likely than controls to have a family history of cancers of the aerodigestive tract (odds ratio 2.78) and a trend toward excess lung cancer incidence (odds ratio 4.14; $p = 0.07$). Previous studies in nonsmokers also demonstrated an increased risk in nonsmoking women, especially for adenocarcinoma of the lung.[53, 55] Another study demonstrated a similar trend in nonsmokers in general with a particularly higher risk in women compared with men (odds ratios, 1.7 versus 0.5).

## Human Papilloma Virus (HPV) Infection

HPV is a well recognized in the pathogenesis of cervical cancer. The most frequently implicated HPV viruses are types 6, 11, 16 and 18. HPV DNA utilizing polymerase chain reaction (PCR) and *in situ* hybridization was detected in the tumors of 49% of women with lung cancer who also had a history of high-grade cervical intraepithelial neoplasia.[56] A study from Taiwan revealed the presence of HPV DNA in the cancer cells of nonsmoking women with lung cancer. Interestingly, the association of HPV infection seems to be with the squamous histology, similar to that seen in the upper aerodigestive tract.[57] A Japanese study detected HPV DNA in well-differentiated squamous cell carcinoma and in adenocarcinoma cells that were adjacent to squamous cell carcinoma.[58] However, the issue of HPV as an etiologic agent in lung cancer is very controversial.[59] An analysis of paraffin-embedded tissue from 32 squamous cell lung carcinomas and 15 cervical cancers utilizing both *in situ* hybridization and PCR techniques was negative for HPV in the lung cancer cases, while 12 of the 15 cervical cases were positive.[60] This association of HPV in lung cancer may be explained by the coexistence of increased/ earlier smoking behavior and more frequent/multiple sexual contacts.

## Conclusion

Lung cancer is the major cause of cancer-related death in women. Available literature suggests that women are inherently more susceptible to lung cancer, although more evidence is necessary for definitive conclusions. However, unambiguous differences in the biology, history, response to therapy and survival exist between men and women diagnosed with lung cancer. Emerging literature sheds some light on these differences, but the understanding is far from complete. Prospective studies are lacking and most of the data are retrospective, the interpretation is fraught with biases, both known and unknown. Currently available therapeutic armamentarium does not take these differences into account. Hence, as new therapeutic interventions are evaluated, the potential for heterogeneous response based on sex must be prospectively sought for in clinical trials. Given the superior prognosis for women in most clinical trials, future studies should stratify according to gender. Prospective data are urgently needed to capitalize on these biologic differences to enhance outcomes.

Once again, to emphasize the point, lung cancer was a rare disease before 1900s. It is the tobacco habit that has led to this epidemic of gigantic proportions. For both men and women, this disease is largely preventable through smoking cessation. Clear and forceful health messages must be effectively conveyed to the masses if the lung cancer epidemic is to be controlled. This is a strategy that has clearly worked in the past and if we persevere to broaden and intensify the impact, there will be light at the end of the tunnel.

## References


[1] Ochsner, A., Corner of history. My first recognition of the relationship of smoking and lung cancer. *Prev. Med,* 1973. 2(4): p. 611-4.

[2] Jemal, A., et al., Cancer statistics, 2006. *CA Cancer J. Clin,* 2006. 56(2): p. 106-30.

[3] Guthrie, E., Smoking and Health: Report of the advisory committee to the Surgeon General of the Public Health Service. U.S. Government Printing Office, Washington, DC., 1964. Public Health Service Publication No. 1103.

[4] Thomas, L., L.A. Doyle, and M.J. Edelman, Lung cancer in women: emerging differences in epidemiology, biology, and therapy. *Chest,* 2005. 128(1): p. 370-81.

[5] Zang, E.A. and E.L. Wynder, Differences in lung cancer risk between men and women: examination of the evidence. *J. Natl. Cancer Inst,* 1996. 88(3-4): p. 183-92.

[6] Fontham, E.T., et al., Environmental tobacco smoke and lung cancer in nonsmoking women. A multicenter study. *Jama,* 1994. 271(22): p. 1752-9.

[7] Nelson, H.H., et al., Implications and prognostic value of K-ras mutation for early-stage lung cancer in women. *J. Natl. Cancer Inst,* 1999. 91(23): p. 2032-8.

[8] Spitz, M.R., et al., Genetic susceptibility to lung cancer: the role of DNA damage and repair. *Cancer Epidemiol. Biomarkers Prev,* 2003. 12(8): p. 689-98.

[9] Moore, K.A., et al., Menopausal effects on presentation, treatment, and survival of women with non-small cell lung cancer. *Ann. Thorac. Surg,* 2003. 76(6): p. 1789-95.

[10] Henschke, C.I., R. Yip, and O.S. Miettinen, Women's susceptibility to tobacco carcinogens and survival after diagnosis of lung cancer. *Jama,* 2006. 296(2): p. 180-4.

[11] Raz, D.J., et al., Bronchioloalveolar carcinoma: a review. *Clin. Lung Cancer,* 2006. 7(5): p. 313-22.

[12] Bray, F., J.E. Tyczynski, and D.M. Parkin, Going up or coming down? The changing phases of the lung cancer epidemic from 1967 to 1999 in the 15 European Union countries. *Eur. J. Cancer,* 2004. 40(1): p. 96-125.

[13] Howe, H.L., et al., Annual report to the nation on the status of cancer (1973 through 1998), featuring cancers with recent increasing trends. *J. Natl. Cancer Inst,* 2001. 93(11): p. 824-42.

[14] Borras, J.M., et al., Lung cancer mortality in European regions (1955-1997). *Ann. Oncol,* 2003. 14(1): p. 159-61.

[15] Patel, J.D., P.B. Bach, and M.G. Kris, Lung cancer in US women: a contemporary epidemic. *Jama,* 2004. 291(14): p. 1763-8.

[16] Cerfolio, R.J., et al., Women with pathologic stage I, II, and III non-small cell lung cancer have better survival than men. *Chest,* 2006. 130(6): p. 1796-802.

[17] Rivera, M.P. and D.E. Stover, Gender and lung cancer. *Clin. Chest Med,* 2004. 25(2): p. 391-400.

[18] Brownson, R.C., J.C. Chang, and J.R. Davis, Gender and histologic type variations in smoking-related risk of lung cancer. *Epidemiology,* 1992. 3(1): p. 61-4.

[19] Risch, H.A., et al., Are female smokers at higher risk for lung cancer than male smokers? A case-control analysis by histologic type. *Am. J. Epidemiol,* 1993. 138(5): p. 281-93.

[20] Prescott, E., et al., Gender and smoking-related risk of lung cancer. The Copenhagen Center for Prospective Population Studies. *Epidemiology,* 1998. 9(1): p. 79-83.

[21] Kreuzer, M., et al., Gender differences in lung cancer risk by smoking: a multicentre case-control study in Germany and Italy. *Br. J. Cancer,* 2000. 82(1): p. 227-33.

[22] Anderson, K.E., et al., Metabolites of a tobacco-specific lung carcinogen in nonsmoking women exposed to environmental tobacco smoke. *J. Natl. Cancer Inst,* 2001. 93(5): p. 378-81.

[23] Zhou, B.S., et al., Indoor air pollution and pulmonary adenocarcinoma among females: a case-control study in Shenyang, China. *Oncol. Rep,* 2000. 7(6): p. 1253-9.

[24] Speizer, F.E., et al., Prospective study of smoking, antioxidant intake, and lung cancer in middle-aged women (USA). *Cancer Causes Control,* 1999. 10(5): p. 475-82.

[25] Michaud, D.S., et al., Intake of specific carotenoids and risk of lung cancer in 2 prospective US cohorts. *Am. J. Clin. Nutr,* 2000. 72(4): p. 990-7.

[26] Seow, A., et al., Diet, reproductive factors and lung cancer risk among Chinese women in Singapore: evidence for a protective effect of soy in nonsmokers. *Int. J. Cancer,* 2002. 97(3): p. 365-71.

[27] Zhong, L., et al., A population-based case-control study of lung cancer and green tea consumption among women living in Shanghai, China. *Epidemiology,* 2001. 12(6): p. 695-700.

[28] Yach, D. and S.A. Bialous, Junking science to promote tobacco. *Am. J. Public Health,* 2001. 91(11): p. 1745-8.

[29] Gupta, P.C., Survey of sociodemographic characteristics of tobacco use among 99,598 individuals in Bombay, India using handheld computers. *Tob. Control,* 1996. 5(2): p. 114-20.

[30] Rom, W.N., et al., Molecular and genetic aspects of lung cancer. *Am. J. Respir. Crit. Care Med,* 2000. 161(4 Pt 1): p. 1355-67.

[31] Ryberg, D., et al., Different susceptibility to smoking-induced DNA damage among male and female lung cancer patients. *Cancer Res,* 1994. 54(22): p. 5801-3.

[32] Mollerup, S., et al., Sex differences in lung CYP1A1 expression and DNA adduct levels among lung cancer patients. *Cancer Res,* 1999. 59(14): p. 3317-20.

[33] Wei, Q., et al., Repair of tobacco carcinogen-induced DNA adducts and lung cancer risk: a molecular epidemiologic study. *J. Natl. Cancer Inst,* 2000. 92(21): p. 1764-72.

[34] Dresler, C.M., et al., Gender differences in genetic susceptibility for lung cancer. *Lung Cancer,* 2000. 30(3): p. 153-60.

[35] Lord, R.V., et al., Low ERCC1 expression correlates with prolonged survival after cisplatin plus gemcitabine chemotherapy in non-small cell lung cancer. *Clin. Cancer Res,* 2002. 8(7): p. 2286-91.

[36] Olaussen, K.A., et al., DNA repair by ERCC1 in non-small-cell lung cancer and cisplatin-based adjuvant chemotherapy. *N. Engl. J. Med,* 2006. 355(10): p. 983-91.

[37] Tang, D.L., et al., Associations between both genetic and environmental biomarkers and lung cancer: evidence of a greater risk of lung cancer in women smokers. *Carcinogenesis,* 1998. 19(11): p. 1949-53.

[38] Bennett, W.P., et al., Environmental tobacco smoke, genetic susceptibility, and risk of lung cancer in never-smoking women. *J. Natl. Cancer Inst,* 1999. 91(23): p. 2009-14.

[39] Leyton, J., et al., Bombesin and gastrin releasing peptide increase tyrosine phosphorylation of focal adhesion kinase and paxillin in non-small cell lung cancer cells. *Cancer Lett,* 2001. 162(1): p. 87-95.

[40] Shriver, S.P., et al., Sex-specific expression of gastrin-releasing peptide receptor: relationship to smoking history and risk of lung cancer. *J. Natl. Cancer Inst,* 2000. 92(1): p. 24-33.

[41] Ardizzoni, A., et al., Study of pretreatment serum levels of HER-2/neu oncoprotein as a prognostic and predictive factor in patients with advanced nonsmall cell lung carcinoma. *Cancer,* 2001. 92(7): p. 1896-904.

[42] Potti, A., et al., Identification of HER-2/neu overexpression and the clinical course of lung carcinoma in non-smokers with chronic lymphocytic leukemia. *Lung Cancer,* 2001. 34(2): p. 227-32.

[43] Hirsch, F.R., W.A. Franklin, and P.A. Bunn, What is the role of HER-2/neu and trastuzumab (Herceptin) in lung cancer? *Lung Cancer,* 2002. 36(3): p. 263-4.

[44] Guinee, D.G., Jr., et al., Gender comparisons in human lung cancer: analysis of p53 mutations, anti-p53 serum antibodies and C-erbB-2 expression. *Carcinogenesis,* 1995. 16(5): p. 993-1002.

[45] Graziano, S.L., et al., Prognostic significance of K-ras codon 12 mutations in patients with resected stage I and II non-small-cell lung cancer. *J. Clin. Oncol,* 1999. 17(2): p. 668-75.

[46] Schiller, J.H., et al., Lack of prognostic significance of p53 and K-ras mutations in primary resected non-small-cell lung cancer on E4592: a Laboratory Ancillary Study on an Eastern Cooperative Oncology Group Prospective Randomized Trial of Postoperative Adjuvant Therapy. *J. Clin. Oncol,* 2001. 19(2): p. 448-57.

[47] Taioli, E. and E.L. Wynder, Re: Endocrine factors and adenocarcinoma of the lung in women. *J. Natl. Cancer Inst,* 1994. 86(11): p. 869-70.

[48] Siegfried, J.M., Women and lung cancer: does oestrogen play a role? *Lancet Oncol,* 2001. 2(8): p. 506-13.

[49] Stabile, L.P., et al., Human non-small cell lung tumors and cells derived from normal lung express both estrogen receptor alpha and beta and show biological responses to estrogen. *Cancer Res,* 2002. 62(7): p. 2141-50.

[50] Adami, H.O., et al., Risk of cancer in women receiving hormone replacement therapy. *Int. J. Cancer,* 1989. 44(5): p. 833-9.

[51] Schabath, M.B., et al., Hormone replacement therapy and lung cancer risk: a case-control analysis. *Clin. Cancer Res,* 2004. 10(1 Pt 1): p. 113-23.

[52] Ganti, A.K., et al., Hormone replacement therapy is associated with decreased survival in women with lung cancer. *J. Clin. Oncol,* 2006. 24(1): p. 59-63.

[53] Schwartz, A.G., P. Yang, and G.M. Swanson, Familial risk of lung cancer among nonsmokers and their relatives. *Am. J. Epidemiol,* 1996. 144(6): p. 554-62.

[54] Mayne, S.T., J. Buenconsejo, and D.T. Janerich, Familial cancer history and lung cancer risk in United States nonsmoking men and women. *Cancer Epidemiol. Biomarkers Prev,* 1999. 8(12): p. 1065-9.

[55] Wu, A.H., et al., Family history of cancer and risk of lung cancer among lifetime nonsmoking women in the United States. *Am. J. Epidemiol,* 1996. 143(6): p. 535-42.

[56] Hennig, E.M., et al., HPV positive bronchopulmonary carcinomas in women with previous high-grade cervical intraepithelial neoplasia (CIN III). *Acta Oncol,* 1999. 38(5): p. 639-47.

[57] Cheng, Y.W., et al., The association of human papillomavirus 16/18 infection with lung cancer among nonsmoking Taiwanese women. *Cancer Res,* 2001. 61(7): p. 2799-803.

[58] Tsuhako, K., et al., Human papillomavirus DNA in adenosquamous carcinoma of the lung. *J. Clin. Pathol,* 1998. 51(10): p. 741-9.

[59] Gorgoulis, V.G., et al., Human papilloma virus (HPV) is possibly involved in laryngeal but not in lung carcinogenesis. *Hum. Pathol,* 1999. 30(3): p. 274-83.

[60] Welt, A., et al., Human papillomavirus infection is not associated with bronchial carcinoma: evaluation by in situ hybridization and the polymerase chain reaction. *J. Pathol,* 1997. 181(3): p. 276-80.

In: Lung Cancer in Women
Editor: Varetta N. Torres, pp.131-146
ISBN: 978-1-60021-659-6


*Chapter VI*

# SMOKING CESSATION: DIFFERENT INTERVENTION TECHNIQUES BETWEEN SEXES

***Ioannis Gkiozos, Georgios Papaetis and Kostas Syrigos****
Oncology Unit, 3rd Department of Medicine, Athens Medical School,
Sotiria General Hospital, Athens, Greece

## ABSTRACT

With 4.9 million people being killed each year due to smoking worldwide, tobacco is the only product that kills half its consumers. Across the E.U. countries, it is estimated that around 106.000 women die prematurely each year as a result of smoking. Women are affected by the main smoking-related diseases in the same way as men, but are also at risk of developing a number of gender-specific problems including cancer of cervix and problems related to reproductive health and osteoporosis.

An important question regarding quitting smoking is whether men and women should receive different cessation treatments. Although smoking cessation clinical trials reveal that the same pharmacotherapy treatments (Bupropion SR, Nicotine Replacement Therapies) benefit both men and women, there is strong evidence that the approach should be different towards female smokers. In fact, women may face different stressing parameters and barriers to quitting that may be useful to address in treatment decisions. These include greater likelihood of depression, greater weight control concerns, and hormonal cycle abnormalities. This suggests that women may benefit from tobacco dependence treatments that address these topics, although only few studies have examined programs targeted to one gender.

* Address for Correspondence: Konstantinos N. Syrigos, MD, PhD; Assistant Professor of Oncology in Medicine; Athens University School of Medicine; Head, Oncology Unit, Third Department of Medicine; Building Z, Sotiria General Hospital; Mesogion 152; 115 27 Athens, Greece; Tel: +30 210 7475 034 / Fax: +30 210 7781 035; Email: knsyrigos@usa.net / ksyrigos@med.uoa.gr

With regard to motivation in a smoking cessation program for females, one should underline benefits such as physical appearance and lower incidence of osteoporosis. In particular, women, who are candidates to become pregnant, may be more receptive to stop smoking because of the serious risks imposed on the fetus.

In conclusion, different smoking cessation treatment strategies with augmented psychosocial interventions and more intensive counseling about weight gain, osteoporosis, physical appearance, depression, and pregnancy may be needed for female smokers in order to achieve better abstinence rates.

## INTRODUCTION

According to the *2001 Report of the Surgeon General on Women and Smoking,* smoking is the leading known cause of preventable death and disease among women [1]. In addition, a woman's annual risk for death more than doubles among continuing smokers compared with persons who have never smoked in all age groups from 45 to 74 years [1].

Although women are affected in the same way as men regarding the main smoking-related diseases, they do face specific gender-related health problems such as increased risks for conception delay, decreased fertility, moderate risk for ectopic pregnancy, spontaneous abortion, osteoporosis, cancer of cervix and vulvae. Moreover, female smokers are a target-group of the tobacco industry marketing which influences there susceptibility to and initiation of smoking especially among girls.

In the world of women-smokers, it is understood that there are many gender-related differences concerning health problems, as well as differences in the reasons of smoking and in the risk rates of developing smoking-related diseases. A reasonable question which is raised is if there are any different interventional techniques in smoking cessation programs between the two sexes in order to achieve better abstinence rates among women.

Research on gender differences in smoking cessation was initiated partially in response to the *1980 Report of the Surgeon General on Women and Smoking*, which stated, 'women have more difficulty in giving up smoking than men, both at the end of treatment and at long-term points of measurement," and partially in response to national survey (NHIS, AUTS) findings from the mid-1960s to mid-1980s which indicated that women had lower quit ratios than men. The quit ratio describes the proportion of ever smokers who are now former smokers (former smokers/ever smokers). Gender differences in the quit ratio have always existed: for men, rising from 31.4% (1965) to 48.7% (1987) to 51.6% (1991); and for women, rising from 24.6% (1965) to 40.1% (1987) to 44.7% (1991) [2,3]. On the other hand, gender differences in the pattern of quitting do not exist, as demonstrated by changes in average quit ratios. According to the 1990 *Surgeon General's Report on the Health Benefits of Smoking Cessation*, quit ratios were reported to increase 0.70% per year for men and 0.76% per year for women over the time period from 1965 to 1987.

Thus, the average annual rate of increase in quitting is similar for men and women. However, do these studies of the previous years reveal any differences between the two sexes and, if so, in which fields? Which are the differences between the two sexes regarding the abstinence rates and the type of pharmacotherapy? Do any specific physiological, psychological, and behavioral factors for women exist that influence the quit ratios? Are there any gender differences in smoking cessation associated with employment and joblessness? Can pregnancy-specific programs enable women to increase cessation rates? Are female-smokers more concerned about physical appearances and body-weight than male-smokers? Do tobacco-control programs with gender-sensitive approaches need to be developed for adolescent boys and girls? All these issues of the last decade have been questioned in regards to implementing effective, possible gender-sensitive, smoking cessation programs.

## Different Pharmacologic Approaches to Smoking Cessation between Two Sexes

Generally, men and women have responded similarly to smoking cessation attempts and interventions [4] but, differences in abstinence or relapse rates have been reported for women [5,6] in unaided quit attempts [7], community interventions [8], and large clinical trials [9,10]. The US National Clinical Practice Guideline for the treatment of nicotine dependence recommends the use of pharmacotherapy with behavioral treatments, but does not make treatment recommendations based on gender with the exception with pregnant women [11]. Nicotine plays an integral role in the vicious circle between the continuous use of tobacco and a steady level of carcinogenic exposure for both sexes [12]. Nicotine Replacement Therapy (NRT) is effective in both men and women as demonstrated by a recent meta-analysis [13], and there is no clinical rational for not using these products in both genders.

However, there are reports of significant differences in women's responses to pharmacotherapies [9-11]. The most common pharmacotherapy using NRT shows that women often, but not always, respond more poorly than men. This suggests that non-nicotinic therapies may be more effective for women [14] than men or that NRT is more effective for men [15,16] than women.

What may partially account for the relatively better outcomes for women in these trials may be the suppression of several important factors related to smoking for women. For example, olfactory and taste stimuli are associated with smoking pleasure for women but not for men and bupropion may change the taste in cigarettes. A change in cigarette taste may result in negatively reinforced smoking behavior, especially for women, by reducing pleasure stimuli. While efficacy of bupropion for smoking cessation is independent of a history of depression, bupropion seems to reduce cessation-related depression, post-cessation appetite, weight gain, irritability and a negative affect [17,18].

Another trial [19] did not reveal any evidence for gender differences either in response to 7 weeks 300 mg bupropion treatment plus brief counseling or after 52 weeks of bupropion vs. placebo for relapse prevention. The authors suggested that bupropion is a promising pharmacotherapy for preventing relapse.

A recent placebo-controlled trial of bupropion with behavioral counselling [20] demonstrated that although women have more difficulty than men in quitting smoking, bupropion may attenuate this gender disparity particularly among females who are lighter smokers. According to the prolonged abstinence data, women tended to respond more poorly than men on placebo plus behavioral counselling but female lighter smokers had better abstinence rates to men on bupropion plus counselling.

In another study [21], women and elderly tobacco users were much less likely to receive prescriptions for cessation medications, while patients requesting treatment for tobacco-cessation and those with tobacco-caused diagnoses were more likely. Women using the Veterans Health Administration (VA) Smoking Cessation Services [22] were less likely to receive a prescription for nicotine patches, probably due to gender differences in knowledge, attitudes, or beliefs on the part of either the patient or the provider. Women may be less willing to use a medication to address a habit compared to men. It was seen that a year after the first attempt to quit, female smokers were less likely to have successfully quit smoking. On the other hand, male veterans were more likely to report problems associated with quitting, which is an important piece of information for providers to initiate pharmacotherapy [23].

A recent study [24] assessed the efficacy of two forms of pharmacotherapy (nicotine and phenylpropanolamine gums in addition to a 13-week cognitive behavioral smoking cessation program targeted for women. The results suggested that although the pharmacological interventions had no effect on cessation rates and post-cessation weight gain, the behavioral component of the intervention was effective in increasing the odds of quitting smoking in weight-concerned women.

A double-blinded, placebo-controlled trial [25] evaluated the efficacy of naltrexone (a primary mu-opioid receptor antagonist that is currently FDA-approved for the treatment of opioid and alcohol dependencies) as an adjunct to standard smoking cessation treatments. A preliminary study showed that naltrexone produced an overall modest improvement in smoking cessation rates. Potentially interesting sex differences were also observed (women showing a worse outcome compared to men) in the placebo group but not in the naltrexone group. Although this finding was statistically significant at 8 weeks, it was no longer significant at the 6-month follow-up, which may suggest a need for longer durations of treatment.

Regarding the type of Nicotine Replacement Therapy, individual NRT formulations have proven efficacy in smokers motivated to make a quit attempt, and there is little direct evidence that one nicotine product is more effective than another. Thus the decision about which product to use should be guided by individual preferences [26].

In conclusion, despite the evidence from various studies that differ in design, sample characteristics and intensity of the interventions, researchers to date have not found consistent gender-specific differences in the effectiveness of pharmacotherapy treatment in smoking cessation programs. Further investigation is still needed.

## The Role of Physiological Factors between Two Sexes in a Smoking Cessation Program

Smoking has a multifactorial dependence: physical, psychological and social. The interaction between nicotine addiction, sociodemographic characteristics and behavioral factors is relevant to the success of smoking cessation [27]. The exploration of differences in nicotine sensitivity, tolerance and dependence as a function of gender began only the last decade.

Although there is no clear consensus, some interesting findings have emerged showing gender differences in nicotine-induced thermogenesis, satiety, heart rate, tolerance and perception of muscle tension. Therefore, the experience of smoking and the withdrawal distress may be somewhat different for women than to men.

A study [28] showed that nicotine enhanced thermogenesis during moderate physical activity for men but not for women and that among women, energy expenditure did not increase when nicotine consumption preceded exercise. In another study, female smokers were noted to work harder than male smokers to obtain food reinforces when they were deprived of cigarettes [29]. This is consistent with the idea that nicotine may enhance feelings of satiety, thus reducing food consumption and this may contribute to lower weight among smokers.

Women also experienced significantly more impairment than men in the detection of forearm muscle tension in smoking versus non-smoking conditions [30]. Thus, in some women, nicotine may be used to block the perception of muscle tension. This may encourage smoking in situations that often result in increased muscle tension (for example: anxiety, pain, headaches, depression). It was also noted that smoking may reduce fatigue or improve concentration to a greater extent for women than for men [31].

Regarding the withdrawal distress, studies have shown that there are significantly more symptoms in women than in men and that females were more likely than males to report that relapses were associated with anxiety or craving [32]. Moreover, gender differences were reported in the severity of withdrawal symptoms among nicotine users. Over an eight-week period, women experienced more severe withdrawal symptoms than men, particularly those who received the lowest doses of nicotine gum (2mg) [33]. On the other hand, the Transdermal Nicotine Study Group reported no differences in nicotine withdrawal symptoms between men and women [34].

Women also face unique biological processes which may affect the course and outcome of cessation. Commonly reported symptoms of smoking withdrawal include depression, irritability, anxiety, lethargy, tension, decreased concentration and weight changes [35]. These symptoms are similar to those reported by many women during menstrual distress. A study reported that women who quit smoking in the luteal phase (ovulation to day prior to menses) of their menstrual cycle experienced greater withdrawal than women who quit during the follicular phase (day 1 of the menses to day 15). When withdrawal scores of men were compared to women who quit in the luteal phase, women reported significantly more withdrawal symptoms [36]. These findings imply that the phase of a woman's menstrual cycle should be considered when selecting a quit day, especially if she experiences a high level of premenstrual distress.

Female smokers are more prone to early menopause than nonsmokers and may also experience more menopausal symptoms. Moreover, postmenopausal women who smoke have lower bone densities and an increased risk for hip fractures compared to women who do not smoke. As a result of these hormonal changes, menopausal women may experience fluctuations in affect, greater difficulties in weight control and changes in body image. Cumulatively, these factors may negatively influence the likelihood of cessation.

# The Role of Behavioral and Psychological Factors between Two Sexes in a Smoking Cessation Program

Concerning the behavioral level, a number of psychological and socially-mediated factors may affect cessation among women. These factors include: fear of weight gain, need for social support, and reliance on cigarettes for control of negative affect or stress management, confidence in ability to quit (self-efficacy).

More women than men fear weight gain if they quit smoking [37,38]. However, few studies have found a relationship between weight gain concerns and smoking cessation among either women or men. Further actual weight gain during cessation does not predict relapse to smoking [39].

A large population-based prospective study (n=4,981) evaluated current and previous weight loss efforts and smoking behavior at baseline and at a two-year follow-up [40]. The researchers found that a change in weight and current or previous dieting were not related to relapse or cessation in men or women. Nevertheless, women who had a history of participation in weight loss programs were significantly more likely to quit smoking than men who also had a history of attending weight loss programs.

In clinical trials, attempts to suppress post-cessation weight gain have been generally unsuccessful [38,41] leading some investigators to conclude that, instead of developing intensive interventions to prevent weight gain, a more prudent strategy might be followed to help smokers to accept this relatively small weight gain[42].

On the other hand, another study revealed that if smoking cessation is followed by a moderate increase in the level of physical activity, then weight gain is minimized [43].

Further interventional trials are warranted to confirm that physical activity or incorporating a weight control program into a smoking cessation program are attractive options for women considering quitting. Additionally, weight control programs may be particularly important for the subgroup of women who use smoking to manage weight [44].

Smoking cessation and the social support derived from family and friends improve cessation rates, but it is inconclusive whether there are gender differences in the role of social support on long-term smoking cessation [39]. While women report that social support (behaviors or acts provided by others that include emotional, instrumental, informational and appraisal support) is of great importance to them, studies that incorporate social support components have not generally shown significant gender differences in cessation outcomes[45].

However, a population-based survey of smokers [46] revealed that the importance of social support in quitting was rated higher among women than men. This means that among women, successful quitters were significantly more likely to report greater social support than those who relapsed, whereas this difference was only marginally significant among men. Finally, women rated empathetic support (encouragement, listening) as more helpful than instrumental support (for example: suggesting alternatives to smoking).

A recent study investigated the effect of the partner smoking status on the success of a cessation program. Significant differences were found in the abstinence rates at 12 months by the partner smoking status: abstinence was achieved by 28.3% of patients with a smoking partner and by 46.5% of patients without a smoking partner. The subjects whose partner was smoking at the beginning of the program appeared to be more likely to relapse than the subjects without smoking partners and this was more pronounced in women than in men [47].

Women tend to use social support more than men to cope with stress and when making lifestyle behavioral changes. Findings from two population-based surveys [48,49] revealed that women making quit attempts are more likely than men to use cessation programs that provide some type of assistance, such as from mental health professionals and prefer formal smoking cessation groups or help from health professionals.

Moreover, there are specific socioeconomic conditions for subgroups of female smokers, like African-American women, which face stressing parameters for smoking cessation, such as a different cultural norm for smoking or a lack of social support and isolation. These women stated that smoking cessation would be feasible if it where a component of broader social support efforts to improve their lives [50]. Detailed research needs to clearly conceptualize social support and examine which types of support are beneficial for men and women.

Regarding the role of the negative affects (stress, anxiety, anger, fear, sadness, depression) on both sexes to smoking habit, few studies have evaluated gender differences. Women smoke more often in stressful and "high arousal" situations [45] and are more likely to relapse in the face of stressful life events, particularly health and financial stressors [51], whereas men relapse more often in positive situations such as social events or as part of relaxation. Studies which support these findings also report that women are more likely than men to expect that smoking will improve their mood [52] and they are more likely to relapse at home when they report a negative mood (in contrast to men who are more likely to report relapses outside of the home, when their mood is positive) [53] .

Special attention should be paid to the assessment and treatment of depressed female smokers, particularly with the use of pharmacological and behavioral therapies. Studies have shown that smokers with major depression, who were more nicotine-dependent, were less successful in quitting, experienced more withdrawal symptoms and were more likely to relapse compared to non-depressed smokers [54, 55, 56. These findings are significant for women given that the incidence of depression is higher in women than in men.

A recent study [57] evaluated the gender differences in smoking cessation associated with employment and joblessness through young adulthood in the US. There were findings that joblessness is more strongly associated with persistence in smoking among women than it is among men and that the lower likelihood of cessation among women who have exited the labor force is due to the associated reductions in social and economic resources. One explanation for that lower likelihood may be the combined strains of material deprivation and parenthood, to which women are unwilling to add to the stress associated with smoking cessation. Women may indeed benefit from a smoking cessation program designed to deal with negative affects and how to cope with them in a different way than men.

Women smokers also seem to be less self-confident than men to attempt to quit smoking. It was found [58] that men were significantly more likely to report plans to quit completely in the next 12 months, while women were significantly more likely to report intentions to cut down on the number of cigarettes smoked in the next 12 months. Although the above study did not find significant differences between the two sexes concerning their self-confidence in making a quit attempt, the researchers noted that women seemed to be less committed to quitting and responded more negatively than men to cessation failures. Therefore, it is critical to help females view relapse as a learning experience for future quit attempts and not as a sign of failure.

## Pregnancy: A Unique Chance for a Successful Smoking Cessation Program

Women who smoke have increased risk for conception delay and for both primary and secondary infertility. Female smokers during pregnancy also risk pregnancy complications, premature birth, low-birth weight infants, stillbirth infant mortality and have a modest increase in risks for ectopic pregnancy (fallopian tube or peritoneal cavity pregnancy) and spontaneous abortion. Moreover, studies show a link between smoking and the risk of sudden infant death syndrome (SIDS) among the offspring of women who smoke during the pregnancy [1]. Despite increased knowledge of the adverse health effects of smoking during pregnancy, it is estimated that pregnant women continue to smoke throughout their pregnancies ranging from 12% (based on birth certificate data) up to 20% (based on survey data). If they manage to quit during pregnancy, most return to smoking after pregnancy- up to 67% by the 12th month after delivery. However, smoking during pregnancy appears to have decreased from 1989 to 2000. *According to the Treating Tobacco Use and Dependence clinical practise guideline* [11] an evidence-based recommendation for brief pregnancy-tailored counselling for routine use in prenatal care has been found to double or triple pregnant smokers' quit rates compared with simply advising them to quit.

Pregnant smokers who are unable to quit with the help of the five A's (Ask, Advise, Assess, Assist, Arrange) may benefit from other clinical practise guidelines and intensive counselling from a provider with special training in the treatment of tobacco dependence and the appropriate use of effective pharmacotherapies. Pharmacotherapies are recommended for consideration only among pregnant women who smoke heavily and are unable to quit using counselling alone and when the potential benefits and likelihood of quitting outweigh the potential risks [59]. Bupropion is specifically contraindicated in pregnancy as well as other antidepressants which are subject to special caution. The treatment of choice for pregnant women is nicotine replacement therapy (NRT). Any safety concerns about this treatment can be discounted by the fact that the alternative for most women is continued smoking and hence, continued fetal exposure to nicotine and other toxins. In order to avoid unnecessary exposure of the fetus to nicotine, it is probably advisable to avoid the longer-acting NRT formulations, such as 24 hour transdermal patches [60]. Additionally, further research is still needed to evaluate the safety of $NRT_S$ during pregnancy.

Programs that encourage women to stop smoking before, during and after pregnancy deserve high priority for two reasons: during pregnancy women are highly motivated to stop smoking and they still have many remaining years of potential life.

## SMOKING CESSATION BETWEEN YOUNG PEOPLE

While smoking has declined among adults in Europe over recent years, there has been little decline among 11 to 15 year olds [61,62]. In addition, smoking among young people has become increasingly gendered, with regular (weekly) smoking in girls being higher than boys in 19 out of 31 European countries. It is now widely accepted that tobacco control strategies aimed at reducing smoking among young people need to adopt a more gender-sensitive approach [63-66], although their development is hampered by our limited understanding of the reasons behind gender differences in youth smoking.

A wide range of factors influence young people to start and continue smoking. These are related to young people's individual characteristics (e.g. attitudes, beliefs, self-esteem, risk-taking, age, educational attainment), their close personal environment (e.g. family and friends' smoking, school ethos) and their wider social and cultural environment (e.g. social norms, tobacco promotion, access to cigarettes) [67,68].

Several studies have found gender differences in relation to some of these factors. These include differences relating to body image (girls are more concerned about body image and believe that smoking can control weight), affect control (girls more likely to smoke so as to cope with negative feelings) and self-esteem (poor self-esteem being more influential in girls' smoking) [69]. Girls who initiate smoking are also more likely to have parents or friends who smoke and have weaker attachments to parents and family and stronger attachments to peers and friends.

A study of Scottish 11- and 13- years olds [70] found that smoking was most common among 'top girls' who were described as 'good-looking', 'loud' and 'cool' and used smoking as a marker of their membership of this group, and by 'bottom girls' who smoked to be like 'top girls' and attain their status. In contrast, high status boys were less vulnerable to smoking as it conflicted with their wish to be fit and they could secure a cool identity through other activities, notably sports.

A recent qualitative study [71] which used single-sex focus groups to explore the gendered nature of the meaning and function of smoking among Scottish 15- to 16- years old smokers found that young people were ambivalent about their smoking and that this was somewhat different for boys and girls. These differences related to their social worlds, pattern of social relationships, interests, activities and concerns, the meanings they attached to smoking, and the role smoking played in dealing with the everyday experience of being a boy or girl in their mid-teens. Of particular importance was how different, according to gender, smoking was identified as, in reference to the working image/status, where adolescents had to go through in order to achieve a socially and culturally acceptable image.

Research evidence on sex-linked differences is unclear or inconsistent for the most of these factors and there is a need for further evaluation in order to achieve better abstinence rates or to avoid smoking in adolescence. In conclusion, tobacco-control programs need to develop broader gender-sensitive approaches to health promotion which are congruent with adolescent boys' and girls' experiences of smoking and their wider social worlds. Moreover, health professionals could consider becoming involved in anti-tobacco educational programs at schools that promote acquisition of social influence skills for young people. This is best achieved by involving young people in the development and evaluation of such programs. It is also important that such interventions occur before smoking (and being a smoker) becomes fully integrated into young people's notions of self.

## Marketing Cigarettes to Women

Tobacco advertising gearing towards women began in the 1920$_s$ and the number of women aged 18 to 25 years who began smoking increased significantly in the mid-1920$_s$. In 1960, about 10% of all cigarette advertisements appeared in popular women's magazines and by 1985 cigarette this increased by 34%. In 1999, expenditures for domestic cigarette advertising and promotion reached $8.24 billion increasing 22.3% from the $6.73 billion spent in 1998 [72].

Tobacco marketing targets women and men smokers in different ways: messages to women tend to link smoking with maturity, confidence, sexual attractiveness, and beauty, particularly in developing countries [73]. Advertising is used in part to reduce women's fear of the health risks from smoking by presenting information on nicotine and tar content or by using positive images (e.g. models engaged in exercise or pictures of white capped mountains against a background of clear blue skies). The promotion of 'mild' and 'light' cigarettes has typically involved associations with weight control with the connotation that there is a benefit in smoking with less of the 'bad' effects. In fact, this is far from the truth and bans on the use of these terms as well as a global control on tobacco advertising are being sought.

## Conclusion

Even though it is known that smoking cessation clinical guidelines and treatments benefit both men and women, further insight raises the reasonable question as to whether or not the approaches should be tailored to suit the sexes, in particular by altering the intervention techniques towards female smokers. There are many studies that have evaluated different pharmacotherapeutic treatments between the two sexes, but there is still conflicting evidence about gender-specific differences in the effectiveness of pharmacotherapy treatment in smoking cessation.

Female smokers experience different withdrawal symptoms than male smokers which may be because of the different role of physiological factors which interact during smoking. Women also seem to smoke for different reasons than men e.g. to cope with negative feelings, control weight, in response to depression and the need for 'time out' in caring responsibilities. Pregnancy is a unique chance for women for a successful smoking cessation attempt knowing the adverse health effects of smoking to fetal and neonatal growth and development. Of particular importance are young girls smokers who are not smoking for the same reasons as the older female smokers. Tobacco-control programs in schools with the involvement of young smokers are needed for these adolescents. Gendered differences between women and men in smoking triggers and associations (in the form of tobacco advertising) also affect the likelihood of successful quits.

It is essential that all the above differences between women/men and girls/boys are factors underling smoking initiation and continuation and are fully understood in order to achieve better abstinence rates in a smoking cessation program for female smokers.

# REFERENCES


[1] US Department of Health and Human Services. *The Health Consequences of Smoking for Women, A Report of the Surgeon General*. US Public Health Service, Office of the Assistant Secretary for Health, Office on Smoking and Health; 2001.

[2] Syrigos KN, Nutting C, Roussos C, Tumors of the chest. Biology, Diagnosis and Management. Verlag, New York, May 2006.

[3] CDC. Cigarette smoking among adults-United States, 1991.*MMWR*. 1993;42:230-233.

[4] Whitlock EP, Vogt TM, Hollis, JF, Lichtenstein E. Does gender affect response to a brief clinic-based smoking intervention? *American Journal of Preventive Medicine*. 1997;13:159-66.

[5] Pomerleau CS. Smoking and nicotine replacement treatment issues specific to women. *Am. J. Health Behav*. 1996;20:291-9.

[6] Escopedo LG, Peddicord JP.Smoking prevalence in US birth cohorts: the influence of gender and education. *American Journal of Public Health*. 1996;86:231-6

[7] Ward KD, Klesges RC, Zbikowski SM, Bliss RE, Garvey AJ. Gender differences in the outcome of an unaided smoking cessation attempt. *Addict. Behav*. 1997;22:521-33.

[8] Royce JM, Corbett K, Sorensen G, Ockene J. Gender, social pressure and smoking cessation: the Community Intervention Trial for Smoking Cessation (Commit) at baseline. *Soc. Sci. Med*. 1997:44:359-70.

[9] Bjornson WM, Rand C, Connett JE, et al. Gender differences in smoking cessation after three years in the Lung Health Study. *Am. J. Public Health*. 1995;85:223-30.

[10] Nides MA, Rakos RF, Gonzales D, Murray RP, Tashkin DP, Bjornson-Benson WM. Predictors of initial smoking cessation and relapse through the first 2 years of the Lung Health Study. *Journ. Consult. Clin. Psychol*. 1995;63:60-69.

[11] Fiore MC, Baile WC, Cohen SJ, et al. Treating tobacco use and dependence: clinical practice guideline. Rockville, MD: *US. Department of Health and Human Services, Public Health Service*, June 2000.

[12] Mauer C, Syrigos KN. Biology of tobacco and smoking. In Tumors of the Chest : Biology, Diagnosis and Management. Eds : Syrigos KN, Nutting C, Roussos Ch. Springer-Verlang, New York, 2006, pp 23-39.

[13] Cepeda-Benito A, Reynoso JT, Erath S. Meta-analysis of the efficacy of nicotine replacement therapy for smoking cessation: differences between men and women. *Journ. Consult. Clin. Psychol.* 2004;72:712-22.

[14] Perkins KA.Nicotine discrimination in men and women.*J Pharmacol Biochem Behav* 1999;64:295-9.

[15] Killen JD, Fortmann SP, Newman B,Varady A. Evaluation of a treatment approach combining nicotine gum with self-guided behavioural treatments for smoking relapse prevention. *Journal of Consulting and Clinical Psychology.* 1990;58:85-92.

[16] Hatsukami D, Skoog K, Allen S,Bills R. Gender and the effects of different doses of nicotine gum on tobacco withdrawal symptoms. *Experimental and Clinical Psychopharmacology.* 1995;3:163-173.

[17] Shiffman S, Johnston JA, Khayrallah M, et al. The effect of bubropionn on nicotine craving and withdrawal. *Psychopharmacologia.* 2000;148:33-40.

[18] Borrelli B, Spring B ,Niaura R, Hitsman B, Papandonatos G. Influences of gender and weight gain on short-term relapse to smoking in a cessation trial. *Journal of Consulting and Clinical Psychology*, 2001;69 *3,511/515.

[19] Gonzales D, Bjornson W, Durcan MJ, White JD, Johnston JA, Buist AS, Sachs DPL, Rigotti NA, Niaura R, Hays T, Hurt RD. Effects of Gender on Relapse Prevention in Smokers Treated with Bubropion SR. *American Journal of Preventive Medicine.* 2002;22:234-239.

[20] Collins BN, Wileyto EP, Patterson F, Rukstalis M, Audrain/McGovern J, Kaufmann V, Pinto A, Hawk L, Niaura R, Epstein LH, Lerman C. Gender differences in smoking cessation in a placebo/controlled trial of bupropion with behavioral counselling. *Nicotine and Tobacco Research.* 2004,6:27/37

[21] Steinberg MB, Akincigil A, Delveno CD, Crystal S, Garson JL. Gender and Age Disparities for Smoking-Cessation Treatment. *American Journal of Preventive Medicine.* 2006;30(5)405-412.

[22] Sherman SE, Fu SS, Joseph AM, Lanto AB, Yano EM. Gender differences in smoking cessation services received among veterans. *Women's Health Issues.* 2005;15:126-133.

[23] Chernof BA, Sherman SE, Lanto AB, Lee ML, Yano EM, Rubenstein LV. Health habit counselling amidst competing demands: effects of patient health habits and visit characteristics. *Medical Care.* 1999;37:738-747.

[24] Cooper TV, Klesges RC, DeBon MW, Zbikowski SM, Johnson KC, Clemens LH. A placebo controlled randomised trial of the effects of phenylpropanolamine and nicotine gum on cessation rates and post-cessation weight gain in women. *Addictive Behaviours.* 2005;30:61-75.

[25] King A, De Wit H, Riley RC, Cao D, Niaura R, HatsukamiD. Efficacy of naltrexone in smoking cessation: A preliminary study and an examination of sex differences. *Nicotine and Tobacco Research.* 2006;8(5):671-682.

[26] Gratziou C, Roussos Ch.Smoking Prevention and Cessation Policies. In Tumors of the Chest : Biology, Diagnosis and Management. Eds : Syrigos KN, Nutting C, Roussos Ch. Springer-Verlang, New York, 2006, pp 627-639.

[27] Kottke T, Battista R, De Friese G. Attributes of successful smoking cessation interventions in medical prectise. A meta-analysis of 39 controlled trials. *The Journal of the American Medical Association.* 1988;259:2883-2889.

[28] Perkins K, Sexton J, Epstein L, Fonte C, DiMarco A. Thermogenic effects of nicotine plus caffeine during light activity in male and female smokers. *Annals of Behavioural Medicine.* 1994;16:S060.

[29] Perkins KA, Epstein LH, Fonte C,Grobe JE. The reinforcing value of food during brief smoking abstinence in male and female smokers. *Annals of Behavioral Medicine.* 1994;16:S110.

[30] Epstein LH, Dickson BE, McKenzie S, Russel PO. The effects of smoking on perception of mulcle tension. *Psychopharmacology.* 1984;83:107-113.

[31] Knott V. Neurophysiological aspects of smoking behavioural: Aneuroelectric percspective. *Br. J. Addict.* 1991;86:511-515.

[32] Shiffman S. The tobacco withdrawal syndrome. In: Kresnegor NM, ed. Cigarette smoking as a Dependence Process. Rockville, Md: Nationale Institute on Drug Abuse, Unitred States Department of bHealth, Education and Welfare;1979:158-184.

[33] Hatsukami D. Effects of nicotine gum on withdrawal symptoms in females versus males. Paper presented at American Phychological Association, Psychosocial and Behavioral Factors in Women's Health: Creating an Agenda for the 21st Century, Washington, DC,1994.

[34] Repsher LH, Group TTNS. Smoking cessation by women and older persons: Results from the Trandermal Nicotine Study Group. *Mod. Med.* 1994;62:34-38.

[35] Gritz ER, Carr CR, Marcus AC. The tobacco withdrawal syndrome in unaided quitters. *Br. J. Addict.* 1991;86:57-69.

[36] O' Hara P, Poster SA, Anderson BP. The influence of menstrual cycle changes on the tobacco withdrawal syndrome in women. *Addict. Behav.* 1989;14: 595-600.

[37] Pomerlau CS, Zucker AN, Steward AJ. Characterizing concerns about post-cessation weight gain: results from a national survey of women smokers. *Nicotine Tob. Res.* 2001;3: 51-60.

[38] Piri PL, McBride CM, Hellerstedt W et al. Smoking cessation in women concerned about weight . *American Journal of Public Health.* 1992;82:1238-43.

[39] US Department of Health and Human Services.Efforts to Reduce Tobacco Use Among Women and Girls, *A Report of the Surgeon General.* US Public Health

Service, Office of the Assistant Secretary for Health, Office on Smoking and Health; 2001.

[40] French SA, Jeffrey RW, Klesges LM, Forster JL. Weight concerns and change in smoking behaviour over two years in a working population. *American Journal of Public Health.* 1995;85: 720-721.

[41] Hall SM, Tunstall CD, Vila KL, Duffy J. Weight ain prevention and smoking cessation: cautionary findings. *American Journal of Public Health.* 1992;82: 799-803.

[42] Pekings KA, Weight gain following smoking cessation. *J. Consult. Clin. Psychol.* 1993;61:768-777.

[43] Kawachi I, Troisi RT, Rotnitzky AG, Coakley EH, Colditz GA. Can Physical Activity Minimize Weight Gain in Women After Smoking Cessation? *Amer. Journal of Public Health.* 1996;86:999-1004.

[44] Pinto BM, Marcus BH, Audrian JE, Taylor ER, Eating habits and weight management in women smokers. Paper presented at American Phychological Association, Psychological and Behavioral Factors in Womens's Health: Creating an Agenda for the 21st Century, Washinton, DC, 1994.

[45] Gritz ER, Nielsen IR, Brooks LA. Smoking Cessation and Gender: The Influence of Physiological, Psychological, and Behaviral Factors. *Journal Amer. Med. Women Assos.* 1996;51: 35-42.

[46] Fisher EB, Auslander WF, Sussman LJ, et al. Community organization and social support among African American women. Paper presented at Workshop on Recruitment and Retention of Women in Clinical Studies, St. Louis, Missuri, 1993.

[47] Walsh PM, Carrili P, Flores G, Masuet C, Morchon S, Ramon JM. Effects of partner smoking status and gender on long term abstinence rates of patients receiving smoking cessation treatment. *Addictive Behaviors.* 2006;xx:xxx-xxx.

[48] Fiore MC, Novotny TE, Pierce JP, et al. Methods used to quit smoking in *the USA. JAMA. 1990;263:2760-2765.*

[49] Owen N, Davies MJ. Smokers' preferences for assistance with cessation. *Preventive Medicine* .1990;19: 424-431.

[50] Lacey LP, Manfredi C, Balch G, Warnecke RB, Allen K, Edwards C. Social support in smoking cessation among black women in Chicago public housing. *Public Health Rep.* 1993;108: 387-394.

[51] McKee SA, Maciejewski PK, Falba T, Mazure CM. Sex differences in the effects of stressful life events on changes in smoking status. *Addiction.* 2003; 98: 847-855.

[52] Brandon TH, Baker TB. The smoking consequences questionnaire: the subjective expected utility of smoking in college students. *Psychological Assessments.* 1991; 3: 484-491.

[53] Borland R. Slip-ups and relapse in attempts to quit smoking. *Addictive Behaviours.* 1990;15: 235-245.

[54] Glassman A, Helzer JE, Covey LS, et al. Smoking, smoking cessation and major depression. *JAMA.* 1990;264: 1546-1549.

[55] Breslau N, Kilbey MM, Andreski P, Nicotine dependence major depression and anxiety in young adults. *Arch. Gen Psychiatry.* 1991; 48: 1069-1074.

[56] Hall SM, Munoz RF, Reus VI,. Cognitive-behavioral intervention increases abstinence rates for depressive-history smokers. *J. Consult. Clin. Psychol.* 1994;62: 141-146.

[57] Weden MM, Astone NM, Bishai D. Racial, ethnic and gender differences in smoking cessation associated with employment and joblessness through young adulthood in the US. *Social Science and Medicine.* 2006;62: 303-316

[58] Sorenson G, Pechacek TF. Attitudes toward smoking cessation among men and women. *J Behav Medicine* 1987;10: 129-137.

[59] Orleans CT, Melvin CL, Marx JF, Maibach E, Vose KK. National action plan to reduce smoking during pregnancy: *The National Partnership to Help Pregnant Smokers Quit. Nicotine and Tobacco Research.* 2004; 6: S269-S277.

[60] Coleman T. ABC of smoking cessation. *BMJ.* 2004; 328: 575-576.

[61] ASPECT Consortium. *Tobacco or Health in the European Union: Past, Present and Future.* Luxembourg: Office for Official Publications of the European Communities, 2004.

[62]

[63] Currie C, Roberts C, Morgan A et al. Young People's Health in Context, Health Behaviour in School-aged Children Study: International Report from the 2001/2002 Survey. Copenhagen: WHO Regional Office for Europe, 2004.

[64] INWAT Europe. Part of the Solution? Tobacco Control Policies and Women. London: Health Development Agency, 2000.

[65] Bostock Y. Searching for the Solution: Women, Smoking and Inequalities in Europe. London: Health Development Agency/INWAT, 2003.

[66] Samet JM, Yoon S-Y. Women and the Tobacco Epidemic, Challenges for the 21st Century. Geneva: WHO, 2001.

[67] WHO. WHO Framework Convention on Tobacco Control. Geneva: WHO, 2003.

[68] Kobus K. Peers and adolescent smoking. Addiction 2003; 98 (Suppl. 1):s37-55.

[69] Pierce JP, Distefan JM, Hill D. Adolescent smoking. In: Boyle P et al. (eds). *Tobacco and Public Health: Science and Policy.* Oxford: Oxford University Press, 2004, 315-328.

[70] Lambert M, Hublet A, Verduyckt et al. *Gender Differences in Smoking in Young People.* Belgium: Flemish Institute for Health Promotion, 2002.

[71] Michell L, Amos A. Girls, pecking order and smoking. *Soc. Sci. Med.* 1997;44: 1861-1869.

[72] Amos A, Bostck Y. Young people, smoking and gender-a qualitative exploration Health Education Research Theory and Practice 2006;August:1-12.

[73] US Department of Health and Human Services. *Marketing Cigarettes to Womenl.* US Public Health Service, Office of the Assistant Secretary for Health, Office on Smoking and Health; 2001.

[74] Department of Gender, Women and Health Family and Community Health. *Gender in Lung Cancer and Smoking Research.* World Health Organization; 2004.

In: Lung Cancer in Women
Editor: Varetta N. Torres, pp. 147-170
ISBN: 978-1-60021-659-6


*Chapter VII*

# The Role of Female Hormones in Lung Cancer Development

***Chee-Keong Toh****

National Cancer Center, Singapore; 11 Hospital Drive;
Singapore 169610; Singapore

## Abstract

Lung cancer is the leading cause of cancer deaths in women. There is increasing evidence to suggest that lung cancer develops and behaves differently between men and women based on the genetic profile of the tumor, as well as the outcome and responses to treatment. It is highly plausible that female hormones play a part in lung cancer development as the two sexes are inherently exposed to different hormonal environment. The female sex hormones, in particular estrogen, have been shown to affect the metabolism of substances, including nicotine and possibly other tobacco carcinogens. In addition, studies in rodents have demonstrated that estrogen or their catechol metabolites can be carcinogenic in various tissues. Estrogen receptors (ER) mediate the cellular response to estrogen and two ERs have been identified, ERα and ERβ. Recent studies suggest that the ERα protein present in the lung are mainly splice variants that may or may not be functional while ERβ may be a more important receptor in lung cancer development. Estrogen receptors, when activated, are known to cause transcriptional activation of several growth factor genes. Laboratory studies have found that estrogen can induce lung tumor growth and the effect of which can be blocked by anti-estrogen therapy. Clinical studies further support the role of female hormones in lung cancer development as early age at menopause has been shown to be associated with a reduced risk while the use of estrogen replacement therapy is associated with a higher risk of adenocarcinoma of the lung. It is possible that the estrogen metabolites and ER-mediated genomic and nongenomic signaling could affect cellular proliferation, which can then contribute to the development of lung cancer in women.

# INTRODUCTION

Lung cancer is one of the most common malignancies in the world [1] and is the leading cause of cancer deaths in both men and women in western [2] as well as asian [3] countries. The association of smoking as a risk factor for lung cancer has been well established from epidemiological evidence since the 1950's.[4,5] As tobacco smoking remains the main etiologic agent for lung cancer, it is of increasing concern that smoking prevalence among women did not show any signs of significant decline over the past years, unlike that of men. Figure 1. This trend is similarly observed among women in asian countries such as Singapore.[6] In addition, there is an increasing proportion of younger women picking up the smoking habit, spurred on by social and psychological reasons such as an increased sense of independence and desirability. Compounding the concern for the women is the cumulating evidence that suggest a sex difference in susceptibility to the carcinogenic effects of tobacco smoke. Several studies have suggested that women smokers may be more susceptible to lung cancer as compared to men.

Some epidemiological studies have suggested the involvement of factors other than smoking in the development of lung cancer. [7,8,9,10] This evidence abound mainly among the asian countries as there appears to be more non-smokers afflicted with lung cancer in this region. This spells further concern for the women as they represent a high 75% among the never-smokers with lung cancer in one of these studies.[11] Thus, women may not just be susceptible to the carcinogenic effects of tobacco smoke but also other environmental factors that are yet to be identified. As one obvious difference between men and women is the hormonal environment, the link between women and lung cancer could possibly involve the female hormones. The discussion in this chapter will focus on the evidence for the possible role of female hormones with regards to the suggested increased susceptiblity of women to the carcinogenic effects of tobacco smoke, as well as how female hormones could possibly contribute to the differences in characteristics seen between men and women with lung cancer.

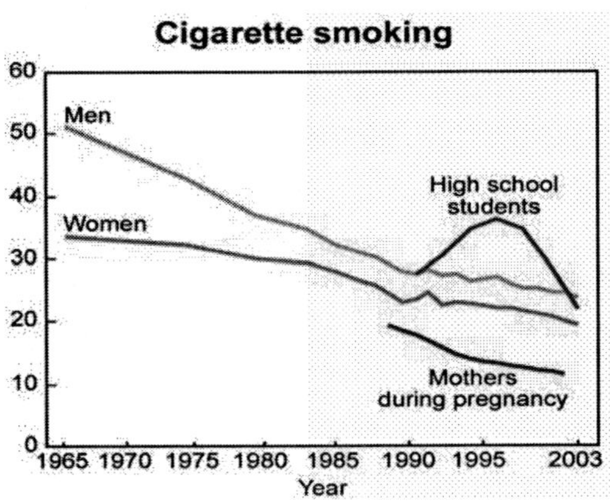


Source: Centers for Disease Control and Prevention, National Center for Health Statistics, Health, United States, 2005, figure 10.

Figure 1. Time trends in cigarette smoking among men and women in the United States.

* Chee-Keong Toh: Tel: 65-6436 8113; Fax: 65-6227 2759; Email: dmotck@nccs.com.sg

# ARE WOMEN MORE SUSCEPTIBLE TO THE CARCINOGENIC EFFECTS OF TOBACCO SMOKE?

## Epidemiological Evidence

### *Positive Studies*

About 2 decades ago, McDuffie et al [12] from North America reported that 'women developed primary lung cancer at an earlier age while smoking for fewer years than men'. In their study based on retrospective review of chart records as well as responses to mailed questionnaires, they also noted that there were significantly more lifetime non-smokers among affected women compared to men. At that time, lung cancer had surpassed breast cancer as the leading cause of cancer deaths among women and concerns arose about women being more susceptible to lung cancer. Several other groups also reported a higher risk of lung cancer among women based on case-control studies. Brownson et al [13] conducted a registry-based case-control study analysing 14,596 cases and 36,438 age-matched controls and reported that the relative risk associated with smoking was consistently higher in women than men for all lung cancer combined (odds ratio (OR) 12.7 for women and 9.1 for men). The increased risk was largest for small-cell-lung carcinoma (SCLC) and lowest for adenocarcinoma. Risch et al [14] performed a case-control study from 1981 to 1985 comparing male-female differences in smoking and lung cancer. The study included 442 women and 403 men cases versus 410 women and 362 men controls matched by age and area of residence. They found an elevated risk of developing lung cancer associated with smoking and this association was stronger for women. The OR for women was 27.9 (95% CI 14.9-52) and that for men was 9.60 (95% CI 5.64-16.3) at a history of 40 pack-years relative to lifelong non-smoking. Harris et al [15] also found a higher relative risk for women (RR of 1.7) than men for a given level of smoking using case-control data. Osann et al [16] reviewed medical records for 1,153 men and 833 women lung cancer cases and 1,851 men and 1,656 women cancers not associated with smoking for the period 1984 to 1986. They found that men and women who smoked 2 or more packs per day experienced about equal risks (OR for men was 19.7 and women was 15.0), but the OR for women was significantly higher for SCLC than for squamous cell carcinoma (SCC). Zang and Wynder [17], in an American Heath Foundation case-control study that involved 1,108 men and 781 women cases and 1,122 men and 948 women controls, found that the OR for women was 1.2 to 1.7 fold higher than men for the same level of exposure to cigarette smoke. They also noted that women were more likely to be non-smokers than men. As one would have noticed, most of the evidence above hinged upon case-control studies which do not provide the most robust clinical evidence.

There are studies with other designs that support the view that women are more susceptible to the carcinogenic effects of tobacco smoke. This includes a population-based study from Norway [18] analysing smoking-associated cancers during the period 1954 to 1993. They found that the lung cancer incidence increased more rapidly relative to the other smoking-associated cancers in women than in men, suggesting that women may be more susceptible than men in developing lung cancer. The other two reports stem from baseline computed tomography (CT) lung cancer screening of men and women smokers. The first was reported by Henschke [19] which was based on two data sources from the lung screening project involving 1,202 women and 1,288 men who were at least 40 years of age, with at least 10 pack-years of cigarette smoking. The prevalence OR of lung cancer for women was significantly higher at 2.7 (95% CI 1.6-4.7), as compared to men after controlling for age and smoking history. The second report based on 7,498 women and 9,427 men, was a further update of the data and was reported by the International Early Lung Cancer Action Program Investigators [20]. They found that the prevalence OR of lung cancer for women remained higher at 1.9 (95% CI 1.5-2.5), as compared to men.

### *Negative Studies*

Just as there are studies with evidence that women are more susceptible to cigarette smoke, there are also studies that refute this stand. Some of the earlier studies performed in the 1960s have demonstrated a higher risk among men smokers compared to women smokers [21,22]. The American Cancer Society's Second Cancer Prevention Study (CPS-II), in a report released in 1964, [23] also found that men smokers were twice as likely to die from lung cancer as women smokers. More recent studies include a report from Copenhagen [24] that was based on 3 prospective population-based studies on 30,874 subjects of which 44% were women. They did not find any difference in rate ratio (RR) of developing lung cancer between men and women (RR was 0.8; 95% CI 0.3-2.1). A multicenter case-control study performed in Germany and Italy [25] also did not find any differences in the relative risk estimates of lung cancer due to smoking. The study was based on 3,723 men and 900 women cases and 4,075 men and 1,095 women controls. Thun et al [26] also did not find that women are at a higher predisposition for lung cancer. In developing a model to estimate lung cancer risk among smokers based on the 18,172 subjects enrolled in the Carotene and Retinol Efficacy Trial (CARET), Bach et al [27] also did not find any association between sex and lung cancer risk. A large recent analysis of prospective data from former and current-smokers in 2 large cohorts – the Nurses' Health Study of women and the Health Professional Follow-up Study of men were reported. [28] This was based on 60,296 women and 25,397 men from 1986 through 2000. The hazard ratio in women ever-smokers for lung cancer compared to men was 1.11 (95% CI 0.95-1.31) which did not support an increased risk for women. Perneger [29] reasoned that the case-control studies that reported a higher relative risk of lung cancer in female smokers may have been interpreted wrongly, due to the substitution of 'risk' for 'relative risk, as compared with nonsmokers of the same sex'. The statistically significant interaction in the studies means that the relative risk of cancer associated with smoking are different between men and women when compared to non-smokers of the same sex and do not compare the men and women.

Several reasons could underlie the different results of the various studies. This includes different baseline risks among men and women due to factors such as occupational exposure. Women were mostly confined in the house to be home-makers several decades ago. Thus, any occupational exposure of the men could increase the risk of them getting lung cancer due to possible positive interaction between tobacco smoke and an occupational carcinogen. This could explain the earlier studies that did not find women to be at higher risk of lung cancer compared to men. As women move into the workforce in the recent years, environmental exposures for both sexes also begin to equalise. Alternatively, if women non-smokers are indeed more susceptible to lung cancer due to unknown factors, the baseline risks of controls would be different between the sexes and would confound the results of the case-control studies looking at differences in susceptibility of the sexes to tobacco smoke. Other reasons include selective recall bias present in case-control studies, as women could under-report their smoking behaviour due to social pressures, although Donato et al [30] found a high reliability for responses relating to smoking with no gender differences. Furthermore, factors such as the depth of inhalation of tobacco smoke and the tar content of the cigarette could affect the risk but these factors are difficult to account or adjust for. Lastly, the type of population studied would make a difference as it is known that there are variations in the risk of lung cancer among different racial populations [31].

## DO HORMONAL FACTORS AFFECT THE RISK OF LUNG CANCER AMONG WOMEN?

### Epidemiological Evidence

Although smoking shows a dose-response relationship with all the major lung cancer histological subtypes, the strength of relationship is the weakest for adenocarcinoma. [32] Epidemiologically, there is a greater proportion of women among the non-smokers with lung cancer and the vast majority of women develop adenocarcinoma. [33, 34] There may be an interaction between the female sex, adenocarcinoma and a non-smoking status. As a result, most of the studies examining the role of hormonal status have focused on the non-smoking women who developed adenocarcinoma of the lung.

Using case-control data, Taioli et al [35] showed that early age at menopause was associated with a reduced risk while the use of estrogen replacement therpay was associated with a higher risk of adenocarcinoma of the lung. There was a positive interaction between estrogen replacement therapy, smoking and adenocarcinoma. Gao et al [36], in a case-control study on 672 female lung cancer patients and 735 population-based controls, found an increased risk of adenocarcinoma (OR 2.9, 95% CI 1.5-5.7) associated with a short menstrual cycle. Futhermore, there was a trend to increased risk for women with late menopause at age 50 yrs or later (OR 1.3, 95% CI 0.9-1.7). Brenner et al [37], however, found a lower risk of lung cancer with later age at menopause (trend, p=0.074) in a case-control study involving 109 lung cancer cases and 435 controls. In another case-control study with 303 Chinese women non-smokers [38], women with 3 or more live births and a menstrual cycle length of more than 30 days had a significantly reduced risk of lung cancer (adjusted OR 0.65, 95% CI 0.44-0.96 and OR 0.46, 95% CI 0.25-0.84 respectively). A case-control study among Czech women [39] involving 145 adenocarcinoma, 221 lung cancer of other cell types and 1624 controls showed a statistically significant inverse relationship of risk of SCC, SCLC and large-cell lung cancer combined with the quantity of menstrual flow ( OR 0.63, 95% CI 0.4-0.99) and pains or mental tension related to menses (OR 0.61, 95% CI 0.42-0.89). Similar to the epidemiological evidence that supports an increased susceptibility among women smokers, all the above evidence are from case-control studies.

There are a few earlier studies which showed an increased risk of lung cancer among female survivors of a primary cancer of the reproductive organs [40-42]. Whether this represents a genetic susceptibility to cancer, the hormonal environment or is simply treatment (eg, radiotherapy) related may be difficult to differentiate. In one study, Kabat GC [43] found that, among females, both a history of a reproductive primary and a history of radiotherapy were associated significantly with lung cancer (OR 4.9, 95% CI 1.4-17.7 and OR 4.4, 95% CI 1.3-15.1 respectively) and he could not determine the effect of one exposure independent of the other. However, one must note that this was a relative small study involving 47 female lung cancer patients. Taking into consideration the epidemiological evidence available, there is likely an interaction between hormonal factors and the risk of lung cancer among women.

## Are There Differences between Men and Women with Lung Cancer?

Differences in epidemiological characteristics between men and women with lung cancer, the putative increased susceptibility of women to lung cancer as well as the possible role of hormonal factors among women has prompted many molecular studies to identify the biological basis for the differences between the sexes. Before I dwell into some of the studies, it is worthwhile to briefly mention the interaction between tobacco carcinogens, DNA adducts and lung cancer.

The pathogenesis of lung cancer involves the interaction of DNA with putative carcinogens present in tobacco smoke. Among the major carcinogens involved include polycyclic aromatic hydrocarbons (PAH), nitrosamines and aromatic amines [44]. There are many studies focusing on PAH and nitrosamines. Benzo(a)pyrene, a type of PAH, was the first carcinogen to be detected in cigarette smoke [45] and thus was one of the most researched PAH. The metabolically activated diol epoxide, Benzo(a)pyrene diol epoxide (BPDE) has been shown to be the cause of mutations in the TP53 gene. Denissenko MF et al [46] mapped the distribution of BPDE adducts within the TP53 gene and found that the adducts preferentially form at lung cancer mutational hotspots. They continued their studies on other PAH adducts and found that other adducts can also form at certain hotspots confirming that other PAH can also induce changes in TP53 gene, although not as frequent as BPDE [47]. The tobacco specific nitrosamines 4-(methylnitrosamino)-1-(3-pyridyl)-1-butanone (NNK) and N`-nitrosonornicotine (NNN) are the most prevalent strong carcinogens in unburned tobacco products [44, 48]. NNK has been shown to induce lung tumors in rodents [49] and DNA adducts from NNK are present in higher levels in lung tissue from lung cancer patients than in controls. Other than PAH and the nitrosamines, there are multiple other carcinogens, co-carcinogens and tumor promoters present in tobacco smoke which can lead to lung cancer.

The presence of DNA adducts in lung tissues has been shown to be associated with increased risk of lung cancer [50]. Most of the carcinogens require metabolic activation before they can form DNA adducts. Metabolic activation is generally initiated by cytochrome P450 enzymes. Most of the activated compounds are excreted, but some react with DNA. At the same time, the cellular repair systems remove the unwanted DNA adducts. However, if the adducts persist and escape repair, mutations will arise and if the mutations occur in crucial areas of oncogenes or tumor suppressor genes, then the result can be tumor growth [51]. Thus, the carcinogens effect through the formation of DNA adducts and mutations in genes. [52] As a result, DNA adducts are often used as a form of carcinogen biomarker in many studies as they provide the most direct measure of tobacco-induced DNA damage [53].

## Studies on DNA Adducts Relating to Differences between Men and Women with Lung Cancer

Toyooka et al [54] found significant difference in the frequencies of G:C to T:A transversions between ever-smokers and never-smokers. When comparing by gender, they found that female smokers tend to have a higher frequency of G:C to T:A transversions compared to female never-smokers. Ryberg et al [55] analyzed normal lung tissue from 63 lung cancer patients. They found that adduct levels were significantly higher in smokers than nonsmokers and that women had higher DNA adduct levels than men when adjusted for smoking dose. In a Taiwanese study on non-smokers [56] involving 62 lung cancer and 20 non-cancer controls, DNA adducts were significantly higher among cancer than non-cancer patients. In addition, DNA adducts were greater in women than men, suggesting that women non-smokers may be at higher risk for lung cancer than men non-smokers. These studies point to the evidence that women have higher DNA adducts than men, which indirectly suggest that they are at a higher risk for lung cancer.

## Studies on Phase I Enzymes (CYP1A1) Relating to Differences between Men and Women

Individuals handle and metabolize carcinogens differently resulting in differences in cancer risk when exposed to similar agents. Many studies have focused on this difference in metabolism of carcinogens to explain the differences in susceptibility between men and women smokers. The following studies support the increased risk among women as the expression and activity of activating enzymes are higher among women.

There is evidence of inter-individual differences in the activity of P-450 cytochrome enzymes. [57] Shimada T et al [58] compared 30 Japanese and 30 Caucasian patients and found differences in activities of some of the cytochrome enzymes between the 2 ethnic groups. There were no clear sex-related differences in carcinogen metabolizing activities, except that P450 1A2 dependent activities were found to be higher in men than women among the Caucasian population only. Sex differences in drug metabolism by these cytochrome enzymes have been described. [59,60,61]. In a study on mice, Lee RP et al [62] found that the bioactivation of 1,1-dichloroethylene was greater in lung microsomes from females compared to males, which suggested that females may be at a higher risk for drug-induced toxicity. The expression of cytochrome P450 enzymes in liver [63] and hair follicles [64] has been found to be different between the sexes.

Mollerup et al [65] examined the CYP1A1 and hydrophobic DNA adducts expression of 29 female and male smokers with lung cancer. They found that female smokers had a significantly higher level of adducts/pack-year (females 0.95+/-0.82 and males 0.46+/-0.46; p=0.0004) and adducts/cigarette/day (1.48+/-1.29 and 0.89+/-0.74; p=0.015). They also found that female smokers had a significantly higher lung expression of CYP1A1 compared to males and there was a positive correlation between CYP1A1 expression and DNA adduct level for both sexes (r=0.50; p=0.009). Recently, they updated their findings [66] on 121 patients and they continued to find that among current smokers, females had a 3.9 fold higher median level of CYP1A1 compared to males (p=0.011). They did not find any differences in CYP1B1 expression between the sexes. This suggests that differences in DNA adduct levels between sexes may be due to differences in CYP1A1 expression and thus CYP1A1 may play a significant role in lung DNA adduct formation and also influence the higher susceptibility among females.

## Studies on Phase II Enzymes (GSTM 1) Relating to Differences between Men and Women with Lung Cancer

The GSTM1 gene encodes for the carcinogen detoxification enzyme glutathione S-transferaseM1. About 50% of humans inherit 2 deleted copies of GSTM1 gene. Bell et al [67] found that the absence of the GSTM1 gene significantly increased the risk of bladder cancer in people with exposure to tobacco smoke (OR 1.8, 95% CI 1.2 -3.0; p=0.01). People with smoking exposure of more than 50 pack-years and had GSTM1 null/null genotype had a six fold increased risk relative to the lowest risk group which are the nonsmokers with GSTM1 +/+ genotype. Although this study pertains to bladder cancer, the same rationale may extend to lung cancer risk as well.

In a study on mutant CYP1A1 and GSTM1 null genotypes in lung cancer [68], Dresler et al found that female cancer patients were more likely than controls to have both the CYP1A1 mutation and GSTM1 null genotypes. The combined genotypes gave an OR of 6.54 for lung cancer in women compared to 2.36 in men, independent of age or smoking history. In a molecular epidemiological case control study [69], Tang et al studied GSTM1 null genotypes and PAH-DNA adducts on 136 NSCLC patients and 115 controls. The OR for GSTM1 null genotype and lung cancer in female smokers was 3.03 (95% CI 1.09 – 8.40) compared with 1.42 (95% CI 0.53 – 4.06) in male smokers. The combined effect of elevated PAH-DNA adducts and GSTM1 null genotype appeared multiplicative (16.19, 95% CI 1.2-115) and the effect of GSTM1 null genotype was greatest in female smokers. All these suggest that the GSTM1 genotype may play a role in determining the susceptibility of women to carcinogens.

## Studies on DNA Repair Capacity Relating to Differences between Men and Women with Lung Cancer

Not many studies had evaluated the role of DNA repair capacity in the susceptibility to lung cancer. The largest study so far [70] was conducted on 316 lung cancer patients and 316 cancer-free controls. A lower DNA repair capacity was found in case patients compared to controls and was associated with a greater than 2-fold increased risk of lung cancer. Patients who were younger at diagnosis, females, lighter smokers, family history of cancer had the lowest DNA repair capacity and the highest risk among the subgroup. This suggests that a low DNA repair capacity may be associated with a higher susceptibility to lung cancer in a subgroup of patients, including women.

## Studies on Factors Affecting Proliferative Capacity Relating to Differences between Men and Women

Willey et al [71] found that bombesin and the C-terminal portion of gastrin-releasing peptide (GRP) can increase the clonal growth rate of human bronchial epithelial cells in the presence or absence of an epidermal growth factor. These peptides may act as autocrine growth factors in lung tumors. DeMichele et al [72] found expression of mRNA for 3 bombesin-like peptide receptor subtypes including neuromedin B receptor, GRP receptor (GRPR) and bombesin receptor subtype 3 in human NSCLC cell lines and biopsies. In a further study, Siegfried et al [73] correlated the mRNA expression with the smoking history of the subjects. They found that GRPR mRNA expression was associated with a long smoking history. The role of GRPR in relation to women's susceptibility to cancer has been postulated as the gene for GRPR is X linked and located on chromosome Xp22, near a cluster of genes that can escape X inactivation.[74] Thus, women can have 2 actively transcribed alleles of the GRPR gene compared with 1 in men. Shriver et al [75] analyzed GRPR mRNA expression in lung tissues and cultured airway cells from 40 males and 38 females. They found that GRPR mRNA expression was detected in airway cells and tissues of more women than men nonsmokers (55% versus 0%). Female smokers showed expression of GRPR mRNA at a lower mean pack-year exposure than male smokers (37.4 pack-years versus 56.3 pack-years; p=0.037). These data suggest that the GRPR gene may play a part in the increased susceptibility of women to tobacco-induced lung cancer.

The epidermal growth factor receptor (EGFR) is frequently expressed in non-small-cell lung cancer (NSCLC). Binding of ligands to the extracellular domain of EGFR results in downstream activation of events that lead to proliferation, reduced apoptosis and enhanced survival. [76] Recently, EGFR-activating mutations in the tyrosine kinase domains were found to be associated with the sensitivity of NSCLC to small molecule tyrosine kinase inhibitors such as gefitinib. [77, 78]. These activating EGFR mutations were found to be more common among never smokers, adenocarcinoma, patients of East Asian ethnicity and women. [79, 80]. Furthermore, in the clinical trials of small molecule tyrosine kinase inhibitors, there was correlation of increased response associated with the female sex. [81,82] In fact, in a case control study on 152 patients comparing the impact of smoking and sex for the risk of NSCLC with or without EGFR mutations, Matsuo et al [83] found that sex was the sole risk factor for EGFR mutant NSCLC (OR for women relative to men, 21.9, 95% CI 1.31-3.39). However, Huang et al [84] did not find any significant difference in the *EGFR* mutation rate between male and female patients with adenocarcinoma (54% versus 55% respectively), and the mutation patterns were also similar between the two sexes. Miller et al

[85] also did not find a gender difference in response rate to gefitinib. Thus, women may be at a higher risk for NSCLC with the EGFR activating mutations, although the causes for these mutations remain unknown.

The K-ras gene encodes a protein that is oncogenic when mutated or overexpressed. Although Nelson et al, [86] in a study on early stage lung cancer, found that NSCLC in women are more likely than men to harbor K-ras mutations, it remains to be contested by other studies. Several studies have found that K-ras mutations are more common in men than in women [87, 88] and are commonly associated with heavy smoking [87, 89, 90] and asbestos exposure. Taken together, differences in K-ras mutations are likely due to differences in tobacco smoking, rather than sex differences as women are more likely to be non-smokers.

The evidence discussed has suggested that women and men with lung cancer may have molecular differences and some are a result of differences in the handling of carcinogens including activation and deactivation of the substances. Whether there are true important differences between the sexes remain to be seen. In the next section, I will discuss the evidence for the role of female hormones contributing to the putative differences between the sexes.

## The Female Hormone and Its Receptors in Lung Cancer

In support of the epidemiological evidence that estrogen may have an interaction with lung adenocarcinoma [35], there is laboratory evidence that estrogen can induce tumor growth in a murine xenograft model. [91] Stabile LP et al reported that mRNA for estrogen receptor (ER)α and ERβ are expressed in cultured human NSCLC, cultured lung fibroblasts and primary cultures of normal bronchial epithelium. The authors also found that beta-estradiol could stimulate the growth of NSCLC cell line as well as tumor xenografts in SCID mice and the effect was blocked by the anti-estrogen fulvestrant. In the 1980s , Khosla SS et al [92] had already demonstrated the ability of estrogen to affect the differentiation and maturation in the lungs of fetal rabbit.

Estrogen receptors mediate the cellular response to estrogen and two ERs have been identified, ERα and ERβ. These receptors possess several distinct functional domains, including a central DNA binding domain that is highly conserved between the 2 receptors. [93] Although there are similarities between the two, the tissue distribution as well as the biologic roles between the 2 are different. [94] There is evidence to suggest that they may actually have functionally opposite roles, at least in breast cancer cell lines. [95] , [96]

There have been many studies looking at the presence of ERs in lung cancer tissues and results have been controversial. The expression of ERα in lung cancer tissue varies between 0% to 98%, depending on the technique used and the patient population.[97-103] Most of these studies comprise small numbers of patients, with the largest being 248 patients with early lung cancer that showed no ER staining at all. [97] In the reports that showed expression of ERα in the lung tumors, women were more likely to express ERα than men.

[101] Unfortunately, a lot of these studies did not stratify the patients by sex or smoking history. In addition, a major limitation of some of these studies were the usage of antibodies that did not distinguish between ERα or ERβ. This was expected as several of them were performed in the earlier year when the role of ERβ in lung cancer was not considered important.

It is believed that ERα protein present in the lungs are mainly splice variants that may or may not be functional and ERβ may be a more important receptor in lung cancer. In their study on NSCLC tumor tissues, Kawai et al [104] found no positive staining when they used a monoclonal antibody against the N-terminus of ERα whereas positive staning was observed with antibodies against the C-terminus of ERα. The significance of the ERα variant that lacks the N-terminus is unknown. The authors also found that 51% of the tumor samples contained ERβ and that both ERα and ERβ may be prognostic in resected NSCLC. Recent evidence have shown that ERβ are expressed and functional in NSCLC cell lines, cells from normal lung and lung cancer tissues.[91,105,106] Omoto et al [105] found that ERβ can bind to estrogen response element (ERE) and increase transcriptional activity in lung cancer, while Patrone et al [107] showed that ERβ is involved in post-natal lung development and homeostasis. Hershberger et al [108] studied the cellular response of NSCLC cells to ER ligands and found that the ligand-dependent estrogenic responses are probably generated via ERβ and the p160 coactivator GRIP1/TIF2. Schwartz et al [109] found that there are differences in expression of ERβ between men and women. Women were less likely to have ERβ positive tumors compared to men (OR 0.54, 95% CI 0.27-1.08). Dougherty et al [110], on the other hand, found that there are no differences in expression the ER receptors between men and women, but that there were difference in activity of the receptors, with the cell line from femlaes more likely to be stimulated by estradiol.

Estrogen receptors, when activated, are known to cause transcriptional activation of several growth factor genes, including transforming growth factor, epidermal growth factor and insulin-like growth factor and all these growth factors are known to cause mitogenesis in lung tumors.[111] Recently, a major lung cancer susceptibility locus was mapped to chromosome 6q23-25 from linkage analysis [112] and that region happens to harbor the ERα, which provides further support for the role of ER in lung cancer. Thus, several molecular studies support the fact that female hormones may play a role in the stimulation of lung cancer growth and development.

## Effect of Estrogen and Its Receptors on Bioactivation of Carcinogens and Their Interaction with Aryl Hydrocarbon (Arh) Receptors

Besides its role in the activation of growth factor genes, one of the more probable effects of ER that can explain sex differences in risk may hinge on the PAH-bioactivation pathway. I will discus some studies that examined the effect of estrogen and/or its receptors on the activation of carcinogens.

The cytochrome enzymes are involved in the bioactivation of carcinogens, among which cytochrome P450CY1A1 and CY1B1 appear to be the most active [113]. The cytochrome P450 enzymes have been shown to be induced by agonists of the aryl hydrocarbon (Arh) receptor, among them are environmental pollutants such as 2,3,7,8-tetrachlorodibenzo-p-dioxin (TCDD) and PAH. The ligand-bound receptor forms a complex with the Arh nuclear translocator protein which in turn can activate genes including CYP1A1[114]. The Arh receptor level and activity has been shown to be affected not just by chemical agents but also biological agents including hormonal factors such as pituitary factors, adrenal glucocorticoids as well as 17 beta –estradiol. Of relevance to our chapter is the interaction of E2 with the Arh receptors.

Jana et al [115] worked on human endometrial cell lines and found that ERα has a positive modulatory effect on TCDD-inducible genes, while Son et al [116] found that estradiol enhances the expression of CYP1A1 in mouse ovarian cancer cell line while estriol does the opposite. On the other hand, Hoivik et al [117] did not find any effect of estrogen on Arh receptor mediated CYP1A1 expression on MCF-7 or Hepa 1c1c7 cells and Kharat et al [118] found that estradiol treatment blocked TCDD-induced accumulation of CYP1A1 mRNA and Arh receptor mediated activation of CYP1A1 promoter. Klinge et al [119] attempted to understand the molecular mechanisms underlying the cross-talk between the ER and Arh receptor systems and identified COUP-TF as a factor that may be involved. Ohtake et al [120] showed that the agonist-activated Arh receptor and its Arh receptor nuclear translocator protein complex can directly associate with ER alpha and ER beta, resulting in the activation of estrogen-responsive gene promoters. Matthews et al [121] also found that ERalpha can act as a co-regulator of Arh receptor mediated activation and support a role for ERα in TCDD-dependent CYP1A1 expression. However, Beischlag et al [122] found that ER-mediated activities repressed Arh receptor-dependent gene regulation. Although these studies have varying outcome, it is likely that estrogen has an enhancing effect on Arh receptor signaling. Further studies have shown that transient expression of the ER can restore Arh receptor responsiveness in human breast cancer cells [123,234]. Spink DC et al [125] also found that the continued presence of estrogen is required to maintain high levels of Arh receptor expression and inducibility of CYP1Aa and CYP1B1 in MCF7 cells.

## Interaction between Estrogen and Its Receptors with the EGFR Pathways

As a significant proportion of lung tumors over-express EGFR, one of the ways that estrogen and/or its receptors influence lung cancer growth could be through the interaction with the EGFR signaling pathway. Ignar-Trowbridge et al reported that EGF induction of DNA synthesis in the uterus could be prevented by an ER antagonist. [126] Further work from the same group found that this EGF-induced DNA synthesis and transcription were absent in the uteri from ERα knock-out mice. [127] This provides some evidence that certain EGFR signaling is dependent on ER in certain organs, such as the uterus. It has also been reported that EGFR can translocate to the nucleus, where it modulate the transcription of cyclin D1gene.[128] Being a nuclear action, there may be a possibility that EGFR can interact with nuclear ER in this aspect.

Just as EGFR action may be mediated through ER, there is evidence that ER signaling may be effected through EGFR. Due to the evidence of rapidity of action of estrogen, several groups have suggested the presence of ERs outside the nucleus that mediate rapid signals leading to cyclic AMP up-regulation. [129,130] Filardo et al showed that estrogen can transactivate EGFR by G-protein-coupled receptors. [131] This pathway was also described by Prenzel et al. [132]

## Effect of Estrogen and Its Receptors on Nicotine Metabolism

Other possible ways the female hormones may influence lung cancer growth is though its effect on nicotine metabolism. Several old studies have shown that men metabolized nicotine faster than women.[133]. This was also supported by studies in rats [134] and macaques [135]. The consequence of a lower clearance of nicotine among women is uncertain. There are data to show that nicotine can bind to nicotinic-acetylcholine receptors which can lead to the activation of protein kinase B, protein kinase A and other factors that can lead to reduced apoptosis, increased cell proliferation and transformation. [136] Nicotine has also been shown to stimulate angiogenesis which can then promote tumor growth [137]. However, there are conflicting studies to show that nicotine does not promote tumor growth [138] and is more likely to act as co-carcinogens in the presence of other cancer-inducing agents. [139,140,141] A recent study [142] in fact found that female sex and oral contraceptives accelerate nicotine metabolism and may result in females taking in more cigarettes compared to males in order to get the same level of nicotine in the blood. There is evidence that faster metabolizers smoke more cigarettes which would mean that women would smoke more [143], however, others found that that women smoke less cigarettes. Due to the complex nature of tobacco smoke, it is likely that nicotine exposure is a marker of the amount of carcinogens present in that individual as the rate of nicotine metabolism would reflect more the way a person smokes his/her cigarettes. Thus, the female hormones may affect nicotine metabolism but exactly how this may affect lung cancer risk is debatable.

## Possible Effect of Estrogen as Direct Carcinogens

Classically, ER-mediated events have been postulated to be the mechanism by which estrogens could contribute towards carcinogenesis. However, there are studies which suggest that estrogen itself can contribute to carcinogenesis as a result of metabolism to quinones which can form DNA adducts.[144] Estrogens are metabolized to catechol estrogens which can be further oxidized to semiquinones and quinones. These molecules can react with DNA to form predominantly depurinating adducts and these adducts can cause mutational changes in the DNA. [145, 146] In rats, TCDD has been shown to be a more potent hepatocarcinogen in female than in males and the study by Lucier et al [147] suggested that ovarian hormones (probably estrogen) may play a significant part in this hepatocarcinogenicity. This is one of the likely roles that the female hormones may play in the contribution to lung cancer development.

## Conclusion

There is increasing evidence to support epidemiological and biological differences between men and women with lung cancer. Several studies have found an increased susceptibility of women to tobacco smoke as well as provide evidence that the female hormones and/or its receptors can affect lung cancer growth. These hormones most likely exert their effects through influencing the way women metabolize environmental carcinogens. However, the hormones may also interact with other signaling molecules or interfere with nicotine metabolism. A thorough understanding of the role that these female hormones play in the development of lung cancer can provide us with further insights into lung cancer biology as well as help us develop new treatment modalities. This would further support the emphasis of anti-smoking efforts on the female sex. Further research into this area is warranted and urgently needed.

## References

[1] Parkin DM, Bray F, Ferlay J, Pisani P. Global cancer statistics, 2002. *CA Cancer J. Clin.* 2005;55:74-108.

[2] Jemal A, Siegel R, Ward E, Murray T, Xu J, Smigal C, Thun MJ. Cancer statistics 2006. *CA Cancer J. Clin.* 2006;56:106-130.

[3] Chia KS, Seow A, Lee HP, Shanmugatharatnam K. Cancer incidence in Singapore 1998-2002. *Singapore cancer registry report* no. 6, 2004: 7-9.

[4] Wynder EL,Graham EA. Landmark article May 27, 1950: Tobacco smoking as a possible etiologic factor in bronchiogenic carcinoma. A study of six hundred and eighty-four proved cases. By Ernest L. Wynder and Evarts A.Graham. *JAMA.* 1985;253:2986-2994.

[5] Doll R, Hill AB. A study of the aetiology of carcinoma of the lung. *Brit. Med. J.* 1952; 2:1271-1285.

[6] Epidemiology and Disease Control Division, Ministry of Health, Singapore. *National health survey.* 2004: 5-6.

[7] Chen CJ, Wu HY, Chuang YC, Chang AS, Luh KT, Chao HH, et al. Epidemiologic characteristics and multiple risk factors of lung cancer in Taiwan. *Anticancer Res.* 1990;10:971-976.

[8] Koo LC, Ho JH, Lee N. An analysis of some risk factors for lung cancer in Hong Kong. *Int. J. Cancer.* 1985;35:149-155.

[9] Maclennan R, Da Costa J, Day NE, Law CH, Ng YK, Shanmugatharatnam K. Risk factors for lung cancer in Singapore Chinese, a population with high female incidence rates. *Int. J. Cancer.* 1977;20:854-860.

[10] Gao YT, Blot WJ, Zheng W, Ershow AG, Hsu CW, Levin LI. Lung cancer among Chinese women. *Int. J. Cancer.* 1987;40:604-609.

[11] Toh CK, Gao F, Lim WT, Leong SS, Fong KW, Yap SP, et al. Never-smokers with lung cancer: epidemiologic evidence of a distinct disease entity. *J. Clin. Oncol.* 2006;24:2245-2251.

[12] McDuffie HH, Klaassen DJ, Dosman JA. Female-male differences in patients with primary lung cancer. *Cancer.* 1987;59:1825-1830.

[13] Brownson RC, Chang JC, Davis JR. Gender and histologic type variations in smoking-related risk of lung cancer. *Epidemiology.* 1992;3:61-64.

[14] Risch HA, Howe GR, Jain M, Burch JD, Holowaty EJ, Miller AB. Are female smokers at higher risk for lung cancer than male smokers? A case-control analysis by histologic type. *Am. J. Epidemiol.* 1993;138:281-293.

[15] Harris RE, Zang EA, Anderson JI, Wynder EL. Race and sex differences in lung cancer risk associated with cigarette smoking. *Int. J. Epidemiol.* 1993;22:592-599.

[16] Osann KE, Anton-Culver H, Kurosaki T, Taylor T. Sex differences in lung-cancer risk associated with cigarette smoking. *Int. J. Cancer.* 1993;54:44-48.

[17] Zang EA, Wynder EL. Differences in lung cancer risk between men and women: examination of the evidence. *J. Natl. Cancer Inst.* 1996;88:183-192.

[18] Engeland A. Trends in the incidence of smoking-associated cancers in Norway, 1954-93. *Int. J. Cancer.* 1996;68:39-46.

[19] Henschke CI, Miettinen OS. Women's susceptibility to tobacco carcinogens. *Lung Cancer.* 2004;43:1-5.

[20] International Early Lung Cancer Action Program Investigators. Women's susceptibility to tobacco carcinogens and survival after diagnosis of lung cancer. *JAMA.* 2006;296:180-184.

[21] Haenszel W, Taeuber KE. Lung cancer mortality as related to residence and smoking histories. II. White females. *J. Natl. Cancer Inst.* 1964;32:803-838.

[22] Hammond EC. Smoking in relation to the death rates of one million men and women. *Natl. Cancer Inst. Monogr.* 1966;19:127-204.

[23] United States Public Health Service. Reducing the health consequences of smoking: 25 years of progress. A report of the Surgeon General Office on Smoking and Health, DHHS publication no. (CDC) 89-8411.

[24] Prescott E, Osler M, Hein HO, Borch-Johnsen K, Lange P, Schnohr P, et al. Gender and smoking-related risk of lung cancer. The Copenhagen Center for Prospective Population Studies. *Epidemiology.* 1998;9:79-83.

[25] Kreuzer M, Boffetta P, Whitley E, Ahrens W, Gaborieau V, Heinrich J, et al. Gender differences in lung cancer risk by smoking: a multicentre case-control study in Germany and Italy. *Br. J. Cancer.* 2000;82:227-233.

[26] Thun MJ, Henley SJ, Calle EE. Tobacco use and cancer: an epidemiologic perspective for geneticists. *Oncogene.* 2002;21:7307-7325.

[27] Bach PB, Kattan MW, Thornquist MD, Kris MG, Tate RC, Barnett MJ et al. Variations in lung cancer risk among smokers. *J. Natl. Cancer Inst.* 2003;96:470-478.

[28] Bain C, Feskanich D, Speizer FE, Thun M, Hertzmark E, Rosner BA, et al. Lung cancer rates in men and women with comparable histories of smoking. *J. Natl. Cancer. Inst.* 2004;96:826-834.

[29] Perneger TV. Sex, smoking and cancer: a reappraisal. *J. Natl. Cancer Inst.* 2001;93:1600-1602.

[30] Donato F, Boffetta P, Fazioli R, Gelatti U, Porru S. Reliability of data on smoking habit and coffee drinking collected by personal interview in a hospital-based case-control study. *Eur. J. Epidemiol.* 1998;14:259-267.

[31] Haiman CA, Stram DO, Wilkens LR, Pike MC, Kolonel LN, Henderson BE, et al. Ethnic and racial differences in the smoking-related risk of lung cancer. *N. Engl. J. Med.* 2006;354:333-342.

[32] Kabat GC. Aspects of the epidemiology of lung cancer in smokers and nonsmokers in the United States. *Lung Cancer.* 1996;15:1-20.

[33] Toh CK, Lim WT. Lung cancer in never-smokers. *J. Clin. Pathol.* 2006; Aug 17 [Epub ahead of print]

[34] Brownson RC, Alavanja MCR, Caporaso N, Simoes EJ, Chang JC. Epidemiology and prevention of lung cancer in nonsmokers. *Epidemiol. Rev.* 1998;20:218-235.

[35] Taioli E, Wynder EL. Re: Endocrine factors and adenocarcinoma of the lung in women. *J. Natl. Cancer Inst.* 1994;86:869-70

[36] Gao YT, Blot WJ, Zheng W, Ershow AG, Hsu CW, et al. Lung cancer among Chinese women. *Int. J. Cancer.* 1987;40:604-609.

[37] Brenner AV, Wang Z, Kleinerman RA, Lei S, Metayer C, Wang W, et al. Menstrual and reproductive factors and risk of lung cancer among Chinese women, Eastern Gansu Province, 1994-1998. *J. Epidemiol.* 2003;13:22-28.

[38] Seow A, Poh WT, The M, Eng P, Wang YT, Tan WC, et al. Diet, reproductive factors and lung cancer risk among Chinese women in Singapore: evidence for a protective effect of soy in nonsmokers. *Int. J. Cancer.* 2002;97:365-371.

[39] Zatloukal P, Kubik A, Pauk N, Tomasek L, Petruzelka L. Adenocarcinoma of the lung among women: risk associated with smoking, prior lung disease, diet and menstrual and pregnancy history. *Lung Cancer.* 2003;41:283-293.

[40] Harvey EB, Brinton LA. Second cancer following cancer of the breast in Connecticut, 1935-82. *Natl. Cancer Inst. Monogr.* 1985;68:99-112.

[41] Curtis RE, Hoover RN, Kleinerman RA, Harvey EB. Second cancer following cancer of the female genital system in Connecticut 1935-82. *Natl. Cancer Inst. Monogr.* 1985;68:113-137.

[42] Ewertz M, Mouridsen HT. Second cancer following cancer of the female breast in Denmark, 1943-80. *Natl. Cancer Inst. Monogr.* 1985;68:325-329.

[43] Kabat GC. Previous cancer and radiotherapy as risk factors for lung cancer in lifetimen nonsmokers. *Cancer Causes Control.* 1993;5:489-495.

[44] International Agency for Research on Cancer. Tobacco smoking. IARC monograph on the evaluation of the carcinogenic risk of chemicals to humans 1986;38:37-375. *IARC, Lyon.*

[45] Cooper RL, Lindsey AJ. 3:4-Benzpyrene and other polycyclic hydrocarbons in cigarette smoke. *Br. J. Cancer.* 1955;9:304-309.

[46] Denissenko MF, Pao A, Tang M, Pfeifer GP. Preferential formation of benzo[a]pyrene adducts at lung cancer mutational hotspots in P53. *Science.* 1996;274:430-432.

[47] Smith LE, Denissenko MF, Bennett WP, Li H, Amin S, Tang M, et al. Targeting of lung cancer mutational hotspots by polycyclic aromatic hydrocarbons. *J. Natl. Cancer Inst.* 2000;92:803-811.

[48] Hecht SS, Hoffmann D. Tobacco-specific nitrosamines, an important group of carcinogens in tobacco and tobacco smoke. *Carcinogenesis.* 1988;9:875-884.

[49] Hecht SS. Biochemistry, biology and carcinogenicity of tobacco-specific N-nitrosamines. *Chem. Res. Toxicol.* 1998;6:559-603.

[50] Veglia F, Matullo G, Vineis P. Bulky DNA adducts and risk of cancer: a meta-analysis. *Cancer Epidemiol. Biomarkers Prev.* 2003;12:157-160.

[51] Osada H, Takahashi T. Genetic alterations of multiple tumor suppressors and oncogenes in the carcinogenesis and progression of lung cancer. *Oncogene.* 2002;21:7421-7434.

[52] Rom WN, Hay JG, Lee TC, Jiang Y, Tchou-Wong KM. Molecular and genetic aspects of lung cancer. *Am. J. Respir. Crit. Care Med.* 2000;161:1355-1367.

[53] Hecht SS. Tobacco carcinogens, their biomarkers and tobacco-induced cancer. *Nat. Rev. Cancer.* 2003;3:733-744.

[54] Toyooka S, Tsuda T, Gazdar AF. The TP53 gene, tobacco exposure, and lung cancer. *Hum. Mutat.* 2003;21:229-239.

[55] Ryberg D, Hewer A, Phillips DH, Haugen A. Different susceptibility to smoking-induced DNA damage among male and female lung cancer patients. *Cancer Res.* 1994;54:5801-5803.

[56] Cheng YW, Hsieh LL, Lin PP, Chen CP, Chen CY, Lin TS, et al. Gender difference in DNA adduct levels among nonsmoking lung cancer patients. *Environ. Mol. Mutagen.* 2001;37:304-310.

[57] Guengerich FP, Shimada T. Oxidation of toxic and carcinogenic chemicals by human P-450 enzymes. *Chem. Res. Toxicol.* 1991;4:391-407.

[58] Shimada T, Yamazaki H, Mimura M, Inui Y, Guengerich FP. Interindividual variations in human liver cytochrome P-450 enzymes involved in the oxidation of drugs, carcinogens and toxic chemicals: studies with liver microsomes of 30 Japanese and 30 Caucasians. *J. Pharmacol. Exp. Ther.* 1994;270:414-423.

[59] Kato R. Sex-related differences in drug metabolism. *Drug. Metab. Rev.* 1974;3:1-32.

[60] Schenkman JB, Frey I, Remmer H, Estabrook RW. Sex differences in drug metabolism by rat liver microsomes. *Mol. Pharmacol.* 1967;3:516-525.

[61] Piekoszewski W, Brandys J, Lipniak M. Studies on sex related differences in elimination of theophylline in the rat after pretreatment with phenobarbital, chrysene, Arocolor 1254 or lindane. *Acta Pol. Pharm.* 1991;48:9-12.

[62] Lee RP, Forkert PG. Pulmonary CYP2E1 bioactivates 1,1-dichloroethylene in male and female mice. *J. Pharmacol. Exp. Ther.* 1995;273:561-567.

[63] Verma AS, Shapiro BH. Sex-dependent expresson of seven housekeeping genes in rat liver. *J. Gastroenterol. Hepatol.* 2006;21:1004-1008.

[64] Sawaya ME. Biochemical mechanisms regulating human hair growth. *Skin. Pharmacol.* 1994;7:5-7.

[65] Mollerup S, Ryberg D, Hewer A, Phillips DH, Haugen A. Sex differences in lung CYP1A1 expression and DNA adduct levels among lung cancer patients. *Cancer Res.* 1999;59:3317-3320.

[66] Mollerup S, Berge G, Baera R, Skaug V, Hewer A, Phillips DH, et al. Sex differences in risk of lung cancer: expression of genes in the PAH bioactivation pathway in relation to smoking and bulky DNA adducts. *Int. J. Cancer.* 2004;119:741-744.

[67] Bell DA, Taylor JA, Paulson DF, Roberstson CN, Mohler JL, Lucier GW. Genetic risk and carcinogen exposure: a common inherited defect of the carcinogen-metabolism gene glutathione S-transferase M1(GSTM1) that increases susceptibility to bladder cancer. *J. Natl. Cancer Inst.* 1993;85:1159-1164.

[68] Dresler CM, Fratelli C, Babb J, Everley L, Evans AA, Clapper ML. Gender differences in genetic susceptibility for lung cancer. *Lung Cancer.* 2000;30:153-160.

[69] Tang DL, Rundle A, Warburton D, Santella RM, Tsai WY, Chiamprasert S, et al. Associations between both genetic and environmental biomarkers and lung cancer: evidence of a greater risk of lung cancer in women smokers. *Carcinogenesis.* 1998;19:1949-1953.

[70] Wei Q, Cheng L, Amos CI, Wang LE, Guo Z, Hong WK, et al. Repair of tobacco carcinogen-induced DNA adducts and lung cancer risk: a molecular epidemiologic study. *J. Natl. Cancer Inst.* 2000;92:1764-1772.

[71] Willey JC, Lechner JF, Harris CC. Bombesin and the C-terminal tetradecapeptide of gastrin-releasing peptide are growth factors for normal human bronchial epithelial cells. *Exp. Cell Res.* 1984;153:245-248.

[72] DeMichele MA, Davis AL, Hunt JD, Landreneau RJ, Siegfried JM. Expression of mRNA for three bombesin receptor subtypes in human bronchial epithelial cells. *Am. J. Respir. Cell Mol. Biol.* 1994;11:66-74.

[73] Siegfried JM, DeMichele MA, Hunt JD, Davis AG, Vohra KP, Pilewski JM. Expression of mRMA for gastrin-releasing peptide receptor by human bronchial

epithelial cells. Association with prolonged tobacco exposure and responsiveness to bombesin-like peptides. *Am. J. Respir. Crit. Care Med.* 1997;156:358-366.

[74] Ishikawa-Brush Y, Powell JF, Bolton P, Miller AP, Francis F, Willard HF, et al. Autism and multiple exostoses associated with an X;8 translocation occurring within the GRPR gene and 3' to the SDC2 gene. *Hum. Mol. Genetics.* 1997;6:1241-1250.

[75] Shriver SP, Bourdeau HA, Gubish CT, Tirpak DL, Davis AL, Luketich JD, et al. Sex-specific expression of gastrin-releasing peptide receptor: relationship to smoking history and risk of lung cancer. *J. Natl. Cancer Inst.* 2000;92:24-33.

[76] Olayioye MA, Neve RM, Lane HA, Hynes NE. The ErbB signaling network: receptor heterodimerization in development and cancer. *EMBO J.* 2000;19:3159-3167.

[77] Lynch TJ, Bell DW, Sordella R, Gurubhagavatula S, Okimoto RA, Brannigan BW, et al. Activating mutations in the epidermal growth factor receptor underlying responsiveness of non-small-cell lung cancer to gefitinib. *N. Engl. J. Med.* 2004;350:2129-2139.

[78] Paez JG, Janne PA, Lee JC, Tracy S, Greulich H, Gabriel S, et al. EGFR mutations in lung cancer: correlation with clinical response to gefitinib therapy. *Science.* 2004;304:1497-1500.

[79] Shigematsu H, Lin L, Takahashi T, Nomura M, Suzuki M, Wistuba II, et al. Clinical and biological features associated with epidermal growth factor receptor gene mutations in lung cancers. *J. Natl. Cancer Inst.* 2005;97:339-346.

[80] Tokumo M, Toyooka S, Kiura K, Shigematsu H, Tomii K, Aoe M, et al. The relationship between epidermal growth factor receptor mutations and clinicopathologic features in non-small-cell lung cancers. *Clin. Cancer Res.* 2005;11:1167-1173.

[81] Kris MG, Natale RB, Herbst RS, Lynch TJ Jr, Prager D, Belani CP. Efficacy of gefitinib, an inhibitor of the epidermal growth factor receptor tyrosine kinase, in symptomatic patients with non-small cell lung cancer: a randomized trial. *JAMA.* 2003;290:2149-2158.

[82] Fukuoka M, Yano S, Giaccone G, Tamura T, Nakagawa K, Douillard JY, et al. Multi-institutional randomized phase II trial of gefitinib for previously treated patients with advanced non-small-cell lung cancer (The IDEAL 1 Trial) [corrected] *J. Clin. Oncol.* 2003;21:2237-2246.

[83] Matsuo K, Ito H, Yatabe Y, Hiraki A, Hirose K, Wakai K, et al. Risk factors differ for non-small-cell lung cancers with and without EGFR mutation: assessment of smoking and sex by a case-control study in Japanese. *Cancer Sci.* 2006 Oct 19;[Epub ahead of print]

[84] Huang SF, Liu HP, Li LH, Ku YC, Fu YN, Tsai HY, et al. High frequency of epidermal growth factor receptor mutations with complex patterns in non-small cell

lung cancers related to gefitinib responsiveness in Taiwan. *Clin. Cancer Res.* 2004;10:8195-8203.

[85] Miller VA, Kris MG, Shah N, Patel J, Azzoli C, Gomez J, et al. Bronchioloalveolar pathologic subtype and smoking history predict sensitivity to gefitinib in advanced non-small-cell lung cancer. *J. Clin. Oncol.* 2004;22:1103-1109.

[86] Nelson HH, Christiani DC, Mark EJ, Wiencke JK, Wain JC, Kelsey KT. Implications and prognostic value of K-ras mutation for early-stage lung cancer in women. *J. Natl. Cancer Inst.* 1999;91:2032-2038.

[87] De Gregorio L, Manenti G, Incarbone M, Pilotti S, Pastorino U, Pierotii MA, et al. Prognostic value of loss of heterozygosity and KRAS2 mutations in lung adenocarcinoma. *Int. J. Cancer.* 1998;79:269-272.

[88] Lung ML, Wong M, Lam WK, Lau KS, Kwan S, Fu KH, et al. Incidence of ras oncogene activation in lung carcinomas in Hong Kong. *Cancer.* 1992;70:760-763.

[89] Kern JA, Slebos RJ, Top B, Rodenhuis S, Lager D, Robinson RA, et al. C-erb-B2 expression and codon 12 K-ras mutations both predict shortened survival for patients with pulmonary adenocarcinomas. *J. Clin. Invest.* 1994;93:516-520.

[90] Slebos RJC, Hruban RH, Dalesio O, Mooi WJ, Offerhaus GJA, Rodenhuis S. Relationship between K-ras oncogene activation and smoking in adenocarcinoma of the human lung. *J. Natl. Cancer Inst.* 1991;83:1024-1027.

[91] Stabile LP, Davis Al, Gubish CT, Hopkins TM, Luketich JD, Christie N, et al. Human non-small cell lung tumors and cells derived from normal lung express both estrogen receptor alpha and beta and show biological responses to estrogen. *Cancer Res.* 2002;62:2141-2150.

[92] Khosla SS, Brehier A, Eisenfeld AJ, Ingleson LD, Parks PA, et al. Influence of sex hormones on lung maturation in the fetal rabbit. *Biochim. Biophy. Acta.* 1983;1:112-126.

[93] Enmark E, Pelto-Huikko M, Grandien K, Lagercrantz S, Lagercrantz J, Fried G, et al. Human estrogen receptor beta-gene structure, chromosomal localization, and expression pattern. *J. Clin. Endocrinol. Metab.* 1997;82:4258-4265.

[94] Taylor AH, Al-Azzawi F. Immunolocalisation of oestrogen receptor beta in human tissues. *J. Mol. Endocrinol.* 2000;24:145-155.

[95] Lewandowski SA, Thiery J, Jalil A, Leclercq G, Szczylik C, Chouaib S. Opposite effects of estrogen receptors alpha and beta on MCF-7 sensitivity to the cytotoxic action of TNF and p53 activity. *Oncogene.* 2005;24:4789-4798.

[96] Paech K, Webb P, Kuiper GG, Nilsson S, Gustafsson J, Kushner PJ, et al. Differential ligand activation of estrogen receptors ERalpha and ERbeta at AP1 sites. *Science.* 1997;277:1508-1510.

[97] Di Nunno L, Larsson LG, Rinehart JJ, Beissner RS. Estrogen and progesterone receptors in non-small cell lung cancer in 248 consecutive patients who underwent surgical resection. *Arch. Pathol. Lab. Med.* 2000;124:1467-1470.

[98] Cagle PT, Mody DR, Schwartz MR. Estrogen and progesterone receptors in bronchogenic carcinoma. *Cancer Res.* 1990;50:6632-6635.

[99] Su JM, Hsu HK, Chang H, Lin SL, Chang HC, Huang MS, et al. Expression of estrogen and progesterone receptors in non-small cell lung cancer: immunohistochemical study. *Anticancer Res.* 1996;16:3803-3806.

[100] Canver CC, Memoli Va, Vanderveer PL, Dingivan CA, Mentzer RM Jr. Sex hormone receptors in non-small cell lung cancer in human beings. *J. Thorac Cardiovasc. Surg.* 1994;108:153-157.

[101] Kaiser U, Hofmann J, Schilli M, Wegmann B, Klotz U, Wedel S, et al. Steroid-hormone receptors in cell lines and tumor biopsies of lung cancer. *Int. J. Cancer.* 1996;67:357-364.

[102] Chaudhuri PK, Thomas PA, Walker MJ, Briele HA, Das Gupta TK, Beattie CW. Steroid receptors in human lung cancer cytosols. *Cancer Lett.* 1982;16:327-332.

[103] Beattie CW, Hansen NW, Thomas PA. Steroid receptors in human lung cancer. *Cancer Res.* 1985;45:4206-4214.

[104] Kawai H, Ishii A, Washiya K, Konno T, Kon H, Yamaya C, et al. Estrogen receptor alpha and beta are prognostic factors in non-small cell lung cancer. *Clin. Cancer Res.* 2005;11:5084-5089.

[105] Omoto Y, Kobayashi Y, Nishida K, Tsuchiya E, Eguchi H, Nakagawa K, et al. Expression , function and clinical implications of the estrogen receptor beta in human lung cancers. *Biochem. Biophys. Res. Commun.* 2001;285:340-347.

[106] Mollerup S, Jorgensen K, Berge G, Haugen A. Expression of estrogen recptors alpha and beta in human lung tissue and cell lines. *Lung Cancer.* 2002;37:153-159.

[107] Patrone C, Cassel TN, Pettersson K, Piao YS, Cheng G, Ciana P, et al. Regulation of postnatal lung development and homeostasis by estrogen receptor beta. *Mol. Cell Biol.* 2003;23:8542-8552.

[108] Hershberger PA, Vasquez AC, Kanterewicz B, Land S, Siegfried JM, Nichols M. Regulation of endogenous gene expression in human non-small cell lung cancer cells by estrogen receptor ligands. *Cancer Res.* 2005;65:1598-1605.

[109] Schwartz AG, Prysak GM, Murphy V, Lonardo F, Pass H, Schwartz J, et al. Nuclear estrogen receptor beta in lung cancer: expression and survival differences by sex. *Clin. Cancer Res.* 2005;11:7280-7287.

[110] Dougherty SM, Mazhawidza W, Bohn AR, Robinson KA, Mattingly KA, Blankenship KA, et al. Gender difference in the activity but not expression of estrogen receptors alpha and beta in human lung adenocarcinoma cells. *Endocr. Relat. Cancer.* 2006;13:113-134.

[111] Osborne CK, Schiff R. Estrogen-Receptor biology: continuing progress and therapeutic implications. *J. Clin. Oncol.* 2005;23:1616-1622.

[112] Bailey-wilson JE, Amos CI, Pinney SM, Petersen GM, de Andrade M, Weist JS, et al. A major lung cancer susceptibility locus maps to chromosome 6q23-25. *Am. J. Hum. Genet.* 2004;75:460-474.

[113] Wilson NM, Christou M, Turner CR, Wrighton SA, Jefcoate CR. Binding and metabolism of benzo[a]pyrene and 7,12-dimethylbenz[a]anthracene by seven purified forms of cytochrome P-450. *Carcinogenesis.* 1984;5:1475-1483.

[114] Nebert DW, Jones JE. Regulation of the mammalian cytochrome P1-450(CYP1A1) gene. *Int. J. Biochem.* 1989;21"243-252.

[115] Jana NR, Sarkar S, Ishizuka M, Yonemoto J, Tohyama C, Sone H. Role of estradiol receptor-alpha in differential expression of 2,3,7,8-tetrachlorodibenzo-p-dioxin-inducible genes in the RL95-2 and KLE human endometrial cancer cell lines. *Arch. Biochem. Biophys.* 1999;368:31-39.

[116] Son DS, Roby KF, Rozman KK, Terranova PF. Estradiol enhances and estriol inhibits the expression of CYP1A1 induced by 2,3,7,8-tetrachlorodibenzo-p-dioxin in a mouse ovarian cancer cell line. *Toxicology.* 2002;176:229-243.

[117] Hoivik D, Willett K. Wilson C, Safe S. Estrogen does not inhibit 2,3,7,8-tetrachlorodibenzo-p-dioxin-mediated effects in MCF-7 and Hepa 1c1c7 cells. *J. Biol. Chem.* 1997;272:30270-30274.

[118] Kharat I, Saatcioglu F. Antiestrogenic effects of 2,3,7,8-tetrachlorodibenzo-p-dioxin are mediated by direct transcriptional interference with the liganded estrogen receptor. Cross-talk between aryl hydrocarbon- and estrogen-mediated signaling. *J. Biol. Chem.* 1996;271:10533-10537.

[119] Klinge CM, Kaur K, Swanson HI. The aryl hydrocarbon receptor interacts with estrogen receptor alpha and orphan receptors COUP-TFI and ERRalpha1. *Arch. Biochem. Biophys.* 2000;373:163-174.

[120] Ohtake F, Takeyama K, Matsumoto T, Kitagaw H, Yamamoto Y, Nohara K, et al. Modulation of estrogen receptor signalling by associaton with the activated dioxin receptor. *Nature.* 2003;423:545-550.

[121] Matthews J, Wihlen B, Thomsen J, Gustafsson JA. Aryl hydrocarbon receptor-mediated transcription: ligand-dependent recruitment of estrogen receptor alpha to 2,3,7,8-tetrachlorodibenzo-p-dioxin-responsive promoters. *Mol. Cell Biol.* 2005;25:5317-5328.

[122] Beischlag TV, Perdew GH. ER alpha-AHR-ARNT protein-protein interactions mediate estradiol-dependent transrepression of dioxin-inducible gene transcription. *J. Biol. Chem.* 2005;280:21607-21611.

[123] Thomsen JS, Wang X, Hines RN, Safe S. Restoration of aryl hydrocarbon (Ah) responsiveness in MDA-MB-231 human breast cancer cells by transient expression of the estrogen receptor. *Carcinogenesis.* 1994;15:933-937.

[124] Wang WL, Thomsen JS, Porter W, Moore M, Safe S. Effect of transient expression of the oestrogen receptor on constitutive and inducible CYP1A1 in Hs578T human breast cancer cells. *Br. J. Cancer.* 1996;73:316-322.

[125] Spink DC, Katz BH, Hussain MM, Pentecost BT, Cao Z, Spink BC. Estrogen regulates Ah responsiveness in MCF-7 breast cancer cells. *Carcinogenesis.* 2003;24:1941-1950.

[126] Ignar-Trowbridge DM, Nelson KG, Bidwell MC, Curtis SW, Washburn TF, McLachlan JA, et al. Coupling of dual signaling pathways: epidermal growth factor action involves the estrogen receptor. *Proc. Natl. Acad. Sci. USA.* 1992;89:4658-4662.

[127] Curtis SW, Washburn T, Sewall C, DiAugustine R, Lindzey J, Couse JF, et al. Physiological coupling of growth factor and steroid receptor signaling pathways: estrogen receptor knockout mice lack estrogen-like response to epidermal growth factor. *Proc. Natl. Acad .Sci .USA.* 1996;93:12626-12630.

[128] Lin SY, Makino K, Xia W, Matin A, Wen Y, Kwong KY, et al. Nuclear localization of EGF receptor and its potential new role as a transription factor. *Nat. Cell Biol.* 2001;3:802-808.

[129] Pietras RJ, Szego CM. Specific binding sites for oestrogen at the outer surfaces of isolated endometrial cells. *Nature.* 1977;265:69-72.

[130] Losel RM, Falkenstein E, Feuring M, Schultz A, Tillmann HC, Rossol-Haseroth K. Nongenomic steroid action: controversies, questions and answers. *Physiol. Rev.* 2003;83:965-1016.

[131] Filardo EJ. Epidermal growth factor receptor (EGFR) transactivation by estrogen via the G-protein-coupled receptor, GPR30: a novel signaling pathway with potential significance for breast cancer. *J. Steroid Biochem. Mol. Biol.* 2002;80:231-238.

[132] Prenzel N, Zwick E, Daub H, Leserer M, Abraham R, Wallasch C, et al. EGF receptor transactivation by G-protein-coupled receptors requires metalloproteinase cleavage of proHB-EGF. *Nature.* 1999;402:884-888.

[133] Benowitz NL, Jacob P 3rd. Daily intake of nicotine during cigarette smoking. *Clin. Pharmacol. Ther.* 1984;35:499-504.

[134] Kyerematen GA, Owens GF, Chattopadhyay B, deBethizy JD, Vesell ES. Sexual dimorphism of nicotine metabolism and distribution in the rat. Studies in vivo and in vitro. *Drug Metab. Dispos.* 1988;16:82-828.

[135] Seaton M, Kyerematen GA, Morgan M, Jeszenka EV, Vesell ES. Nicotine metabolism in stumptailed macaques, Macaca arctoides. *Drug Metab. Dispos.* 1991;19:946-954.

[136] West KA, Brognard J, Clark AS, Linnoila IR, Yang X, Swain SM, et al. Rapid Akt activation by nicotine and a tobacco carcingen modulates the phenotype of normal human airway epithelial cells. *J. Clin. Invest.* 2003;111:81-90.

[137] Heeschen C, Jang JJ, Weis M, Pathak A, Kaji S, Hu RS, et al. Nicotine stimulates angiogenesis and promotes tumor growth and atherosclerosis. *Nat. Med.* 2001;7:833-839.

[138] Berger MR, Petru E, Habs M, Schmahl D. Influence of perinatal nicotine administration on transplacental carcnogenesis in Sprague Dawley rats by N-methylnitrosourea. *Br. J. Cancer.* 1987;55:37-40.

[139] Chen YP, Squier CA. Effect of nictoine on 7,12-dimethylbenz[a]anthracene carcinogenesis in hamster cheek pouch. *J. Natl. Cancer Inst.* 1990;82:861-864.

[140] Gurkalo VK, Volfson NI. Nictoine influence upon the development of experimental stomach tumors. *Arch. Geschwulstforsch.* 1982;52:259-265.

[141] Schuller HM, McGavin MD, Orloff M, Riechert A, Porter B. Simultaneous exposure to nicotine and hyperoxia causes tumors in hamsters. *Lab. Invest.* 1995;73:448-456.

[142] Benowitz NL, Lessov-Schlaggar CN, Swan GE, Jacob III P. Female sex and oral contraceptive use accelerate nicotine metabolism. *Clin. Pharmacol. Ther.* 2006;79:480-488.

[143] Tyndale RF, Sellers EM. Genetic variation in CYP2A6-mediated nicotine metabolism alters smoking behavior. *Ther. Drug Monit.* 2002;24:163-171.

[144] Raftogianis R, Creveling C, Weinshilboum R, Weisz J. Estrogen metabolism by conjugation. *J. Natl. Cancer Inst. Monogr.* 2000;27:113-124.

[145] Cavalieri EL, Li K, Balu N, Saeed M, Devanesan P, Higginbotham S, et al. Catechol ortho-quinones: the electrophilic compounds that form depurinating DNA adducts and could initiate cancer and other diseases. *Carcinogenesis.* 2002;23:1071-1077.

[146] Cavalieri EL, Rogan EG. A unifying mechanism in the initiation of cancer and other diseases by catechol quinones. *Ann. NY Acad. Sci.* 2004;1028:247-257.

[147] Lucier GW, Tritscher A, Goldsworthy T, Foley J, Clark G, Goldstein J, et al. Ovarian hormones enhance 2,3,7,8-tetrachlorodibenzo-p-dioxin-mediated increases in cell proliferation and preneoplastic foci in a two-stage model for rat hepatocarcinogenesis. *Cancer Res.* 1991;51:1391-1397.

In: Lung Cancer in Women
Editor: Varetta N. Torres, pp. 171-193

ISBN: 978-1-60021-659-6


*Chapter VIII*

# TARGETED THERAPIES FOR LUNG CANCER: DIFFERENCES AMONGST SEXES

***Georgios Papaetis, Ioannis Giozos and Kostas N. Syrigos****

Oncology Unit, 3rd Department of Medicine, Athens Medical School,
Sotiria General Hospital, Athens, Greece

## ABSTRACT

We are now living in an exciting new era that the understanding of tumor biology and oncogenesis has begun to evolve. Molecular techniques have allowed insight into specific biological pathways involved in tumorigenesis and these same techniques have developed a cascade of novel therapies directed towards molecular factors critical to the pathogenesis of cancer growth and survival. With lung cancer being the leading cause of world-wide cancer mortality, and with a fourfold increase of incidence in women, the need for new treatment strategies is obvious. In fact, the epidermal growth factor receptor (EGFR) autocrine pathway has a major contribution to a number of processes which are essential for tumor progression and that somatic mutations of the EGFR gene, which are associated with clinical response to the EGFR oral tyrosine kinase inhibitors gefitinib and erlotinib, are more frequently detected in women. At the same time women are three times more likely to have K-ras mutation than men and often express HER-2/neu (one of the four members of EGF receptors). HER-2/neu is also most commonly expressed in the adenocarcinoma histology, the most common subtype in women. All these data raise an issue about the different pathobiology of lung cancer in women and the emerging role of targeted therapies designed specifically for female lung cancer patients.

---

* Address for Correspondence: Konstantinos N. Syrigos, MD, PhD; Assistant Professor of Oncology in Medicine; Athens University School of Medicine; Head, Oncology Unit, Third Department of Medicine; Building Z,

# INTRODUCTION

Lung cancer still remains the leading cause of worldwide cancer mortality despite all recent improvements in surgery, radiotherapy and chemotherapy [1]. Over the past 30 years there has been a fourfold increase in lung cancer in women and it is estimated that this rise will not reach a plateau before 2010 [2]. Non-small cell lung cancer (NSCLC) constitutes about 80% of all lung cancer cases and approximately 60% of these patients have advanced disease at the time of diagnosis with a 5 year survival rate being below 5% in stage IIIB/IV [3,4]. At the same time, a woeful minority of NSCLC patients who will present with stage I and II and are radically resected, may experience a recurrence within two years which is more frequent in distal sites [5]. Under these circumstances, the development of new treatment strategies is mandatory.

We are now living in an exciting new era where the understanding of tumor biology and oncogenesis has begun to evolve. Molecular techniques have allowed insight into specific biological pathways involved in tumorigenesis and these same techniques have developed a cascade of novel therapies directed towards molecular factors critical to the pathogenesis of cancer growth and survival [6]. Due to the targeted mechanism of action, these therapies are more specific, more sensitive and less toxic to non-cancerous cells.

In fact, the epidermal growth factor receptor (EGFR) autocrine pathway has a major contribution to a number of processes which are essential for tumor progression and somatic mutations of the EGFR gene, which are associated with clinical response to the EGFR oral tyrosine kinase inhibitors gefitinib and erlotinib, and which are more frequently detected in women. At the same time, women are three times more likely to have K-*ras* mutation than men and often express HER-2/neu (one of the four members of EGF receptors) [7]. HER-2/neu is more commonly expressed in adenocarcinoma histology, the most common subtype in women [8]. All these data raise an issue about the different pathobiology of lung cancer in women and the emerging role of targeted therapies designed specifically for female lung cancer patients.

We have thoroughly reviewed the existing evidence of novel agents now studied in clinical trials targeting epidermal growth factor receptor family as well as farnesyl transferase inhibitors.

# A. EPIDERMAL GROWTH FACTOR RECEPTOR (EGFR) FAMILY INHIBITORS

The EGF family of receptors consists of four structurally similar members including EGFR- (ErbB1/HER-1), HER-2/neu (erbB2), HER3 (erbB3) and HER4 (erbB4) [9]. EGFR is the first receptor discovered which has two predominant ligands, the EGF and the transforming growth factor-a (TGF-a) [10]. This receptor crosses the cell membrane and has two portions; an extracellular portion that is the ligand-binding side and an intracellular

Sotiria General Hospital; Mesogion 152; 115 27 Athens, Greece; Tel: +30 210 7475 034 / Fax: +30 210 7781 035; Email: knsyrigos@usa.net / ksyrigos@med.uoa.gr portion that has a tyrosine kinase activity [11]. Activation of the receptor by the ligand leads to an autophosphorylation of the tyrosine residues in the intracellular portion. This, in turn, leads to a sequential activation of molecules that mediate the transduction of a signal downstream towards the nucleus and activate gene transcription and consequently, oncogenesis. Three major pathways are involved in the HER-1 signal transduction: (i) The mitogen-activated protein kinase (MAPK) which is strongly connected with the transduction of proliferation signals, (ii) The phosphatidylinositol –3-OH kinase (PI3K/Akt) which is a major anti-apoptotic pathway and (iii) The signal transducer and activator of transcription (STAT) - mediated pathways. These multi-complex signal cascades involve the interaction or dimerization with other erbB-receptor types, the interactions with signals from heterologous pathways such as stress inducers, hormones and lymphokines, and the complex activation and inhibition of all intermediate molecules. It is suggested that there is both an overexpression and an abnormal activation of EGFR in many solid tumors which enhance their growth and survival, leading to a poorer outcome [12].

Overexpression of EGFR has been observed in 43-83% of NSCLC [13]. The lack of a gold standard method in detecting EGFR expression can explain the variety of levels reported [14]. Most of the available data are based on immunohistochemistry (IHC) in which direct evaluation of the target can be achieved on resected surgical specimens. In addition, EGFR promotes invasiveness through activation or downregulation of matrix metalloproteinases (MMPs) and interacts with the integrin pathway which is crucial for the tumor to invade local tissues [15,16].

## 1. Anti-EGFR Monoclonal Antibodies

Monoclonal antibodies directed against the extracellular portion of EGFR, block ligand binding and inhibit the activation of the EGFR pathway [17]. Cetuximab and panitumumab (ABX-EGF) are the major monoclonal antibodies against EGFR, studied in clinical trials [3].

### *Cetuximab (IMC-C225, ERBITUX)*

Cetuximab is a monoclonal chimeric human-mouse IgG1 monoclonal antibody which has a higher binding affinity to HER-1 than other ligands (EGF, TGF-a). Cetuximab competes with ligands for receptor binding causing internalization of the receptor and promoting inhibition of angiogenesis and enhancement of apoptosis [18]. When this antibody was tested in preclinical models, an interesting antitumor activity was reported causing EGFR antagonism and tumor regression [19]. Synergistic tumor growth inhibition was also demonstrated when cetuximab was combined with chemotherapy and radiotherapy in preclinical models [20,21].

Two phase I pharmacokinetic studies in patients with solid tumors supported a weekly regimen between 250 and 400 mg/m$^2$ [22,23]. Most of the patients developed grade 1 or 2 skin rash. In another multicenter phase I trial in patients with EGFR-expressing tumors, cetuximab was examined with or without cisplatin [24]. There was no pharmacokinetic alteration of cetuximab from cisplatin and only one of the 52 patients developed antibodies to cetuximab. Grade 3 toxicities of the above combination were dyspnea, diarrhea, epiglottitis, and anaphylaxis. In a phase I/II study, cetuximab was administered with paclitaxel and carboplatin in 31 untreated patients with stage IV NSCLC [25]. The most common toxicity observed was rash in 84% of the patients (grade 3 in 13%). Objective response (OR) was seen in 8 patients (26%), median time to progression was 5 months, median overall survival was 11 months and the first- and second- year survival rates were 40% and 16%, respectively. In another phase I/IIa study, cetuximab was combined with carboplatin and gemcitabine in 35 chemotherapy-naïve patients with stage IV NSCLC [26]. The major toxicities related to cetuximab were mild to moderate, presenting either as an acne-like rash (88.6%), skin disorders, dry skin, asthenia, mucositis, fever, chills, or nausea and vomiting. Partial responses (PRs) were observed in 28.6% of the patients. In addition, 60% of the patients had stable disease (SD). The median time to progression was 165 days and the median overall survival was 310 days.

A randomized phase II trial studied the combination of cisplatin and vinorelbine with and without cetuximab in the first-line setting of patients with advanced NSCLC [27]. Forty-three patients were randomized in each arm and 90% of the patients had EGFR-expressing tumors. There was a higher incidence of acneiform rash, diarrhea, asthenia, leukopenia, thrombocytopenia, and infection in the cetuximab arm. The response rate (RR) and median survival time were 31.7% versus 20% and 8.3 months versus 7.0 months in favor of cetuximab, with no statistical significance reported. Patients younger than 60 with normal lactate dehydrogenase (LDH) level and adenocarcinoma histology had a better benefit from the addition of cetuximab to cisplatin/vinorelbine. The combination of cetuximab with docetaxel in EGFR-positive patients with recurrent NSCLC was examined in another phase II study [28]. The most common grade 3 toxicities were rash, infection, and fatigue. The RR was 28% and in one patient, a complete response (CR) was achieved. Nearly 66% of the patients had SD with this combination regimen. Finally, in another single-arm phase II trial, cetuximab was examined in 66 patients with relapsed NSCLC who had failed at least one regimen [29]. The RR was 3.3% and 28% had SD. The median survival was 8.1 months and median time to progression was 2.3 months. Cetuximab was well-tolerated with rash being the most common adverse effect reported (77%, 6.1% with grade 3). The cetuximab-related acneiform rash, which is the commonest adverse effect observed so far, possibly predicts response and prolonged survival [30]. The dosing regimen of cetuximab in clinical studies is a loading dose of 400 mg/m$^2$ followed by a maintenance dose of 250 mg/m$^2$/weekly. The role of cetuximab combination with radiotherapy for local disease control is being studied in the RTOG phase II trial 0324 [3]. Another phase II study (the NEAR protocol-NCT00115518) is currently examining the combination of cetuximab with logo-regional irradiation in 30 patients with stage III NSCLC who are not eligible for a radiochemotherapy, with primary endpoint in the feasibility and safety of the combined treatment.

### *Panitumumab (ABX-EGF)*

Panitumumab is a fully humanized IgG2 monoclonal antibody which has a higher affinity for EGFR than cetuximab [31]. Activity of panitumumab, in combination with cytotoxic agents or as a single agent, has been documented for a wide range of human cancer cell lines in vivo and in vitro [32]. Its action in xenograft tumor models is quite promising but without any effect on EGFR-negative tumors [33].

In a phase I study, ABX-EGF was well-tolerated and its biologic activity, evidenced by a dose-dependent acneiform reversible rash, was observed at a dose level of 1.0 mg/kg [34]. The most common adverse effect which occurred in another phase I trial also involved skin toxicity [35]. Among the 43 patients of this study, two PRs and one minor response (MR) were demonstrated. From the 4 patients who experienced SD, two had NSCLC. The combination of ABX-EGF with paclitaxel and carboplatin in 19 EGFR-overexpressing patients with advanced NSCLC is currently under study in a phase II trial. Until now, one CR and four PRs have been observed [36]. Skin rash was the most common toxicity reported, which did not appear to be dose-related. There was no pharmacokinetic interaction between chemotherapy and this novel agent.

## 2. EGFR Oral Tyrosine Kinase Inhibitors (EGFR-TKIs)

Two agents are mainly available for clinical trials in this class of tyrosine kinase inhibitors (TKIs), gefitinib and erlotinib. Both agents belong to the quinazolamine class and inhibit the EGFR by directly blocking the phosphorylation of the intracellular receptor tyrosine kinase, preventing its activity and subsequently, decreasing cellular proliferation, increasing apoptosis and inhibiting angiogenesis [3]. After failure of chemotherapy, gefitinib and erlotinib are able to induce responses in approximately 10% of Caucasian patients and 25-30% of Japanese patients (gefitinib only) with NSCLC tumors [37].

### *Erlotinib (OSI-774, Tarceva)*

Erlotinib showed in vivo and in vitro activity when tested in preclinical trials in several human cancer cell lines, including NSCLC [38,39]. In two phase I trials, an interesting antitumor activity was demonstrated and erlotinib was evaluated using different doses and schedules [40,41]. The regimen that was selected for further evaluation was the daily administration of 150mg. Higher doses resulted in a dose-limiting acneiform rash and diarrhea [41]. Other adverse effects reported were mild to moderate nausea and vomiting, headaches, mucositis, and elevation in bilirubin. At the same time, encouraging results were observed in an erlotinib phase II trial [42]. The overall response rate was 12.54% (26.3% had an additional SD), the median survival was 9 months and the one-year survival rate was 40%, with EGFR expression being a requirement for entry into the study. Response to erlotinib was not associated with EGFR expression level. Erlotinib was generally well-tolerated and the most common toxicity was an acneiform rash (78% of the patients). In another phase II trial of erlotinib in patients with bronchoalveolar carcinoma (BAC), 26% of the patients experienced an objective response [43]. The presence of rash in erlotinib patients may indicate response and improved survival, like cetuximab patients [44].

Of vital importance is the result of a phase III randomized placebo-control trial (BR.21 study) in which erlotinib was administered to patients with advanced NSCLC (stage III/B and IV) after failing one or two lines of chemotherapy [45]. In this study, 731 patients were randomly assigned in a 2:1 ratio for erlotinib, to receive either oral erlotinib or placebo. The overall response rate to erlotinib was 8.9% and less than 1% in the placebo group ($p<0.001$) with a median duration of response 7.9 months and 3.7 months, respectively. Overall survival was 6.7 months for the erlotinib group versus 4.7 months in the placebo group ($p<0.001$). The most common adverse effects in the erlotinib group were skin toxicity, diarrhea, and infections. Twenty-six patients (5%) discontinued erlotinib due to drug-related toxic effects compared to four patients (2%) who received placebo. In a multivariate analysis, objective response was significantly associated with never-smoking status, adenocarcinoma histology and expression of EGFR by IHC. This is the first study demonstrating that EGFR-TKIs may prolong survival after chemotherapy in NSCLC and brought erlotinib to registration by the US Food and Drug Administration (November 2004) and by the European Union (September 2005) as a second- and third-line treatment of advanced NSCLC.

A phase I/II study explored the combination of erlotinib and bevacizumab (a recombinant antibody against vascular endothelial growth factor-VEGF) in patients with advanced NSCLC with one or more chemotherapeutic failures [46]. Erlotinib was administered at the full dose of 150 mg/daily orally and bevacizumab at 15 mg/kg/intravenously every 3 weeks without any dose limiting toxicities (DLTs) observed in the phase I part of the study. A total of 40 patients were enrolled in the study with 34 treated at phase II of whom 21 were female. The most common toxicities were diarrhea, a mild to moderate rash and proteinuria. Eight patients (20%) experienced PRs and 26 patients (65%) had disease stabilization as their best response. The progression-free survival was 6.2 months and the median overall survival 12.6 months.

### *Gefitinib (ZD1839, Iressa)*

When gefitinib was studied in a wide range of human tumor xenografts, an antitumor activity was postulated [47]. In phase I trials, gefitinib was well-tolerated achieving objective antitumor responses when used as a single agent in refractory NSCLC patients [48-50]. An acneiform skin rash, diarrhea, asthenia, nausea and vomiting were the most common toxicities. DLTs including reversible rash and diarrhea occurred at daily doses of 700 to 800 mg. In one of these trials, 10% of the 100 NSCLC patients achieved PRs and 13% had disease stabilization [49]. Antitumor activity was reported in all dose levels, without a clear dose-response relationship, and 28% of the patients remained on gefitinib for at least 3 months and 20% for at least 6 months. Based on these encouraging results, two large phase II trials, IDEAL 1 and IDEAL 2, were conducted in patients with advanced disease who exhibited progression with standard platinum chemotherapy [3].

In the IDEAL 1 trial 210 patients with advanced disease received either 250 mg or 500 mg of gefitinib without EGFR expression being a requirement for entry into the study [51]. The overall RR was 18.4% and 19% and disease stabilization was observed in 36% and 32% of patients, respectively. Approximately 40% of all the patients enrolled experienced symptomatic improvement, which was higher in patients who had an objective response. The median progression-free survival times were 2.7 months and 2.8 months and median overall survival times 7.6 and 8.0 months, respectively. Side effects were mild and included rash, pruritus, and diarrhea, which were more commonly seen in the higher dose group. In a multivariate analysis, it became apparent that patients with adenocarcinoma histology, female sex and patients who had previously received immunologic or hormonal therapies had a higher possibility for response.

In the IDEAL 2 study, a total of 221 unselected patients were randomized to receive either 250 or 500 mg of gefitinib [52]. PRs were observed in 12% and 9% and symptomatic improvement in 43% and 35% of patients treated with 250mg and 500mg, respectively. The one year-overall survival rate was 25%. A greater toxicity was also observed with the higher dose of gefitinib. Given the similar response rates of the two dose level groups, the recommended dosage for gefitinib was established at 250 mg/daily.

The possible role of gefitinib as a second- or third-line treatment for patients with advanced NSCLC who were refractory or intolerant to their latest chemotherapy regimen was recently examined in a phase III clinical trial (ISEL trial) [53]. In this study, 1692 patients were randomized to receive either gefitinib (n=1129) or a placebo (n=563). After a median follow-up of 7 months, the investigators reported no difference in overall survival (5.6 months for gefitinib and 5.1 months for placebo). Longer survival on the gefitinib arm was observed in patients with Asian ethnicity (n=342, hazard ratio [HR]=0.66, p=0.01) or who were nonsmokers (n=375, HR=0.67, p=0.01). The use of gefitinib as a maintenance therapy after systemic therapy has been completed in the phase III trial SWOG (South-West Oncology Group) 0023 [54]. This study involved patients with stage IIIA/B NSCLC which were randomized to receive either gefitinib or placebo after completing the SWOG 9504 phase II study [55]. In the SWOG 9504 regimen, patients received cisplatin plus etoposide with concurrent thoracic radiation therapy followed by docetaxel in stage IIIB patients. The study was designed to demonstrate a 33% increase in median survival time in the gefitinib group over the estimated 21-month survival of the control group. SWOG 0023 was closed early, after the results of the ISEL trial, with 575 patients of the planned 840 who registered. An interim analysis of 263 patients suggested that gefitinib maintenance could not have possibly improved survival (p=0.0015) even if this trial was completed to accrual. Grade 3 or 4 pneumonitis was more common during docetaxel treatment (8% of the patients) as well as in the gefitinib arm (3% of the patients compared with 0% in the placebo arm).

The role of gefitinib, as a monotherapy, in preventing brain metastasis was also investigated and showed promising anticancer activity [56,57]. Patients with poor performance status may also benefit from gefitinib therapy with very promising results in Chinese patients [58,59]. Clinical activity and a low toxicity profile were reported in elderly patients with NSCLC [60].

Gefitinib can be also administered safely with the cyclooxygenase inhibitors celecoxib and rofecoxib [61,62]. When gefitinib was combined with cetuximab, a synergistic effect was demonstrated on apoptosis, cell proliferation and HER1/EGFR-dependent pathway, compared with either agent alone [63]. Enhanced antitumor antiangiogenic effect was observed when gefitinib was combined with ZD 6126, an antivascular microtubule-destabilizing agent [64,65].

The worldwide incidence of interstitial lung disease after gefitinib treatment is approximately 1% and about one-third of the cases were fatal.

### *Combinations of Gefitinib and Erlotinib with Chemotherapy*

Based on the results of phase II trials, two phase III clinical trials (INTACT1 and INTACT2) were launched to study the combination of gefitinib with chemotherapy. In the INTACT 1 study, 1,093 chemotherapy-naïve patients with advanced NSCLC were randomized to receive gefitinib in combination with cisplatin and gemcitabine or cisplatin/gemcitabine with placebo [66]. All patients received up to 6 cycles of chemotherapy with either 250mg gefitinib, 500mg gefitinib, or a placebo. No significant toxicity was reported. Median survival times were identical between the two gefitinib groups (9.9 and 9.9 months) and even slightly better in the placebo group (10.9 months). Median times to progression were also insignificantly different (5.8 months for the 250mg/d dosing, 5.5 for the 500 mg/d dosing, and 6.0 months for the placebo). Response rates varied slightly at 50.3%, 49.7%, and 44.8%, respectively. In the INTACT 2 study, 1,037 patients with advanced NSCLC were randomized to receive paclitaxel and carboplatin plus either gefitinib 250 mg/d, or gefitinib 500 mg/d, or a placebo [67]. Again, there was also no difference in overall survival (median 9.8, 8.7, and 9.9 months, respectively). In gefitinib patients, dose-related diarrhea and skin toxicity were observed. A trend towards improved survival in patients with adenocarcinoma histology was also demonstrated. Gefitinib was better tolerated in both trials at a dose regimen of 250 mg/d with fewer dose reductions and treatment interruptions.

Two phase III clinical trials (TALENT and TRIBUTE) studied the possible role of erlotinib in combination with chemotherapy. In the TALENT study, 1172 previously untreated patients with advanced NSCLC patients were treated with six cycles of cisplatin/gemcitabine and either erlotinib or placebo [68]. Erlotinib was continued until disease progression. Unfortunately, the combination of erlotinib with platinum-based chemotherapy did not significantly prolong overall survival. In the parallel study, TRIBUTE, 1059 patients were randomized to receive either erlotinib or placebo combined with carboplatin and paclitaxel followed by maintenance monotherapy with erlotinib [69]. Median survival was 10.6 versus 10.5 months for the erlotinib and placebo group, respectively ($p=0.95$). There was also no difference in OR and median time to progression. Skin toxicity and diarrhea were the main toxicities in the erlotinib group. An interesting observation from the TRIBUTE study was that never smokers in the erlotinib group had a median survival twice as long as those on chemotherapy alone [70].

Several possible explanations have been postulated so as to interpret these negative results of the concurrent combination of both TKIs with conventional chemotherapy: (a) The concurrent use of TKIs with chemotherapy may result in an antagonistic effect, (b) TKIs and chemotherapy may be targeting the same cell population, (c) Neoplastic cells may use alternative pathways as escape mechanisms, or (d) Clinical trials are made in an unselected population [71-73].

An essential breakthrough in the field of EGFR-targeted therapy is the identification of somatic mutations of the EGFR gene, which are associated with clinical response to gefitinib and erlotinib in patients with NSCLC [74-76]. These genetic alterations are mainly frame deletions or point mutations in exons 18-24 which encode the kinase domain of the protein. The most common alterations reported are point mutations in the exon 21 and small deletions in the exon 19 that eliminate amino acids 747-750 (Leu-Arg-Glu-Ala). These mutations are most frequently detected in a subpopulation of patients with NSCLC with characteristics associated with an improved outcome: female sex, never-smokers, East Asian ethnicity and adenocarcinoma histology and in particular, BAC histology [77-79]. In a recent analysis from IDEAL 1, IDEAL 2, and INTACT studies, a RR was seen in 46% of patients with an EGFR mutation versus 10% of those with wild-type EGFR, and in 29% having a high copy number versus 15% with a low copy number [80]. Recent analysis from BR.21 study has suggested that there was an unusually high EGFR mutation rate (23% of the 177 patients for whom tumor tissue was adequate for the study), with a low positive predictive value (16%) and a higher response rate (20% versus 2.4%) in patients with a high versus a low EGFR copy number, respectively [81]. Dr. Paul Gumerlock has also reported a response rate in 23% of patients with an EGFR mutation versus 13% of those with wild-type EGFR, and in 26% of those with a high copy number versus 11% of those with a low one, with K-*ras* mutations being a possible resistance marker for response [82]. At the same time, higher results (53% to 100%) were reported by other groups regarding the positive predictive role of an EGFR mutation [83-85]. K-*ras* gene mutations, which are detected in 30% of NSCLC patients, lead to a resistant form of cancer cells to TKIs and are associated with a lack of response [77,86]. In the TRIBUTE study, k-*ras* mutations detected in 21% of the tumors were associated with decreased time to progression and overall survival in patients treated with erlotinib combined with chemotherapy [87]. The fact that in TRIBUTE study EGFR mutations were detected in 13% of tumors and were associated with longer survival irrespective of treatment may suggest that EGFR mutations may be an independent positive prognostic factor for survival. An acquired resistance to EGFR-TKIs has been suggested to be associated with the prevalence of an additional EGFR mutation [88].

### *Other EGFR-TKIs*

CI-1033 is an irreversible pan-EGFR inhibitor having synergistic action with both chemotherapy and radiotherapy in phase I trials [89,90]. A phase II randomized trial comparing different schedules and doses of CI-1033 in NSCLC patients entering the second-line is ongoing with one-year survival as the primary efficacy parameter. PKI 166 is a selective inhibitor of the tyrosine kinase activities of the EGFR and HER-2/neu which has been recently evaluated in phase I trials [91,92]. GW 572016 (lapatinib) is also a TKI with molecular action on HER-1 and HER-2 having an acceptable toxicity profile as described in phase I trials [93,94]. AEE 788 is a novel agent which inhibits both EGFR/ErbB2 and the vascular endothelial receptor 2 (VEGFR2) now studied on phase I clinical trials [95,96].

## 3. ErbB2(HER) Inhibitors

HER-2/neu functions as a heterodimer with the other members of EGF receptors and has a potent tyrosine kinase activity although it has not a discrete ligand. HER-2/neu overexpression has been associated with a poor prognosis in a variety of malignancies including NSCLC [97].

Trastuzumab (Herceptin) is a chimeric monoclonal antibody that targets HER-2 receptor with activity in metastatic breast cancer. In lung cancer cell lines, antitumor activity was demonstrated in HER-2/neu positive cells with a synergistic activity when combined with cytotoxic agents [98,99]. Unfortunately, all phase II trials of trastuzumab when combined with chemotherapy failed to demonstrate any additional therapeutic benefit [100-103]. In the largest trial performed to date, 619 patients screened to select 103 eligible patients with HER-

2 positive NSCLC who were randomized to receive gemcitabine and cisplatin with or without trastuzumab [103]. No differences were reported in the RR (36% in the antibody arm and 41% in the control arm), median time to progression, and progression-free survival.

Pertuzumab (Omnitarg, rhuMAb 2C4) is a humanized monoclonal antibody which belongs to the new class of targeted therapeutics known as HER dimerization inhibitors [104]. Pertuzumab binds to HER2 and blocks ligand-associated heterodimerization of HER1, HER3 and HER4. When pertuzumab was tested with or without erlotinib in tumor cell lines an additive or greater than additive antitumor activity was observed when these two agents were combined [105]. Pertuzumab has been studied in phase I clinical trials in patients with advanced malignancies having an acceptable toxicity profile [106]. When this agent was studied in a phase II trial in 33 patients with advanced or recurrent NSCLC previously treated with chemotherapy, none of the patients had an objective response [107].

The presence of mutations in the HER-2 kinase domain has been reported in NSCLC patients, although the response to gefitinib seems to be independent of HER-2 levels [108,109]. These mutations are more frequent in patients with clinical characteristics similar to the group of patients bearing EGFR mutations.

The possible role of HER2/neu as a prognostic factor of survival between males and females with NSCLC was recently examined [110]. Tumor samples of 90 NSCLC patients with stage I-IIIA, who underwent a complete resection, were evaluated for HER2/neu gene expression by quantitative reverse-transcriptase polymerase chain reaction (PCR). No significant difference was reported between gene expression levels of men and women. High HER2/neu messenger RNA expression levels were associated with worse survival ($p=0.09$). No significant difference for survival time was established when men with high HER2/neu gene expression were compared with men with low HER2/neu mRNA levels. On the contrary, women with a low expression of HER2/neu had a superior survival time (≥94.7 months) compared with women high HER2/neu levels (26.4 months) ($p=0.043$).

## B. Farnesyl Transferase Inhibitors (FTIs)

The *ras* family of proto-oncogenes encodes proteins that play an essential role in critical cellular process such as proliferation, differentiation and apoptosis. Mammalian cells contain 3 functional *ras* genes (H-*ras*, N-*ras* and K-*ras*) that encode 4 oncoproteins (H-Ras, N-Ras, K-Ras4A and K-Ras4B). K-Ras4A and K-Ras4B are the result of two alternatively spliced K-*ras* gene products [3]. Mutations in the Ras proteins are found in about 30 % of all human cancers and 40 % of NSCLC indicating poor prognosis [111]. Activating mutations in these proteins lead to constitutive signaling, inhibition of apoptosis and promotion of cellular proliferation [112]. When a *ras* protein is being generated a nonpolar farnesyl group is attached to the COOH-terminal, a reaction catalyzed by the enzyme farnesyl tranferase. This reaction enables the *ras* protein to move from the cytoplasm to the cell membrane, as it becomes more hydrophobic, where it cycles from the inactive *ras*-GDP to the activated *ras*-GTP in response to cellular binding of growth promoting factors to its tyrosine kinase receptor. Geranylgeranyl tranferases I (GGTase-I) and II (GGTase-II) can alternatively catalyze the farnesylation of K-*ras* and other proteins. FTIs block this procedure and its cellular consequences. Other proteins, which may have a role in mediating the antitumor activity of FTIs, are the centromeric (CENP-E and CENP-F) proteins, RhoB, and members of the phosphatidylinositol 3'-kinase/Akt pathway [113-115]. FTIs have been shown to inhibit the growth of a broad spectrum of tumor cell lines in vitro and in vivo and it is suggested that tumor cells bearing mutated K-*ras* may be less sensitive to FTIs than those with wild-type *ras* or mutated 11-*ras* genes [116,117]. The combination of FTIs with irradiation and paclitaxel may increase cell cytotoxicity and death [118,119]. A possible suppression of the angiogenic factors expression such as VEGF from FTIs antitumor action is also suggested [120].

L-778,123 was studied in a phase II trial in 23 NSCLC patients with stage IIIB (with pleural effusion) or IV, with a performance status (PS) of 0-1 who have not received chemotherapy before [121]. The DLTs of this agent, when examined in a phase I trial, was fatigue, myelosuppression and neurotoxicity and the recommended dose was 560 mg/m$^2$ i.v. daily [122]. Thromboembolic toxicity was observed in patients with a central venous access. Three patients developed a pulmonary embolism and one patient had a superior vena cava thrombosis. Nineteen of the 23 patients completed at least one cycle without any objective response observed. The development of this compound was then discontinued.

Lonafarnib (SCH 66336) is an oral tricyclic halogenated competitive FTI which is active in tumors having all *ras* mutations as well as wild type *ras* mutations. In a phase I trial, one patient with advanced NSCLC had an objective PR and 8 patients demonstrated disease stabilization for up to 10 cycles of the drug [123]. In another phase I trial, lonafarnib was given in 24 patients with solid tumor in combination with paclitaxel every 3 weeks [124]. Partial remission was demonstrated in 15 patients, including 2 with taxane resistant advanced NSCLC. The DLTs observed were neutropenia, peripheral neuropathy, diarrhea, and hyperbilirubinemia. A phase II trial of lonafarnib combined with paclitaxel in 33 taxane-refractory advanced NSCLC patients was then organized [125]. Toxicities were minimal and included febrile neutropenia, diarrhea and fatigue. Five patients (15%) achieved PR, four patients MR and ten patients sustained disease stabilization. These promising results led to a phase trial III of combinations with carboplatin/paclitaxel versus carboplatin/paclitaxel/placebo in 675 good performance status patients with advanced NSCLC [126]. There was no statistically significant improvement in time to progression (137 versus 152 days) and overall survival (144 versus 168 days) for patients receiving lonafarnib with the placebo arm having numerically superior outcomes.

Tipifarnib (R115777) is an oral methylquinolone analogue of the imidazoles which inhibits the growth of tumors with N-*ras*, H-*ras*, and wild-type mutations being less active against wild-type *ras* mutations. When tipifarnib was investigated in a phase I trial, one patient with platinum-refractory NSCLC who received continuous dosing had a partial remission [127]. The major toxicities observed were hematological with peripheral neuropathy. Fatigue and skin toxicities were also reported. A phase II study of tibifarnib as a single agent therapy in advanced NSCLC was organized in 44 patients with performance status 0-2 who have not received either chemotherapy or radiotherapy to more than 25% of their bone marrow [128]. The regimen schedule was 300 mg orally twice daily for 21 days of a 28-day cycle. The most common grade 3 and 4 toxicities were neutropenia, anemia, and anorexia. There were no objective responses, although 7 patients had SD for more than six months. Evidence of farnesyl transferase inhibition was documented in 83% of the patients.

Median survival was 7.7 months, median time to progression was 2.7 months and 70% of the patients were able to continue with conventional chemotherapy after completing tibifarnib.

BMS-214662 is an imidazole-containing tetrahydrobenzodiazepine with cytotoxic and apoptotic properties that differentiate it from other FTIs [129]. Because of its unacceptable gastrointestinal toxicity profile, intravenous administration is preferred. In a phase I trial of 44 patients with advanced solid tumor malignancies, the dose-limiting toxicities observed after the first cycle of therapy were nausea, vomiting, and diarrhea [130]. Four patients developed reversible transaminitis, which was not dose-limiting. When BMS-214662 was combined with cisplatin in 29 patients with advanced solid tumor malignancies transaminitis, nausea, vomiting, diarrhea and renal failure were the DLTs, with 15 patients having disease stabilization as their best response [131]. In another phase I trial, 30 patients with advanced solid tumor malignancies received escalating doses of this novel agent, followed by the combination of carboplatin/paclitaxel on the first day of a 21-day cycle [132]. Three patients had PR and eight had SD with neutropenia, thrombocytopenia, nausea and vomiting as the most important DLTs.

## Conclusion

The introduction of EGFR TKIs, and especially erlotinib, in the treatment of patients with advanced NSCLC is undoubtedly a major improvement in current clinical oncology practice. As female sex is strongly connected with EGFR mutations in the tyrosine kinase domain and a higher probability for response to these novel agents, the organization of future clinical trials in which patient population will be stratified into sexes, seems necessary. Nonsmoker women with EGFR mutations may have a particular benefit from EGFR TKIs, especially if they lack K-*ras* mutations, but this must be proven in clinical studies especially designed for this purpose.

Moreover, lung cancer is a heterogeneous disease with a variety of mutations thus blocking one molecular pathway each time may permit others to act as escape mechanisms for tumor cells. The combination of novel agents as well as the development of new drugs which target multiple pathways simultaneously may have a better chance of shutting down the oncogenetic process and improving the outcome. Novel agents which inhibit both EGFR and HER2, such as lapatinib, may have an enhanced activity in female patients who overexpress HER2/neu. This activity may not be verified if men and women are grouped together.

Finally, it is crucially anticipated that by continuing to analyze extensively and to integrate fully all of the pertinent information collected from first generation clinical trials, second generation studies will successfully continue to broaden our knowledge in the direction that will, someday, deliver hope to the patient with NSCLC.

# REFERENCES

[1] Syrigos KN, Nutting C, Roussos C, Tumors of the chest. *Biology, Diagnosis and Management.* Verlag, New York, May 2006.

[2] Patel JD, Bach PB, Kris MG. Lung Cancer in US women: a contemporary epidemic. *JAMA.* 2004;291:1763-1768.

[3] Papaetis GS, Roussos C, Syrigos KN. Targeted therapy for Non-Small Cell Lung Cancer. *Current Pharmaceutical Design*, 2006 (in press).

[4] Ginsberg RJ, Vokes EE, Rosenzweig K. Non-small cell lung cancer. In: De Vita VT Jr, Hellman S, Rosenberg SA, eds. *Cancer: Principles and Practice of Oncology, 6th Edition.* Philadelphia: Lippincott, Williams and Wilkins; 2001, p. 925-83.

[5] Feld R, Rubinstein LV, Weisenberger TH. Sites of recurrence in resected stage I non-small-cell lung cancer: a guide for future studies. *J. Clin. Oncol.* 1984;2:1352-8.

[6] Syrigos KN, Harrington KJ. Targeted therapy for cancer. Oxford University Press, October 2002.

[7] Nelson HH, Christiani DC, Mark EJ, et al. Implications and prognostic value of K-ras mutations for early-stage lung cancer in women. *J. Natl. Cancer Inst. (Bethesda)* 1999;91:2032-2038.

[8] Hirsch FR, Varella-Garcia M, Franklin WA, et al. Evaluation of HER-2/neu gene amplification and protein expression in non-small cell lung carcinomas. *Br. J. Cancer.* 2002; 86:1449-56.

[9] Wells A. EGF receptor. *Int. J. Biochem. Cell Biol.* 1999; 31:637-43.

[10] Carpenter G, King L Jr, Cohen S. Epidermal growth factor stimulates phosphorylation in membrane preparations in vitro. *Nature.* 1978; 276:409-10.

[11] Yarden Y, Sliwkowski MX. Untangling the ErbB signaling network. *Nat. Rev. Mol. Cell Biol.* 2001; 2:127-37.

[12] Nicholson RI, Gee JM, Harper ME. EGFR and cancer prognosis. *Eur. J. Cancer.* 2001; 37: 9-15.

[13] Ohsaki Y, Tanno S, Fujita Y et al. Epidermal growth factor expression correlates with poor prognosis in non-small cell lung cancer patients with p53 overexpression. *Oncol. Rep.* 2000; 7: 603-7.

[14] Hortobagyi GN, Sauter G. Challenges and opportunities for Erlotinib (Tarceva): what does the future hold? *Semin. Oncol.* 2003; 30:47-53.

[15] Ellerbroek SM, Halbleib JM, Benavidez M et al. Phosphatidylinositol 3-kinase activity in epidermal growth factor-stimulated matrix metalloproteinase-9 production and cell surface association. *Cancer Res.* 2001; 61: 1855-61.

[16] Hazan R. B., Norton L. The epidermal growth factor receptor modulates the interaction of E-cadherin with the actin cytoskeleton. *J. Biol. Chem.* 1998; 273: 9078-84.

[17] Kawamoto T, Sato JD, Le A et al. Growth stimulation of A431 cells by epidermal growth factor: identification of high-affinity receptors for epidermal growth factor by an anti-receptor monoclonal antibody. *Proc. Natl. Acad. Sci. USA.* 1983; 80:1337-41.

[18] Herbst RS, Langer CJ. Epidermal growth factor receptors as a target for cancer treatment: The emerging role of IMC-C225 in the treatment of lung and head and neck cancers. *Semin. Oncol.* 2002; 29: 27-36.

[19] Sato JD, Kawamoto T, Le AD et al. Biological effects in vitro of monoclonal antibodies to human epidermal growth factor receptors. *Mol. Biol. Med.* 1983; 1:511–29.

[20] Milas L, Mason K, Hunter N et al. In vivo enhancement of tumour radioresponse by C225 antiepidermal growth factor receptor antibody. *Clin. Cancer Res.* 2000; 6:701–8.

[21] Fan Z, Baselga J, Masui H et al. Antitumour effect of anti-epidermal growth factor receptor monoclonal antibodies plus cis-deammine-dichloroplatinum on well established A431 cell xenografts. *Cancer Res.* 1993; 53:4637–42.

[22] Fracasso PM, Garrett C, Burris HA et al. A study to assess the pharmacokinetics (PK) and pharmacodynamics (PD) of a single infusion of cetuximab (IMC-C225) [abstract]. *Proc. Am. Soc. Clin. Oncol.* 2003; 22:196a.

[23] Rubin EH, Doroshow J, Hidalgo M et al. A study to assess the pharmacokinetics (PK) of a single infusion of cetuximab (IMC-C225) [abstract]. *Proc. Am. Soc. Clin. Oncol.* 2004; 23:216a.

[24] Baselga J, Pfister D, Cooper MR et al. Phase I studies of anti-epidermal growth factor receptor chimeric antibody C225 alone and in combination with cisplatin. *J. Clin. Oncol.* 2000; 18:904-14.

[25] Thienelt CD, Bunn PA Jr, Hanna N et al. Multi-centered phase I/II study of cetuximab with paclitaxel and carboplatin in untreated patients with stage IV non-small cell lung cancer. *J. Clin. Oncol.* 2005; 23(34):8786-93.

[26] Robert F, Blumenschein G, Herbst RS et al. Phase I/IIa study of cetuximab with gemcitabine plus carboplatin in patients with chemotherapy-naive advanced non-small cell lung cancer. *J. Clin. Oncol.* 2005; 23(36):9089-96.

[27] Rosell R, Daniel C, Ramlau R et al. Randomized phase II study of cetuximab in combination with cisplatin (C) and vinorelbine (V) vs. CV alone in the first-line treatment of patients (pts) with epidermal growth factor receptor (EGFR)-expressing advanced non-small-cell lung cancer (NSCLC) [abstract]. *Proc. Am. Soc. Clin. Oncol.* 2004; 23:618a.

[28] Kim E, Mauer A, Tran H et al: A phase II study of cetuximab, an epidermal growth factor receptor (EGFR) blocking antibody, in combination with docetaxel in chemotherapy refractory/resistant patients with advanced non-small cell lung cancer: Final report [abstract]. *Proc. Am. Soc. Clin. Oncol.* 2003; 22:642.

[29] Lilenbaum R, Bonomi P, Ansari R. A phase II trial of cetuximab as therapy for recurrent non-small cell lung cancer (NSCLC): Final results [abstract 7036]. *Proc. Am. Soc. Clin. Oncol.* 2005;23 (Suppl):629s.

[30] Saltz L, Kies M, Abbruzzese J et al. The presence and intensity of the cetuximab-induced acne-like rash predicts increased survival in studies across multiple malignancies [abstract 817]. *Proc. Am. Soc. Clin. Oncol.* 2003; 22:204a.

[31] Shridhar SS, Seymour L, Shepherd FA. Inhibitors of epidermal-growth-factor-receptors: a review of clinical research with a focus on non-small cell lung cancer. *Lancet Oncol.* 2003; 4(7):397-406.

[32] Lynch DH, Yang XD. Therapeutic potential of ABX-EGF: a fully human anti-epidermal growth factor receptor monoclonal antibody for cancer treatment. *Semin. Oncol.* 2002; 29:47-50.

[33] Yang XD, Jia XC, Corvalan JR et al. Development of ABX-EGF, a fully human anti-EGF receptor monoclonal antibody for cancer therapy. *Crit. Rev. Oncol. Hematol.* 2001; 38:17-23.

[34] Figlin RA, Belldegrun AS, Crawford J et al. ABX-EGF, a fully human anti-epidermal growth factor receptor (EGFR) monoclonal antibody (mAb) in patients with advanced cancer: phase 1 clinical results [abstract 35]. *Proc. Am. Soc. Clin. Oncol.* 2002; 21:10a.

[35] Foon KA, Yang XD, Weiner LM et al. Preclinical and clinical evaluations of ABX-EGF, a fully human anti-epidermal growth factor receptor antibody. *Int. J. Radiat. Oncol. Biol. Phys.* 2004; 58: 984-90.

[36] Crawford J, Sandler A, Hammond J et al. ABX-EGF in combination with paclitaxel and carboplatin for advanced non-small cell lung cancer (NSCLC) [abstract 7083]. *Proc. Am. Soc. Clin. Oncol.* 2004; 22 (Suppl 14): 21a.

[37] Giaccone G. Epidermal growth factor receptor inhibitors in the treatment of non-small-cell lung cancer. *J. Clin. Oncol.* 2005; 23: 3235–42.

[38] Pollack VA, Savage DM, Baker DA et al. Inhibition of epidermal growth factor receptor-associated tyrosine phosphorylation in human carcinomas with CP-358,774: dynamics of receptor inhibition in situ and antitumour effects in athymic mice. *J. Pharmacol. Exp. Ther.* 1999; 291:739-48.

[39] Moyer JD, Barbacci EG, Iwata KK, et al. Induction of apoptosis and cell cycle arrest by CP-358,774, an inhibitor of epidermal growth factor receptor tyrosine kinase. *Cancer Res.* 1997;57:4838-4848.

[40] Hidalgo M, Siu LL, Neumanitis K et al. Phase I and pharmacology study of OSI-774, an epidermal growth factor receptor tyrosine kinase inhibitor in patients with advanced solid malignancies. *J. Clin. Oncol.* 2001; 119:3267-79.

[41] Karp D, Ferrante KJ, Tensfeldt TG et al. A phase I dose escalation study of epidermal growth factor receptor (EGFR) tyrosine kinase (TK) inhibitor CP-358,774

in patients (pts) with advanced solid tumours [abstract 208]. *Lung Cancer.* 2000;29:72.

[42] Perez-Soler R, Chachoua A, Huberman M et al. A phase II trial of the epidermal growth factor receptor (EGFR) tyrosine kinase inhibitor (OSI-774) following platinum-based chemotherapy in patients with advanced EGFR-expressing non small cell lung cancer (NCSLC) [abstract 1235]. *Proc. Am. Soc. Clin. Oncol.* 2001; 20:210a.

[43] Patel JD, Miller VA, Kris MG et al Encouraging activity and durable responses demonstrated by the EGFR tyrosine kinase inhibitor erlotinib (Tarceva™, OSI-774) in patients with advanced bronchioalveolar (BAC) cell carcinoma. *Lung Cancer.* 2003; 41(Suppl): S56.

[44] Perez-Soler R, Chachoua A, Hammond L et al. Determinants of tumour response and survival with erlotinib in patients with NSCLC. *J. Clin. Oncol.* 2004; 22: 3238-3247.

[45] Shepherd FA, Rodrigues Pereira J et al. Erlotinib in previously treated non-small cell lung cancer. *N. Engl. J. Med.* 2005; 353(2):123-32.

[46] Herbst RS, Johnson DH, Mininberg E et al. Phase I/II trial evaluating the anti-vascular endothelial growth factor monoclonal antibody bevacizumab in combination with the HER-1/epidermal growth factor receptor tyrosine kinase inhibitor erlotinib for patients with recurrent non-small-cell lung cancer. *J. Clin. Oncol.* 2005; 23:2544-55.

[47] Sirotnak FM, Zakowski MF, Miller VA, Scher HI, Kris MG. Efficacy of cytotoxic agents against human tumour xenografts is markedly enhanced by coadministration of ZD1839 (Iressa™), an inhibitor of EGFR tyrosine kinase. *Clin. Cancer Res.* 2000; 6:4885-92.

[48] Herbst RS, Maddox AM, Rothenberg ML et al. Selective oral epidermal growth factor receptor tyrosine kinase inhibitor ZD1839 is generally well-tolerated and has activity in non-small-cell lung cancer and other solid tumours: results of a phase I trial. *J. Clin. Oncol.* 2002; 20:3815-25.

[49] Herbst R. S., Kies M. S. ZD1839 (Iressa™) in non-small cell lung cancer. *Oncologist.* 2002; 7 (Suppl 4): 9-15.

[50] Ranson M, Hammond LA, Ferry D et al. ZD1839, a selective oral epidermal growth factor receptor-tyrosine kinase inhibitor, is well tolerated and active in patients with solid, malignant tumours: results of a Phase I trial. *J. Clin. Oncol.* 2002; 20: 2240-50.

[51] Fukuoka M, Yano S, Giaccone G et al: Multi-institutional randomized phase II trial of gefitinib for previously treated patients with advanced non-small-cell lung cancer. *J. Clin. Oncol.* 2003; 21:2237-46.

[52] Kris MG, Natale RB, Herbst RS et al: Efficacy of gefitinib, an inhibitor of the epidermal growth factor receptor tyrosine kinase, in symptomatic patients with non-small cell lung cancer: A randomized trial. *JAMA.* 2003; 290:2149-58.

[53] Thatcher N, Chaug A, Parikh P et al. Gefitinib plus best supportive care in previously treated patients with refractory advanced non-small-cell lung cancer: results from a randomized, placebo-controlled, multicentre study (Iressa™ Survival Evaluation in Lung Cancer). *Lancet.* 2005; 366(9496):1527-37.

[54] Kelly K, Gaspar LE, Chansky K, et al. Low incidence of pneumonitis on SWOG 0023: a preliminary analysis of an ongoing phase III trial of concurrent chemoradiotherapy followed by consolidation docetaxel and Iressa™/placebo maintenance in patients with inoperable stage III non-small cell lung cancer [abstract 7058]. *Proc. Am. Soc. Clin. Oncol.* 2005;23 (Suppl):634s.

[55] Gandara DR, Chansky K, Albain KS et al; Southwest Oncology Group Study S9504. Consolidation docetaxel after concurrent chemoradiotherapy in stage IIIB non-small-cell lung cancer: phase II. *J. Clin. Oncol.* 2003; 21:2004–10.

[56] Cappuzo F, Ardizzoni A, Soto-Parra H et al. Epidermal growth factor receptor targeted therapy by ZD 1839 (Iressa™) in patients with brain metastases from non-small cell lung cancer. *Lung Cancer.* 2003; 41:227-31.

[57] Namba Y, Kijima T, Yokota S, et al. Gefitinib in patients with brain metastases from non-small-cell-lung cancer: Review of 15 clinical cases. *Clin. Lung Cancer.* 2004; 6(2):123-128.

[58] Gridelli C, Maione P, Castaldo V, et al. Gefitinib in elderly and unfit patients affected by advanced non-small-cell lung cancer. *Br. J. Cancer.* 2003;89(10):1827-1829.

[59] Chang GC, Chen KC, Yang TY, et al: Activity of gefitinib in advanced non-small-cell lung cancer with very poor performance status. *Invest. New Drugs.* 2005; 23(1):73-77.

[60] Copin M, Kommareddy A, Behnken D, et al. Gefitinib in elderly patients with non-small cell lung cancer (NSCLC). *Proc. Am. Soc. Clin. Oncol.* 2003;22:758.

[61] Gadgeel S, Shehadeh N, Ruckdeschel J et al. Gefitinib and celecoxib in patients with platinum refractory non-small cell lung cancer (NSCLC). ASCO Annual Meeting Proceedings (Post-Meeting Edition) *J. Clin. Oncol.* 2004;22 (Suppl 14):7094.

[62] O'Byrne KJ, Clarke L, Dunlop D, Ranson M, Danson S, Botwood N. Clinical evaluation of gefitinib (Iressa,ZD1839) in combination with rofecoxib in cisplatin pre-treated relapsed non-small cell lung cancer [abstract O-113]. *Lung Cancer.* 2003; 41(Suppl 2):S36.

[63] Matar P, Rojo F, Cassia R, et al. Combined epidermal growth factor receptor targeting with the tyrosine kinase inhibitor gefitinib (ZD 1839) and the monoclonal antibody cetuximab (IMC-C225): superiority over single-agent receptor targeting. *Clin. Cancer Res.* 2004; 10:6487-6501.

[64] Raben D, Bianco C, Damiano V, et al. Antitumor activity of ZD6126, a novel vascular-targeting agent, is enhanced when combined with ZD1839, an epidermal growth factor receptor tyrosine kinase inhibitor, and potentiates the effects of

radiation in a human non-small cell lung cancer xenograft model. *Mol. Cancer Ther.* 2004;3(8):977-83.

[65] Bozec A, Lassalle S, Guqenheim J, et al. Enhanced tumour antiangiogenic effects when combining gefitinib with the antivascular agent ZD6126. *Br. J. Cancer.* 2006;95(6):722-8.

[66] Giaccone G, Herbst RS, Manegold C et al. Gefitinib (ZD1839) in combination with gemcitabine and cisplatin in advanced non-small-cell lung cancer: A phase III trial (INTACT 1). *J. Clin. Oncol.* 2004; 22:777-84.

[67] Herbst RS, Giaccone G, Schiller JH et al. Gefitinib (ZD1839) in combination with paclitaxel and carboplatin in advanced non-small-cell lung cancer: A phase III trial (INTACT 2). *J. Clin. Oncol.* 2004; 22:785-94.

[68] Gatzemeier U, Pluzanska A, Szczesna A et al. Results of a phase III trial of erlotinib (OSI-774) combined with cisplatin and gemcitabine (GC) chemotherapy in advanced non-small cell lung cancer [abstract]. *Proc. Am. Soc. Clin. Oncol.* 2004; 22:7010a.

[69] Herbst RS, Prager D, Herman R et al. TRIBUTE-A phase III trial of erlotinib HCI (OSI-774) combined with carboplatin and paclitaxel chemotherapy in advanced non-small cell lung cancer. *J. Clin. Oncol.* 2005; 23(25):5892-9.

[70] Miller VA, Herbst R, Prager D et al. Long survival of never smoking non-small cell lung cancer (NSCLC) patients treated with erlotinib HCI (OSI-774) and chemotherapy: subgroup analysis of TRIBUTE. ASCO Annual Meeting Proceedings (Post-Meeting Edition); *J. Clin. Oncol.* 2004;22 (14 Suppl):7061.

[71] Johnson DH. Gefitinib (Iressa$^{TM}$) trials in non-small cell lung cancer. *Lung Cancer.* 2003; 41 (Suppl 1):S23-S28.

[72] Baselga J. Combining the anti-EGFR agent gefitinib with chemotherapy in non-small-cell lung cancer: how do we go from INTACT to impact? *J. Clin. Oncol.* 2004; 22:759-61.

[73] Dancey JE, Freidlin B. Targeting epidermal growth factor receptor-are we missing the mark? *Lancet.* 2003; 362:62-4.

[74] Lynch TJ, Bell DW, Sordella R et al. Activating mutations in the epidermal growth factor receptor underlying responsiveness for non-small-cell lung cancer to gefitinib. *N. Engl. J. Med.* 2004; 350:2129-39

[75] Paez JG, Janne PA, Lee JC et al. EGFR mutations in lung cancer: Correlation with clinical response to gefitinib therapy. *Science.* 2004; 304:1497-500.

[76] Pao W, Miller V, Zakowski M et al. EGF receptor gene mutations are common in lung cancers from ‘never smokers’ and are associated with sensitivity of tumours to gefitinib and erlotinib. *Proc. Natl. Acad. Sci. USA.* 2004; 101:13306-11.

[77] Pao W, Miller VA. Epidermal growth factor receptor mutations, small-molecule kinase inhibitors and non-small-cell lung cancer: current knowledge and future directions. *J. Clin. Oncol.* 2005; 23:2256-2658.

[78] Janne PA. Epidermal growth factor receptor mutations in non-small-cell lung cancer: implications for treatment and tumour biology. *J. Clin. Oncol.* 2005; 23: 3227–34.

[79] Shah NT, Miller VA, Kris MG et al. Bronchioalveolar histology and smoking history predict response to gefitinib. *Proc. Am. Soc. Clin. Oncol.* 2003; 22:628a.

[80] Lynch TJ, Bell DW, Harber DA et al. Correlation of molecular markers including mutations with clinical outcomes in advanced non small cell lung cancer (NSCLC) patients treated with gefitinib, chemotherapy or chemotherapy and gefitinib in IDEAL and INTACT clinical trials [abstract 7006]. *Proc. Am. Soc. Clin. Oncol.* 2005; 23:622s.

[81] Tsao MS, Sakurada A, Lorimer J et al; National Cancer Institute of Canada Clinical Trials Group (NCIC CTG) trial BR.21. Molecular analysis of the epidermal growth factor receptor (EGFR) gene and protein expression in patients treated with erlotinib [abstract 7007]. *Proc. Am. Soc. Clin. Oncol.* 2005;23(Suppl):622s.

[82] Gumerlock PH, Holland WS, Chen H et al. Mutational analysis of K-RAS and EGFR implicates K-RAS as a resistance marker in the Southwest Oncology Group (SWOG) trial S0126 of bronchioalveolar carcinoma (BAC) patients treated with gefitinib [abstract 7008]. *Proc. Am. Soc. Clin. Oncol.* 2005; 23 (Suppl):623s.

[83] Han SW, Kim TY, Hwagn PG et al. Predictive and prognostic impact of epidermal growth factor receptor mutation in non-small-cell lung cancer patients treated with gefitinib. *J. Clin. Oncol.* 2005; 23:2493-501.

[84] Mitsudomi T, Kosaka T, Endoh H et al. Mutations of the epidermal growth factor receptor gene predict prolonged survival after gefitinib treatment in patients with non-small cell lung cancer with postoperative recurrence. *J. Clin. Oncol.* 2005; 23:2513-20.

[85] Cappuzzo F, Hirsch FR, Rossi E et al. Epidermal growth factor receptor gene and protein and gefitinib sensivity in non-small-cell lung cancer. *J. Natl. Cancer Inst.* 2005; 97:643-55.

[86] Rodenhuis S, Slebos RJ, Boot AJ, et al. Incidence and possible clinical significance of K-ras oncogene activation in adenocarcinoma of the human lung. *Cancer Res.* 1998; 48: 5738–41.

[87] Eberhard DA, Johnson BE, Amler LC, et al. Mutations in the epidermal growth factor receptor and in KRAS are predictive and prognostic indicators in patients with non-small cell lung cancer treated with chemotherapy alone and in combination with erlotinib. *J. Clin. Oncol* .2005; 23(25):5900-5909.

[88] Kobayashi S, Boggon TG, Dayaram T et al. EGFR mutation and resistance of non-small-cell lung cancer to gefitinib. *N. Engl. J. Med.* 2005; 352:786-92.

[89] Garrison MA, Tolcher A, McGreery H et al. A phase I pharmacokinetic study of CI-1033, a pan-erbB tyrosine kinase inhibitor, given orally on days 1,8 and 15 every 28 days to patients with solid tumours [abstract]. *Proc. Am. Soc. Clin. Oncol.* 2001; 21:72a.

[90] Shin DM, Nemunaitis J, Zinner RG et al. A phase I clinical and biomarker study of CI-1033, a novel pan-erbB tyrosine kinase inhibitor in patients with solid tumours [abstract]. *Proc. Am. Soc. Clin. Oncol.* 2001; 20:82a.

[91] Dumez H, Hoekstra R, Eskens F et al. A phase I pharmacologic study of PKI 166 and epidermal growth factor receptor (EGFR) tyrosine kinase inhibitor, administered orally 3 times a week to patients with advanced cancer [abstract]. *Proc. Am. Soc. Clin. Oncol.* 2002; 21:86a.

[92] Murren JTR, Papadimitrakopoulou VA, Sizer KC et al. A phase I, dose-escalating study to evaluate the biological activity and pharmacokinetics of PKI166, a novel tyrosine kinase inhibitor, in patients with advanced cancers [abstract 377]. Program and abstracts of the 38th Annual Meeting of the American Society of Clinical Oncology; 2002 May 18-21; Orlando, Florida.

[93] De Simone PA, Bence AK, Anderson EB et al. A phase I study to investigate the safety, tolerability and pharmacokinetics of single oral escalating doses of GW572016 in healthy volunteers [abstract]. *Proc. Am. Soc. Clin. Oncol.* 2002; 21:94a.

[94] Minami H, Nakagawa K, Kawada K et al. A phase I study of GW572016 in patients with solid tumours; ASCO Annual Meeting Proceedings (Post-Meeting Edition). *J. Clin. Oncol.* 2004; 22:3048.

[95] Traxler P, Allegrini PR, Brandt R, et al. AEE 788: A dual family epidermal growth factor receptor/ErbB2 and vascular endothelial growth factor receptor tyrosine kinase inhibitor with antitumor and antiangiogenic activity. *Cancer Res.* 2004;64(14):4931-4941.

[96] Martinelli E, Takimoto CH, van Oosterom AT, et al. AEE 788, a novel multitargeted inhibitor of ErbB and VEGF receptor family tyrosine kinases: Preliminary phase I results (abstract 3039). *J. Clin. Oncol.* 2005;23(suppl 16):201s.

[97] Tsigris C, Karayiannakis AJ, Syrigos KN et al. Clinical significance of soluble c-erbB-2 levels in the serum and urine of patients with gastric cancer. *Anticancer Res.* 2002; 22(5):3061-5.

[98] Bunn PA, Helfrich B, Soriano AF et al. Expression of HER-2/neu in human lung cancer cell lines by immunohistochemistry and fluorescence in situ hybridization and its relationship to in vitro cytotoxicity by trastuzumab and chemotherapeutic agents. *Clin. Cancer Res.* 2001; 7:3239-50.

[99] Lewis GD, Figari I, Fendly B et al. Differential responses of human tumour cell lines to anti-p185HER2 monoclonal antibodies. *Cancer Immunol. Immunother.* 1993; 37:255-63.

[100] Krug LM, Miller VA, Crapanzano J et al. Randomized phase II trial of trastuzumab (Tras) plus either weekly docetaxel (Dopc) or paclitaxel (Pac) in previously untreated advanced non-small cell lung cancer [abstract]. *Proc. Am. Soc. Clin. Oncol.* 2001; 20:33.

[101] Langer CJ, Adak S, Thor A, Vangel M, Johnson D. Phase II Eastern Cooperative Oncology Group (ECOG) pilot study of paclitaxel (P), carboplatin (C) and trastuzumab (T) in HER-2/neu (+) advanced non-small cell lung cancer [abstract]. *Proc. Am. Soc. Clin. Oncol.* 2001; 20:315a.

[102] Zinner GR, Glisson BS, Pisters KM et al. Cisplatin and gemcitabine combined with herceptin in patients with HER2 overexpressing, untreated, advanced, non-small cell lung cancer (NSCLC): a phase II trial [abstract]. *Proc. Am. Soc. Clin. Oncol.* 2001; 20:328a.

[103] Gatzemeier U, Groth G, Butts C et al. Randomized phase II trial of gemcitabine-cisplatin with or without trastuzumab in HER-2-positive non-small cell lung cancer. *Ann. Oncol.* 2004; 125:19-27.

[104] Franklin MC, Carey KD, Vajdos FF, et al. Insights into ErbB signalling from the structures of the ErbB2-pertuzumab complex. *Cancer Cell.* 2004;5:317-28.

[105] Friess T, Scheuer W, Hasmann M. Combination treatment with erlotinib and pertuzumab against human tumor xenografts is superior to monotherapy. *Clin. Cancer Res.* 2005;11(14):5300-9.

[106] Agus DB, Gordon M, Taylor C, et al. Clinical activity in a phase I trial of HER-2-targeted rhuMAb 2C4 (pertuzumab) in patients with advanced solid malignancies (AST) [abstract 771]. *Proc. Am. Soc. Clin. Oncol.* 2003;22:192.

[107] Johnson Be, Janne PA. Rationale of a phase II trial of pertuzumab, a HER-2 dimerization inhibitor, in patients with non-small cell lung cancer. *Clin. Cancer Res.* 2006; 12(14Pt2):4436s-4440s.

[108] Shigematsu H, Takahashi T, Nomura M, et al. Somatic mutations of the HER2 kinase domain in lung adenocarcinomas. *Cancer Res.* 2006, 65:1642-46.

[109] Cappuzzo F, Gregorc V, Rossi E, et al. Gefitinib in pretreated non-small cell lung cancer (NSCLC): analysis of efficacy and correlation with HER2 and epidermal growth factor receptor expression in locally advanced or metastatic NSCLC. *J. Clin. Oncol.* 2003; 21:2658-63.

[110] Valbohmer D, Brabender J, Yang DY, et al. Sex differences in the predictive power of the molecular prognostic factor HER2/neu in patients with non-small-cell lung cancer. *Clin. Lung Cancer.* 2006;7(5):332-7.

[111] Huncharek M, Muscat J, Geschwind JF. K-ras oncogene mutation as a prognostic marker in non-small cell lung cancer. A combined analysis of 881 cases. *Carcinogenesis.* 1999; 20:1507-10.

[112] Downward J. Ras signaling and apoptosis. *Curr. Opin. Genet Dev.* 1998; 8:9-54.

[113] Liu M, Du W, Liu JP, Jessell TM, Prendergast GC. RhoB alteration is necessary for apoptotic and antineoplastic responses to farnesyltransferase inhibitors. *Mol. Cell Biol.* 2000; 20(16) 6105-13.

[114] Ashar HR, James L. Gray K et al. Farnesyl transferase inhibitors block the farnesylation of CENP-E and CENP-F and alter the association of CENP-E with the microtubules. *J. Biol. Chem.* 2000; 275(39): 30451-7.

[115] Jiang K, Coppola D, Crespo NC et al. The phosphoinisitide 3-OH kinase/AKT2 pathway as a critical target for farnesyltransferase inhibitor-induced apoptosis. *Mol. Cell Biol.* 2000; 20(1): 139-48.

[116] End DW, Smets G, Todd AV et al. Characterization of the antitumour effects of the selective farnesyl protein transferase inhibitor R115777 in vivo and in vitro. *Cancer Res.* 2001; 61(1): 131-7.

[117] Nagasu T, Yoshimatsu K, Rowell C, Lewis MD, Garcia AM. Inhibition of human tumour xenograft growth by treatment with the farnesyl transferase inhibitor B956. *Cancer Res.* 1995; 55(22): 5310-4.

[118] Bernhard EJ, McKenna WG, Hamilton AD et al. Inhibiting Ras prenylation increases the radiosensivity of human tumour cell lines with activating mutations of ras oncogenes. *Cancer Res.* 1998; 58:1754-61.

[119] Moaser MM, Sepp-Lorenzino L, Kohl NE et al. Farnesyl transferase inhibitors cause enhanced mitotic sensivity to Taxol and epothilones. *Proc. Natl. Acad. Sci. USA.* 1998;95:1369-74.

[120] Rak J, Mitsuhashi Y, Bayko L et al. Mutant ras oncogenes upregulate VEG/vPF expression: Implications for induction and and inhibition of tumour angiogenesis. *Cancer Res.* 1995; 55:4574-80.

[121] Evans TL, Fidias P, Scarin A et al. A phase II study of efficacy and tolerability of the farnesyl-protein transferase inhibitor L-778,123 as first-line therapy in patients with advanced non-small cell lung cancer (NSCLC). *Proc. Am. Soc. Clin. Oncol.* 2002; 2:13a.

[122] Britten CD, Rowinsky EK, Soignet S et al. A phase I and pharmacological study of the farnesyl-protein transferase inhibitor L-778,123 in patients with solid malignancies. *Clin. Cancer Res.* 2001; 7(12): 3894-903.

[123] Adjei AA, Erlichman C, David JN et al. A phase I trial of the farnesyl transferase inhibitor SCH66336: evidence for biological and clinical activity. *Cancer Res.* 2000; 60: 1171-7.

[124] Khuri FR, Glisson BS, Kim ES et al. Phase I study of the farnesyl transferase inhibitor lonafarnib with paclitaxel in solid tumours. *Clin. Cancer Res.* 2004; 10:2968-76.

[125] Kim ES, Kies MS, Fossela FV et al. A phase I/II study of the farnesyl transferase inhibitor (FTI) SCH66336 (lonafarnib) with paclitaxel in taxane-refractory/resistant patients with non-small cell lung cancer (NSCLC): final report [abstract]. *Proc. Ann. Meet Assoc. Cancer Res.* 2002; 43:2735.

[126] Blumenschein G, Ludwig C, Thomas G et al. A randomized phase III trial comparing ionafarnib/carboplatin/paclitaxel versus carboplatin/paclitaxel in chemotherapy naive

patients with advanced or metastatic non small cell lung cancer [abstract O-082]. *Lung Cancer.* 2005; 49(Suppl 2):S30.

[127] Schellens JHM, de Klerk G, Swart M et al. Phase I and pharmacologic study of the novel farnesyltransferase inhibitor (FTI) R115777 [abstract 715]. Program and abstracts of the 36th Annual Meeting of the American Society of Clinical Oncology; 2000 May 20-23; New Orleans, Louisiana.

[128] Adjei AA, Mauer A, Bruzek L et al. Phase II study of the farnesyl transferase inhibitor R115777 in patients with advanced non-small cell lung cancer. *J. Clin. Oncol.* 2003; 21:1760-6.

[129] Rose WC, Lee FYF, Fairchild CR et al. Preclinical anitumour activity of BMS-214662, a highly apoptotic and novel farnesyltransferase inhibitor. *Cancer Res.* 2001; 61:7507-17.

[130] Ryan DP, Eder JP Jr, Puchlaski T et al. Phase I clinical trial of the farnesyltranferase inhibitor BMS-214662 given as a 1-hour intravenous infusion in patients with advanced solid tumours. *Clin. Cancer Res.* 2004; 10:2222-30.

[131] Mackay HJ, Hoekstra R, Eskens FA et al. A phase I pharmacokinetic and pharmacodynamic study of the farnesyl transferase inhibitor BMS-214662 in combination with cisplatin in patients with advanced solid tumours. *Clin. Cancer Res.* 2004; 10:2636-44.

[132] Dy GK, Bruzek LM, Croghan GA et al. A phase I trial of a novel farnesyl protein transferase inhibitor, BMS-214662, in combination with paclitaxel and carboplatin in patients with advanced cancer. *Clin. Cancer Res.* 2005; 11:1877-1883.

In: Lung Cancer in Women
Editor: Varetta N. Torres, pp. 195-212
ISBN: 978-1-60021-659-6


*Chapter IX*

# WOMEN AND LUNG CANCER: CLINICAL AND MOLECULAR PROFILING AS A TOOL FOR TREATMENT DECISIONS. A LITERATURE REVIEW

***Rossana Berardi*[*], *Lorena Verdecchia, Mario Scartozzi, Chiara Pierantoni, Paola Mazzanti and Stefano Cascinu***
Clinica di Oncologia Medica, Azienda Ospedaliero-Universitaria Ospedali Riuniti Umberto I – GM Lancisi – G Salesi di Ancona, Italy

## ABSTRACT

In the past decade the incidence of lung cancer among women has risen, whereas among men it has slightly declined. The link between smoking and lung cancer has been well established in both men and women. However, gender-based difference in susceptibility to smoking-related lung cancer have been found, with women showing a higher risk than men of developing lung cancer for a given level of tobacco consumption. An increasing number of lung cancer cases have also been documented in non-smokers and a disproportionate number of these are adenocarcinomas and occur in women. Several case-control studies showed that long-term, regular exposure to either residential or occupational environmental tobacco smoke is associated with increased lung cancer risk in never-smoking women. Exposure to coal fumes, as well as hormonal effects, have been suggested as potential risk factors for lung cancer in non smoking women. Individual susceptibility factors may also be important in the development of lung cancer. These factors may include family history of lung cancer, personal history of lung disease (asthma, chronic bronchitis, pneumonia, or tuberculosis), diet and specific xenobiotic metabolic profiles.

[*] Correspondence to: Rossana Berardi, MD; Clinica di Oncologia Medica; Università Politecnica delle Marche – Azienda Ospedaliero-Universitaria Ospedali Riuniti Umberto I – GM Lancisi – G Salesi di Ancona; Via Conca 71; 60020 Ancona; Italy; Tel.:+39 071 5964169; Fax: +39 071 5964192; E-mail: r.berardi@univpm.it

In never-smoking women several lung cancer susceptibility genes have been proposed, and enzymes activating or detoxifying chemical carcinogens have been investigated. Some studies analyzed germline polymorphisms in genes that have been associated with cancer susceptibility and whose products activate (cytochrome P450 1A1=CYP1A1) and detoxify (glutatione S-transferases M1=GSTM1 and T1=GSTT1) chemical carcinogens found in tobacco smoke.

We extensively reviewed the published scientific literature on this topic in order to investigate the clinical and genetic profiling underlying lung cancer in women and to use this information as a tool for medical therapy.

This review is divided in two parts, in the first one we illustrated the clinical and pathological carachteristics of lung cancer in women and the differences between women and men in terms of results and toxicity to therapies. In the second part we analysed the molecular targets focusing on women and the future perspectives in particular based on target therapies.

## Introduction

Despite the progresses of the last years in the diagnosis and treatment (radio and chemotherapy), Non-Small Cell Lung Cancer (NSCLC) remains the leading cause of death due to tumour worldwide. Actually the incidence and mortality are higher in the developed countries, expecially in Europe and USA, with an increasing in the women. [1]

Female lung cancer mortality rates have dramatically increased since 1950, and in 1987 lung cancer surpassed breast cancer as the leading cause of cancer death among USA women. The epidemiology of this disease in women is different, with tobacco smoking explaining only 70% of the incidence. Moreover, even if smoking is the primary cause of lung cancer, the reported duration and amount smoked is generally lower than in men with equivalent disease. [2-4]

Recent epidemiologic studies demonstrated that risk factors of lung cancer differ according to histological types. Among the major risk factors, cigarette smoking was found to be strongly associated with squamous cell and small cell carcinoma, but less strongly with adenocarcinomas [5, 6]. Some studies indicated that saturated fat intake, familial tumor history, previous lung diseases, specific occupational exposure, cooking practices, and genetic susceptibility are correlated with an elevated risk of adenocarcinoma of the lung. [7, 8]

The cell type distribution of lung cancer differed notably across gender and the frequency of adenocarcinoma is greater in women. This may be partly explained by historic differences in smoking patterns so that a higher proportion of women with lung cancer are non-smokers, but the risk factors between the genders, as well as between histological types, were heterogeneous. Some risk factors such as hormonal factors, radon, passive smoking, diet, pollution and personal history of lung disease, may play a role and have been investigated to define their influence in the development of women lung cancer. [9, 13]

We extensively reviewed the published scientific literature on this topic in order to investigate the clinical and genetic profiling underlying lung cancer in women and to use this information as a tool for medical therapy.

In fact, molecular alterations may constitute a molecular target to innovative therapies that with introduction of new biological agents (i.e. EGFR- or VEGF-targeted antineoplastic molecules) will be hopefully soon available to the practising oncologist.

We used the MEDLINE database, the search was restricted to English-language publications and works in abstract form were considered only if they focused on new target therapies. Where results were reported or updated in more than one publication, only the most recent was used.

This review is divided in two parts, in the first one we illustrated the clinical and pathological characteristics of lung cancer in women and the differences between women and men in terms of results and toxicity to therapies.

In the second part we analysed the molecular targets focusing on women and the future perspectives in particular based on target therapies.

## A. Clinical and Pathological Characteristics of Lung Cancer in Women

In the recent years, several case-control and cohort studies have investigated the role of tobacco and other known or suspected factors responsible for the risk of developing lung cancer in women.

Smoking prevalence is lower among women than men in most countries. Approximately 22% of women in developed countries and 9% of women in developing countries smoke and the prevalence of female smoking is likely to rise 20% by 2025. This would mean that by 2025 there could be 532 million women smokers [3].

Several studies have established that the association between a personal smoking history and lung cancer is stronger with squamous cell carcinoma and small cell carcinoma than with adenocarcinomas [14]

Therefore, it is not surprising that adenocarcinoma has always represented the majority of lung cancers among non-smokers of both genders, and that adenocarcinoma is the least affected by increasing duration of smoking cessation [15]. The greater proportion of adenocarcinomas among non-smokers in comparison to other cell types may suggest that factors other than smoking may be involved in the etiology of this cell type of lung cancer [16].

In order to investigate the role of tobacco and some other known or suspected factors responsible for the risk of developing adenocarcinoma of the lung, and in order to compare with other cell types (squamous-, small- and large-cell cancers) in Czech women, Zatloukal et al. conducted a case-control study. This report, based on 145 cases of adenocarcinoma of the lung, 221 lung cancer cases of other cell types, and 1624 controls, describes the risk associated with smoking habits, passive smoking, previous lung disease or cancer, diet, and menstrual and pregnancy history [17].

The smoking habits of lung cancer patients were different by cell types. Among adenocarcinomas cases more than one-third (34.5%) of patients were never smokers, and 29.7% were current smokers. On the other hand, patients with other cancer cell types had smoking habit more frequently than cases with adenocarcinoma. As much as 39.2% of women with squamous-cell cancer, 51.6% with small-cell cancer, and 38.5% with large-cell cancer were current smokers. Among controls, 23.7% were current smokers while more than one-half (54.7%) were never smokers.

Significant associations of risk with cigarette smoking were found both for adenocarcinoma, and for squamous-, small- and large-cell cancers combined. However, the risk estimates (ORs) were lower for adenocarcinoma. It should be pointed out that the risk estimates among short-term ex-smokers (<10 years ago) and current smokers were higher than among ex-smokers who stopped smoking 10 or more years ago.

Lung cancer risk among female former smokers has been shown to decrease with increasing duration of smoking abstinence. Case-control and cohort studies showed a 50% or greater lung cancer risk reduction in the first decade of smoking abstinence for female former smokers compared with current smokers. However, the time that needs to pass before the risk of lung cancer among former smokers reaches the one of never smokers is less clear. Case-control study data have indicated that a higher lung cancer risk persist beyond 10 to 15 years of smoking abstinence and that this risk may decline more quickly for lighter than heavier smokers [18].

During the last years, epidemiologic studies on the association between exposure to environmental tobacco smoke (ETS) and lung cancer have been conducted [19, 20]. Several authors and regulatory agencies have concluded that a causal link has been established, whereas some authors consider that bias and confounding factors constitute a plausible explanation for the observed association. The available studies are, in most cases, too small to adequately assess the magnitude of the effect and to address specific aspects, such as the shape of the dose-response relationship, the effect of cessation of exposure, the importance of multiple source of ETS exposure, and the interaction of ETS exposure with other risk factors of lung cancer.

Over 40 compounds in environmental tobacco smoke (ETS) are known or probable human carcinogens and several studies indicated that exposure to environmental tobacco smoke from spouses who smoke, is associated with an increased risk of lung cancer. However, evidence for a causal association between ETS and lung cancer has been inconsistently reported across studies. Stockwell et al. observed that lung cancer risk increases with the amount of years exposed to ETS with an odds ratio of 1.1 (95% confidence interval (CI): 0.5—2.6) when exposed to ETS for 18-21 years and an odds ratio of 2.4 (95% CI: 1.1—5.4) when exposed for 22 years or more [21]. However, most previous ETS epidemiological studies have based risk assessment on spousal smoking or co-worker history, potentially underestimating the true risk of lung cancer associated with ETS exposure especially if occurring during childhood [22]. De Andrade et al. in a descriptive study, analyzed the relationships between smoking history, ETS exposure, and lung cancer histological subtypes, 810 women with lung cancer were interviewed to obtain data including the source, intensity, and duration of ETS exposure [23]. Among the 810 patients, 773 (95.4%) reported personal smoking or ETS exposure including 170 of 207 (82%) never smokers. Among the never smokers with a history of ETS exposure, the mean years of exposure were 27 from a smoking spouse, 19 from parents, and 15 from co-workers.

There were 207 (25%) never smokers, 361 (45%) former smokers, and 242 (30%) current smokers. The distribution of a positive history of ETS exposure for never, former, and current smokers, is shown in Table 1 [23].

Among the 810 total patients, only 37 (4.6%) reported no tobacco smoke exposure either through a personal smoking history or ETS exposure.

**Table 1. Smoking status and ETS exposure in 810 female lung cancer patients, Mayo Clinic (1997—2001)**

| Smoking status | ETS exposure (%/%[a]) | | |
|---|---|---|---|
| | No | Yes | Total |
| Never | 37 (18/56) | 170 (82/23) | 207 (100/25) |
| Former | 18 (5/27) | 343 (95/46) | 361 (100/45) |
| Current | 11 (5/17) | 231 (95/31) | 242 (100/30) |
| Total | 66 (8/100) | 744(92/100) | 810 (100/100) |

[a] Row %/column %.

Accurate measurements of ETS are important for establishing dose-response relationships between levels of tobacco smoke exposure and lung cancer. This may be useful for never smokers, former smokers, and light smokers with a history of heavy ETS exposure. ETS exposure has been estimated to be equivalent to personal smoking of 0.1-1 cigarettes per day. Thus, the potential for underestimating the risk of lung cancer with ETS is similar to underestimating the risk from smoking by misclassifying a light smoker as a never smoker [24].

A meta-analysis of six case-control studies on the relationship between reported exposure to environmental tobacco smoke (ETS) and lung cancer in non-smoking Chinese women was performed [19].

This meta-analysis showed no association between exposure to ETS and the risk of lung cancer in non-smoking women. Also, no statistically significant association between the amount or the duration of exposure and risk for lung cancer was found.

It should be noted, however, that non-smoker lung cancer risk factors differ markedly between Chinese and American women. In Chinese women, in addition to ETS, exposure to other potential risks, such as cooking oil vapors, coal-burning smoke, and air pollution must be considered; whereas in American women, research usually concentrates on exposure to ETS.

Many studies have shown that ETS biomarkers, such as urinary nicotine and cotinine, and two urinary metabolites of NNK (tobacco- specific nitrosamine, a tobacco specific lung carcinogen) are higher in non-smokers exposed to tobacco smoke than in unexposed non-smokers.

A recent study was conducted in non-smoking women to test the hypothesis that urinary levels of nicotine, cotinine and the tobacco specific nitrosamine metabolites, NNAL and NNAL-Gluc, would be higher in women exposed to tobacco smoke from their male partner than in unexposed women [25]. The results of this case-control study showed that urinary levels of NNAL and NNAL-Gluc, are statistically significantly higher in women who are exposed to their partner's cigarette smoke than in unexposed women. The geometric mean level of NNAL plus NNAL-Gluc was approximately six fold higher in the exposed women than in unexposed women. This is a small case-control study, but such considerations may be of interest for future studies.

It should be noted about ETS that the actual dose received by individuals is complex and depends on many factors, including smoking behaviour, room size, and ventilation. Even when the conditions are identical, different people exposed to the same concentrations of ETS, receive different doses due to the following factors: age, activity level, and breathing rate. In addition to differences in ETS exposure, functional polymorphisms in enzymes that metabolize carcinogens may cause inter-individual variation in the mutagenic dose.

Recently, a study focusing on the characteristics of non-smoking women living in four areas of Italy was conducted in order to evaluate whether certain risk factors (socio-demographic factors, medical conditions, preventive behaviours and dietary habits) potentially associated with cardiovascular or respiratory diseases and lung cancer could differ among women with and without exposure to ETS from their husbands [26]. The results of this study do not support previous claims of more frequent risk factors for cardiovascular and pulmonary diseases among ETS-exposed subjects, in fact the authors found a few differences in socio-economic and dietary characteristics among non-smoking Italian women exposed and not exposed to spouses who smoke. Such differences would likely to be controlled for when investigating health effects of passive smoking.

Other clinical factors may be associated to the risk of developing lung cancer in women. In a hospital based case-control study, data collected by inperson interviews from 569 female lung cancer cases and 2120 controls were analyzed using unconditional logistic regression stratifying by appropriate factors. Protective effects were observed for intake of milk/dairy products (OR=0.57, 95%CI 0.35-0.94), vegetables (OR=0.60, 95%CI 0.40-0.91), apples (OR=0.69), wine (OR=0.77), and physical exercise (OR=0.59, 95%CI 0.42-0.83) among smokers only, while no similar effects were found among nonsmokers. In contrast, the intake of black tea was associated with a protective effect (OR=0.66, 95%CI 0.47-0.94) among nonsmokers only [27]. Radzikowska et al. analysed data regarding demographics, smoking, histology, treatment and survival obtained from 20561 lung cancer patients diagnosed in Poland from 1995 to 1998.

Lung cancer was six times more frequent in men than in women. Women with lung cancer were younger than men and smoked less intensively. Over-representation of adenocarcinoma and small cell lung cancer (SCLC) was observed in the women. Women with lung cancer had a better prognosis than men [28]. Recently another study evaluated the risk factors and trends of lung cancer between genders.

A prospective cohort of consecutive patients with non-small cell lung cancer (NSCLC) who were carefully clinically and pathologically staged with stage I, II, or III disease underwent homogenous treatment algorithms and were followed up over a period of 7 years. There were 1,085 patients (671 men and 414 women). Groups were similar for race, pulmonary function, smoking history, comorbidities, neoadjuvant therapy, histology, and resection rates. Women were younger ($p = 0.014$), had a higher incidence of adenocarcinoma ($p = 0.01$), and presented at an earlier pathologic stage ($p = 0.01$) than men. The overall age-adjusted and stage-adjusted 5-year survival rate favored women (60% vs 50%, respectively; $p < 0.001$). Women had better stage-specific 5-year survival rates (stage I disease, 69% vs

64%, respectively [p = 0.034]; stage II disease, 60% vs 50%, respectively [p = 0.042]; and stage III disease, 46% vs 37%, respectively [p = 0.024]). Women who received neoadjuvant chemotherapy alone (n = 76) were more likely to be a complete or partial responder than men (n = 142; p = 0.025) [29].

In never-smoking women several lung cancer susceptibility genes have also been proposed, and enzymes activating or detoxifying chemical carcinogens have been investigated. Some studies analyzed germ line polymorphisms in genes that have been associated with cancer susceptibility and whose products activate (cytochrome P450 1A1=CYP1A1) and detoxify (glutationeS-transferases M1=GSTM1 and T1=GSTT1) chemical carcinogens found in tobacco smoke.

CYP1A1 is a phase I enzyme that catalyzes key reactions in the metabolic activation of polycylic aromatic hydrocarbons [30], and functional studies suggest that the variant genotypes of this enzyme are associated with greater CYP1A1 activity or inducibility [31-33]. While CYP1A1 is involved with the activation of pre-carcinogens, enzymes of the glutathione S-transferase (GST) family, including GSTM1 and GSTT1, are involved in the detoxification of such activated pre-carcinogens, including PAH-derived epoxides, by converting them to water-soluble conjugates [34]. The accumulated evidence suggests that individuals null for GSTM1 are at increased risk of lung cancer [35] and those who also possess CYP1A1 polymorphisms appear to have an even higher risk implying possible gene–gene interactions [36].

In a case-control study, the authors examined whether polymorphisms of CYP1A1, confer an increased risk of lung cancer in lifetime non-smoking Chinese women [37].

A total of 126 incident lung cancer cases, of which 87.7% were pathologically confirmed, and 162 ages matched hospital controls were included. CYP1A1 MspI and Ile462Val polymorphisms were genotyped and tested for association with this disease. An elevated risk of lung cancer was observed among individuals with the MspI CC (OR=1.7, 95% CI=0.9–3.3) and Ile462Val ValVal genotypes (OR=2.8, 95% CI=1.1–7.6). After stratifying by environmental tobacco smoke (ETS) exposure, the risk of lung cancer associated with both polymorphisms was higher among individuals with lower exposure to ETS, compared with those who reported at least weekly exposure. Individuals with the MspI CC genotype showed a two-fold higher risk of lung cancer if they were also null for either glutathione S-transferase M1 (GSTM1) or T1 (GSTT1).

In another case-control study, Bennett et al. [38] find that the GSTM1 homozygous null genotype is associated with a statistically significant lung cancer risk in never-smoking women exposed to high levels of ETS which suggests that the observed excess lung cancer risk among never-smoking women results from cancers in two distinct groups: one that is genetically at high risk and one that is genetically at lower risk of lung cancer from exposure to ETS. Additional studies are needed to confirm these observations and to investigate the contributions of other detoxification pathways to lung cancer risk.

# B. Molecular Targets and Future Therapeutics Perspectives in Women Lung Cancer

In the last few years, clinical and translational research in oncology has focused on the development of new anticancer agents, targeting the unique molecular profile of tumor cells with the aim to improve both the efficacy and specificity of cancer therapies and to decrease toxicity and side effects.

Several molecular targets have been suggested in NSCLC; and in this part of the review we will focus on those that were more extensively analysed in NSCLC, with particular regard to women.

## EGFR Expression and EGFR Mutations

The Epidermal growth factor receptor (EGFR) gene is frequently expressed in solid tumours, and in some tumours the expression of the gene correlates with a poor clinical outcome.

EGFR is over expressed in 40 to 80% of NSCLC patients and is therefore an important target of interest for therapy in this disease.

The kinase inhibitors erlotinib (Tarceva) and gefitinib (Iressa) have been studied most extensively in clinical trials.

In the IDEAL trials, the EGFR tyrosine kinase inhibitor gefitinib (Iressa) showed antitumor activity in 10% to 20% of patients with previously treated advanced NSCLC. Another 20% of patients had stable disease as their best response. In both patients with stable disease and response, tumor-related symptoms improved. Accordingly, gefitinib has been approved for the treatment of advanced NSCLC in the United States by the Food and Drug Administration and in Japan [39, 40]. The INTACT trials, however, failed to find a benefit in the first-line setting for gefitinib added to standard chemotherapy regimens (cisplatin/gemcitabine or carboplatin/paclitaxel) [41, 42]. These major negative findings raised questions regarding the preclinical models that had shown synergistic or additive effects of chemotherapy and gefitinib. Although response to gefitinib did not correlate with EGFR expression, in the IDEAL trials [43] a rapid improvement in disease related symptoms was observed in patients who went on to respond, an observation that, if confirmed, may be useful in clinical decision-making. Women, patients with adenocarcinomas histology, and never-smokers were more likely to respond to gefitinib. No correlation between treatment response and the degree of skin toxicity was reported in the IDEAL studies, in contrast to the studies with erlotinib. Patients with bronchioalveolar carcinoma appear to constitute a distinct subpopulation that have only limited response to chemotherapy but possibly superior response rates to EGFR tyrosine kinase inhibitors.

It is worth noting that adenocarcinoma is the most frequent histological type in women, and bronchioalveolar carcinoma is also more common in women [44].

Studies of response in these patients may serve to identify predictive markers of efficacy for the anti-EGFR agents in other patient subgroups.

The National Cancer Institute of Canada Clinical Trials Group (NCIC CTG) conducted a trial (BR.21) to compare erlotinib with placebo after the failure of standard chemotherapy for non–small-cell lung cancer. In this study, the authors found that the overall response rate was higher among women ($p=0.006$), non-smokers ($p<0.001$), patient with adenocarcinomas ($p<0.001$) and patient in whom 10 percent or more of the tumor cell expressed EGFR ($p=0.10$) [45].

Median overall survival in the erlotinib group was 6.7 months, and in the placebo group it was 4.7 months (adjusted hazard ratio, 0.70; 95% confidence interval, 0.58 to 0.85; $P<0.001$). In the Cox regression analysis, erlotinib remained associated with longer survival ($P=0.002$), as did Asian origin ($P=0.01$), adenocarcinoma on histological examination ($P=0.004$), and never having smoked ($P=0.048$ vs. current or past smoking). Although the sample sizes may be inadequate to detect small or moderate differences, a benefit from erlotinib was apparent in most of the subgroups. The interaction between treatment and the covariate defining the subgroup was statistically significant only for smoking status. Median progression-free survival was 2.2 months in the erlotinib group and 1.8 months in the placebo group (adjusted hazard ratio, 0.61; 95 percent confidence interval, 0.51 to 0.74; $P<0.001$). In the Cox model, treatment with erlotinib ($P<0.001$) and never having smoked ($P<0.01$ for the comparison with current or past smoking) were associated with longer progression-free survival.

Exploratory multivariate analyses showed that only Asian origin, adenocarcinoma on histological examination, and a history of not smoking were significant independent predictors of survival after adjustment for treatment and other potential predictors. Erlotinib had a beneficial effect on survival in almost all subgroups tested, but only the interaction between smoking status and treatment was significantly predictive of a differential effect on survival.

Finally, these two oral EGFR TK inhibitors have shown to be effective for relieving symptoms, maintaining stable disease, and improving quality of life without the adverse events that may be associated with cytotoxic cancer therapies.

The frequency of EGFR mutations in NSCLCs were reported 26% to 40% in Asian patients and 2% to 12% in non-Asian patients, and almost all mutations were detected in adenocarcinoma. It was also reported that EGFR mutations were more frequent in females and in never smokers [46-50].

On the other hand, Huang et al. reported that there was no significant association EGFR mutation with gender and smoking history [51]. Specific mutations in the tyrosine kinase domain of EGFR are associated with sensitivity to either gefitinib or erlotinib, but mechanisms of acquired resistance have not yet been reported.

Recent data, reported simultaneously by two research groups, have shown that the presence of mutations within the EGFR gene can distinguish responders from nonresponders. In particular, Lynch et al. [52] found heterozygous mutations within the TK domain of *EGFR* in eight of nine tumors obtained from patients who had responded to gefitinib. On the contrary, no mutations were documented in seven nonresponders. Paez et al. [53] found that five of five tumors from gefitinib-responsive patients harbored EGFR kinase domain mutations, while tumors from patients who progressed on gefitinib were not affected by mutations. In both studies, conducted by mutational analysis of the entire EGFR coding sequence, only genetic alterations in exons 19, 21, and 18 were found.

These results could assist to select patients who should be treated by gefitinib or erlotinib.

Another new drug targeting EGFR is cetuximab, an immunoglobulin G1 monoclonal antibody that binds with high affinity to the extracellular region of human EGFR. Cetuximab prevents endogenous ligands from binding to EGFR and disrupts the cell signaling pathway, leading to tumor proliferation. In preclinical experiments and clinical trials, cetuximab demonstrated antitumor activity in a variety of solid tumors [54]. In NSCLC cetuximad showed promising activity, too, but no definitive data on women are available [55-57]. Furthermore it may be possible to find EGFR tyrosine kinase inhibitors that bind to the EGFR kinase domain in different ways than gefitinib and erlotinib. For example, the crystal structure of another EGFR inhibitor, lapatinib (GW572016), was recently solved bound to EGFR [58]. This study revealed that the quinazoline rings of erlotinib and lapatinib interact differently with the EGFR kinase domain, suggesting that while the mutations may affect inhibition by erlotinib and gefitinib, it may not affect inhibition of EGFR by compounds similar to lapatinib.

A number of other new inhibitors are currently in clinical development with different spectra of activity or mechanisms of receptor inhibition. These include monoclonal antibodies, such as panitumumab and matuzumab; dual inhibitors of EGFR and vascular endothelial growth factor receptor, such as ZD6474 and AEE788 and irreversible inhibitors, such as canertinib and HKI272. Preclinical studies suggest that several of these agents, such us the above mentioned lapatinib, may have activity in tumors refractory to erlotinib or gefitinib. Among these agents, ZD6474 has undergone the most extensive clinical testing.

However, to date, no data on activity in lung cancer female are available.

Research efforts are attempting to identify molecular markers and corresponding clinical features that will allow physicians to individualize patients' therapy and that can predict patients (and in particular female) more likely to respond to anti-EGFR therapy.

## VEGF

The vascular endothelial growth factor (VEGF) is a glycoprotein similar to the platelet-derived growth factor and it is considered as the main angiogenic stimulator [59]. The role of vascular endothelial growth factor in promoting tumor angiogenesis, in maintaining existing vasculature, and in resistance to traditional therapies, together with its negative prognostic significance in NSCLC, make it an appropriate target for therapy. VEGF expression is upregulated in a range of solid tumors and is greatest in hypoxic tumor cells near necrotic areas, suggesting that hypoxia-induced VEGF is vital for the development of tumor vasculature [60]. Moreover, microvessel count, which is an indication of angiogenic effect, is an independent predictor of poor prognosis in patients with NSCLC [61]. Bevacizumab is the recombinant humanized version of the murine antihuman VEGF monoclonal antibody. In phase I trials, bevacizumab was generally well tolerated and was not associated with a dose-limiting toxicity [62]. When combined with classical cytotoxic chemotherapy agents, there was no exacerbation of expected toxicities [63]. Encouraging antitumor activity has also been observed when bevacizumab was combined with paclitaxel plus carboplatin in chemotherapy-naïve patients with advanced NSCLC in a small randomized phase II trial [64]. Again, also in trials employing bevacizumab in NSCLC, data on female are not reported.

## HER-2

The HER-2 proto-oncogene (HER2/neu/c-erbB-2) encodes a transmembrane tyrosine kinase receptor that shares homology with the epidermal growth factor receptor family [65]. Overexpression of this oncogene has been reported in many human carcinomas and it has been shown to represent an independent marker of poor prognosis in primary breast cancer and in pulmonary adenocarcinomas [66, 67]. HER2 overexpression has been reported in approximately 10–15% of NSCLCs, with a reported incidence as high as 30% in adenocarcinomas [68, 69].

This overexpression is associated with poor prognosis and shortened survival [70-72].

The humanized anti-HER2 monoclonal antibody, trastuzumab (Herceptin), the first oncogene-targeted drug for solid tumor therapy, has efficacy only in HER2-positive tumors, i.e., those with amplification/overexpression [73].

Recently, trastuzumab has been investigated in a phase II trial in NSCLC by Krug et al. Weekly docetaxel plus trastuzumab was compared with weekly paclitaxel plus trastuzumab in patients with previously untreated advanced NSCLC. No difference was noted in the median survival (16 months versus 14 months) or 1-year survival (57% vs. 55%) (P=0.998). Toxicities were mild in both treatment arms and no difference with regard to response rates or survival was noted between HER-2-positive (2+ or 3+) and HER-2-negative (0-1+) patients. Results were not considered encouraging enough by the authors to test the regimen in a Phase III trial [74]. Recently, another international, multi-institutional consortium conducted a randomized phase II study of cisplatin and gemcitabine ±trastuzumab. Eligibility stipulated HER-2/neu positivity as defined by one of the following: 2+ or 3+ expression by IHC. Nearly 600 patients were screened at 60 sites. One hundred three patients were enrolled. The response rate and time to progression in the chemotherapy-only group were 41% and 7.2 months, respectively, versus 36% and 6.3 months for patients receiving combination gemcitabine/cisplatin/trastuzumab. Of note, the median PFS was 8.7 months for those whose tumors proved FISH positive or who had 3+ expression and received the three drug combination (six patients total) [75].

In view of the limited target population for HER2 inhibition, the majority of the efforts and resources are currently directed toward molecular targets other than HER2 in NSCLC.

For the above mentioned reason, data on women with lung cancer are not available.

Pertuzumab (rhuMAb 2C4), a humanized HER2 antibody, represents a new class of targeted therapeutics that inhibit dimerization of HER2 with ligand-activated EGFR (HER1), HER3, and HER-4. Pertuzumab can have antitumor activity in patients with HER-2 present on the tumor without gene amplification or 3+ staining by immunohistochemistry.

A phase II trial with pertuzumab was undertaken for patients with relapsed NSCLC. None of the 33 patients enrolled with evaluable disease had a response to the treatment, therefore pertuzumab seems to have an appropriate rationale for therapeutic use in patients with NSCLC [76].

## CONCLUSION

Although several clinical and molecular markers have been studied in women affected by lung cancer, their potential role in the treatment and prognostic stratification of these patients have not been completely defined, yet.

Available data are interesting, showing a different potential use of new drugs in women than in men; but most of them arise from retrospective studies with relatively small number of patients or from exploratory analysis of clinical trials which did not represent objectives of the studies and were performed after the completion of the trials.

Prospective studies in a large number of patients are required to be a diagnostic tool for selection of the treatment method based on molecular classification.

Research efforts should continue to focus on identifying molecular markers and corresponding clinical features that will allow physicians to individualize patients' therapy.

## REFERENCES

[1] Gusterson BA, Gelber RD, Goldhirsch A, Price KN, Save-Soderborgh J, Anbazhagan R, Styles J, Rudenstam CM, Golouh R, Reed R. Prognostic importance of c-erbB2 expression in breast cancer. *J. Clin. Oncol.* 1992;10:1049-1056.

[2] Kern JA, Slebos RJ, Top B, Rodenhuis S, Lager D, Robinson RA, Weiner D, Schwartz DA. C-erbB2 expression and codon 12 k-ras both predict shortened survival for patients with pulmonary adenocarcinomas. *J. Clin. Invest.* 1994;93:516-520.

[3] Kern JA, Slebos R.J, Top B, Rodenhuis S, Lager D, Robinson R A, Weiner D, Schwartz DA. C-erbB-2 expression and codon K-ras mutations both predict shortened survival for patients with pulmonary adenocarcinomas. *J. Clin. Investig.* 1994,93:516-520,.

[4] Tateishi M., Ispida T., Mitsudomi T., Kaneko S., Sugimachi K. Prognostic value of c-erbB-2 protein expression in human lung adenocarcinoma and squamous cell carcinoma. *Eur. J. Cancer.* 1991;27:1372-1375.

[5] Harpole D. H., Jr., Marks J. R., Richards W. G., Herndon J. E., 2nd, Sugarbaker D. J. Localized adenocarcinoma of the lung. Oncogene expression of erbB-2 and p53 in 150 patients. *Clin. Cancer Res.* 1995;1:659-664.

[6] Shi D., He G., Cao S., Pan W., Zhang H. Z., Yu D., Hung M. C. Williams MD, Sandler AB. The epidemiology of lung cancer. Cancer Treat Res. 2001;105:31-52.

[7] Kreuzer M, Boffetta P, Whitley E, Ahrens W, et al. Gender differences in lung cancer risk by smoking: a multicentre case-control study in Germany and Italy. *Br. J. Cancer.* 2000;82(1):227-333.

[8] Zang EA, Wynder EL. Differences in lung cancer risk between men and women: examination of the evidence. *J. Natl. Cancer Inst.* 1996 Feb 21;88(3-4):183-92

[9] Mackay J, Amos A. Women and tobacco. *Respirology,* 2003; 8(2): 123-30.

[10] Boffetta P, Agudo A, Ahrens W, Benhamou E, Benhamou S, Darby SC, et al. Multicenter case–control study of exposure to environmental tobacco smoke and lung cancer in Europe. *J. Natl. Cancer Inst.* 1998;90:1440–50.

[11] Sobue T, Yamamoto S, Hara M, Sasazuki S, Sasaki S, Tsugane S; JPHC Study Group. Japanese Public Health Center. Cigarette smoking and subsequent risk of lung cancer by histologic type in middle-aged Japanese men and women: the JPHC study. *Int. J. Cancer.* 2002;99(2):245-51.

[12] Speizer FE, Colditz GA, Hunter DJ, et al. Prospective study of smoking, antioxidant intake, and lung cancer in middle-aged women (USA). *Cancer Causes Control.* 1999;10:475-482.

[13] Burns DM. Primary prevention, smoking, and smoking cessation: implications for future trends in lung cancer prevention. *Cancer.* 2000;89:2506-2509.

[14] Johnson KC, Hu J, Mao Y; Canadian Cancer Registries Epidemiology Research Group. Lifetime residential and workplace exposure to environmental tobacco smoke and lung cancer in never-smoking women, Canada 1994-97. *Int. J. Cancer.* 2001 Sep;93(6):902-6.

[15] Seow A, Poh Wee-Teng, Teh M, Eng P, Wang Yee-Tang, Tan Wan-Cheng, Yu MC, and Lee Hin-Peng. Fumes from Meat Cooking and Lung Cancer Risk in Chinese Women. *Cancer Epidemiology, Biomarkers and Prevention.* 2000;9:1215–1221.

[16] Blackman JA, Coogan PF, Rosenberg L, Strom BL, Zauber AG, Palmer JR, Langenberg P, Shapiro S. Estrogen replacement therapy and risk of lung cancer. *Pharmacoepidemiol Drug Saf.* 2002;11(7):561-7.

[17] Behera D, Balamugesh T. Indoor air pollution as a risk factor for lung cancer in women. *J. Assoc. Physicians India.* 2005;53:190-2.

[18] Brenner AV, Wang Z, Kleinerman RA, Lei S, Metayer C, Wang W, Lubin JH. Menstrual and reproductive factors and risk of lung cancer among Chinese women, Eastern Gansu Province, 1994-1998. *J. Epidemiol.* 2003;13(1):22-8.

[19] Khuder SA. Effect of cigarette smoking on major histological types of lung cancer: a meta-analysis. *Lung Cancer.* 2001;31:139-48.

[20] Khuder SA, Mutgi AB. Effect of smoking cessation on major histologic types of lung cancer. *Chest.* 120:1577-1583, 2001.

[21] Franceschi S, Bidoli E. The epidemiology of lung cancer. *Ann. Oncol.* 1999;10(l 5):S3-S6.

[22] Zatloukal P, Kubik A, Pauk N, Tomasek L, Petruzelka L. Adenocarcinoma of the lung among women: risk associated with smoking, prior lung disease, diet and menstrual and pregnancy history. *Lung Cancer.* 2003;41(3):283-93.

[23] Ebbert JO, Yang P, Vachon, Vierkant RA, Cerhan JR, Folsom AR, and Sellers TA. Lung Cancer Risk Reduction After Smoking Cessation: Observations From a Prospective Cohort of Women. *J. Clin. Oncol.* 2003,21(5):921-926.

[24] Wang TJ, Zhou BS. Meta-analysis of the potential relationship between exposure to environmental tobacco smoke and lung cancer in non-smoking Chinese women. *Lung Cancer.* 1997;16(2-3):145-50.

[25] Enstrom JE, Kabat GC. Environmental tobacco smoke and tobacco related mortality in a prospective study of Californians, 1960—98. *BMJ.* 2003;326:1057-66.

[26] Stockwell HG, Goldman AL, Lyman GH, Noss CI, et al. Environmental tobacco smoke and lung cancer risk in non-smoking women. *J. Natl. Cancer Inst.* 1992;84(18):1417-22.

[27] National Cancer Institute. Health effects of exposure to environmental tobacco smoke. The Report of the California Environmental Protection Agency. Smoking and Tobacco Control, Monograph no. 10. Bethesda (MD): US Department of Health and Human Services, National Institutes of Health, National Cancer Institute 1999, NIH Publ 99:4645.

[28] de Andrade M, Ebbert JO, Wampfler JA, Miller DL, Marks RS, Croghan GA, Jatoi A, Finke EE, Sellers TA, Yang P. Environmental tobacco smoke exposure in women with lung cancer. *Lung Cancer.* 2004;43(2):127-34.

[29] Lubin JH. Estimating lung cancer risk with exposure to environmental tobacco smoke. *Environ Health Perspect.* 1999;107:879-83.

[30] Anderson KE, Carmella SG, Ye M, Bliss RL, Le C, Murphy L, Hecht SS. Metabolites of a Tobacco-Specific Lung Carcinogen in non-smoking Women Exposed to Environmental Tobacco Smoke. *J. Nat. Cancer Inst.* 2001:93(5).

[31] Forastiere F, Mallone, Lo Presti E, Baldacci S, et al. Characteristics of Nonsmoking Women Exposed to Spouses Who Smoke: Epidemiologic Study on Environment and Health in Women from Four Italian Areas Environmental Health Perspectives 2000;10(12).

[32] Kubik A, Zatloukal P, Toma Ek L, Pauk N, Havel L, Dole Al J, Ple Ko I. Interactions between smoking and other exposures associated with lung cancer risk in women: diet and physical activity. *Neoplasma.* 2007;54(1):83-8.

[33] Radzikowska E, Glaz P, Roszkowski K. Lung cancer in women: age, smoking, histology, performance status, stage, initial treatment and survival. Population-based study of 20 561 cases. *Ann. Oncol.* 2002;13(7):1087-93.

[34] Cerfolio RJ, Bryant AS, Scott E, Sharma M, Robert F, Spencer SA, Garver RI. Women with pathologic stage I, II, and III non-small cell lung cancer have better survival than men. *Chest.* 2006;130(6):1796-80.

[35] Bartsch H, Nair U, Risch A, Rojas M, Wikman H, Alexandrov K Genetic polymorphism of CYP genes, alone or in combination, as a risk modifier of tobacco-related cancers. *Cancer Epidemiol. Biomarkers Prev.* 2000;9: 3–28.

[36] Crofts F, Taioli E, Trachman J, et al. Functional significance of different human CYP1A1 genotypes. *Carcinogenesis.* 1994;15:2961–2963.

[37] Mooney LA, Bell DA, Santella RM, et al. Contribution of genetic and nutritional factors to DNA damage in heavy smokers. *Carcinogenesis.* 1997;18: 503–509.

[38] Nerurkar PV, Okinaka L, Aoki C, et al. CYP1A1, GSTM1,and GSTP1 genetic polymorphisms and urinary 1-hydroxypyrene excretion in non-occupationally exposed individuals. *Cancer Epidemiol. Biomarkers Prev.* 9: 1119–1122(2000).

[39] Hayes JD, Pulford DJ (1995) The glutathione S-transferase supergene family: regulation of GST and the contribution of the isoenzymes to cancer chemoprotection and drug resistance. *Crit. Rev. Biochem. Mol. Biol.* 30: 445–600.

[40] Benhamou S, Lee WJ, Alexandrie AK, et al. (2002) Meta- and pooled analyses of the effects of glutathione S-transferase M1 polymorphisms and smoking on lung cancer risk. *Carcinogenesis.* 23: 1343–1350.

[41] Hung RJ, Boffetta P, Brockmoller J, et al. (2003) CYP1A1 and GSTM1 genetic olymorphisms and lung cancer risk in Caucasian non-smokers: a pooled analysis. *Carcinogenesis.* 24: 875–882.

[42] Ng DPK, Tan Kar-Wai, Zhao B and Seow A. CYP1A1 polymorphisms and risk of lung cancer in non-smoking Chinese women: influence of environmental tobacco smoke exposure and GSTM1/T1 genetic variation. *Cancer Causes and Control.* 2005;16:399–405.

[43] Bennett WP, Alavanja MCR, Blomeke B, Vahakangas KH, et al. Environmental Tobacco Smoke, Genetic Susceptibility, and Risk of Lung Cancer in Never-Smoking Women. *J. Nat. Cancer Inst.* 1999,91(23).

[44] Lynch TJ, Adjei AA, Bunn PA, DuBois RN Novel Agents in the Treatment of Lung Cancer: Conference Summary Statement. *Clin. Cancer Res.* 2004;10:4199s–4204s.

[45] Kris MG, Natale RB, Herbst RS, et al. Efficacy of gefitinib, an inhibitor of the epidermal growth factor receptor tyrosine kinase, in symptomatic patients with non-small cell lung cancer: a randomized trial. *JAMA.* 2003; 290:2149-58.

[46] Herbst RS, Giaccone G, Schiller JH, et al. Gefitinib in combination with paclitaxel and carboplatin in advanced non-small-cell lung cancer: a phase III trial -INTACT 2. *J. Clin. Oncol.* 2004;22:785-94.

[47] Giaccone G, Herbst RS, Manegold C, et al. Gefitinib in combination with gemcitabine and cisplatin in advanced non-small cell lung cancer: a phase III trial - INTACT 1. *J. Clin. Oncol.* 2004;22:777-84.

[48] Fukuoka M, Yano S, Giaccone G, et al. Multi-institutional randomized phase II trial of gefitinib for previously treated patients with advanced non-small-cell lung cancer (the IDEAL Trial). *J. Clin. Oncol.* 2003;21:2237-46.

[49] Rivera, MP, Stover, DE Gender and lung cancer. *Clin. Chest Med.* 2004;25,391-40.

[50] Shepherd FA, Pereira JR, Ciuleanu T, Tan Eng Huat, et al. Erlotinib in Previously Treated Non–Small-Cell Lung Cancer. *N. Engl. J. Med.* 2005;353;2.

[51] Kosaka T, Yatabe Y, Endoh H, Kuwano H, Takahashi T, Mitsudomi T. Mutations of the epidermal growth factor receptor gene in lung cancer: biological and clinical implications. *Cancer Res.* 2004;64:8919–2.

[52] Huang SF, Liu HP, Li LH, et al. High frequency of epidermal growth factor receptor mutations with complex patterns in non-small cell lung cancers related to gefitinib responsiveness in Taiwan. *Clin. Cancer Res.* 2004;10:8195–203.

[53] Marchetti A, Martella C, Felicioni L, et al. EGFR mutations in non-small-cell lung cancer: analysis of a large series of cases and development of a rapid and sensitive method for diagnostic screening with potential implications on pharmacologic treatment. *J. Clin. Oncol.* 2005;23:857–65.

[54] Tokumo M, Toyooka S, Kiura K, et al. The relationship between epidermal growth factor receptor mutations and clinicopathological features in non-small cell lung cancers. *Clin. Cancer Res.* 2005;11:1167–73.

[55] Cappuzzo F, Magrini E, Ceresoli GL, Bartolini S, Rossi E, Ludovini V, Gregorc V, Ligorio C, Cancellieri A, Damiani S, Spreafico A, Paties CT, Lombardo L, Calandri C, Bellezza G, Tonato M, Crino L. Akt phosphorylation and gefitinib efficacy in patients with advanced non-small-cell lung cancer. *J. Natl. Cancer Inst.* 2004;96(15):1133-41).

[56] Huang SF, Liu HP, Li LH, et al. High frequency of epidermal growth factor receptor mutations with complex patterns in non-small cell lung cancers related to gefitinib responsiveness in Taiwan. *Clin. Cancer Res.* 2004;10:8195–203.

[57] Lynch TJ, Bell DW, Sordella R, et al. Activating mutations in the epidermal growth factor receptor underlying responsiveness of non-small-cell lung cancer to gefitinib. *N. Engl. J. Med.* 2004;350:2129–39.

[58] Paez JG, Janne PA, Lee JC, et al. EGFR mutations in lung cancer: correlation with clinical response to gefitinib therapy. *Science.* 2004;304:1497–500.

[59] Baselga J, Arteaga CL. Critical update and emerging trends in epidermal growth factor receptor targeting in cancer. *J. Clin. Oncol.* 2005;23(11):2445-59.

[60] Nasser Hanna, Rogerio Lilenbaum, Rafat Ansari, Thomas Lynch, Ramaswamy Govindan, Pasi A. Jänne, Philip Bonomi. Phase II Trial of Cetuximab in Patients With Previously Treated Non–Small-Cell Lung Cancer. *Journal of Clinical Oncology.* 2006;24(33):5253-5258.

[61] Thienelt C, Bunn P, Hanna N, et al: Multicenter phase I/II study of cetuximab with paclitaxel and carboplatin in untreated patients with stage IV non-small cell lung cancer. *J. Clin. Oncol.* 23 : 8786 -8793, 20.

[62] Rosell R, Daniel C, Ramlau R, et al: Randomized phase II study of cetuximab in combination with cisplatin (C) and vinorelbine (V) vs. CV alone in the first-line

treatment of patients (pts) with epidermal growth factor receptor (EGFR)-expressing advanced non-small cell lung cancer (NSCLC). *J. Clin. Oncol.* 2004;22:620s (abstr 7012).

[63] Wood ER, Truesdale AT, McDonald OB, Yuan D, Hassell A, et al. A unique structure for epidermal growth factor receptor bound to GW572016 (Lapatinib): Relationships among protein conformation, inhibitor off-rate, and receptor activity in tumor cells. *Cancer Res.* 2004;64:6652–6659.

[64] Folkman J. Tumor angiogenesis and tissue factors. *Nature Med.* 1996;2:167-168.

[65] Ferrara N, Davis-Smyth T: The biology of vascular endothelial growth factor. *Endocr. Rev.* 1997;18:4-25.

[66] Fontanini G, Lucchi M, Vignati S, et al: Angiogenesis as a prognostic indicator of survival in non-small-cell lung carcinoma: A prospective study. *J. Natl. Cancer Inst.* 1997;89:881-886.

[67] Gordon MS, Margolin K, Talpaz M, et al: Phase I safety and pharmacokinetic study of recombinant human anti-vascular endothelial growth factor in patients with advanced cancer. *J. Clin. Oncol.* 2001;19:843–850.

[68] Margolin K, Gordon MS, Holmgren E, et al: Phase Ib trial of intravenous recombinant humanized monoclonal antibody to vascular endothelial growth factor in combination with chemotherapy in patients with advanced cancer: Pharmacologic and long-term safety data. *J. Clin. Oncol.* 2001;19:851–856.

[69] Johnson DH, Fehrenbacher L, Novotny WF, Herbst RS, Nemunaitis JJ, Jablons DM, et al. Randomized Phase II Trial Comparing Bevacizumab Plus Carboplatin and Paclitaxel With Carboplatin and Paclitaxel Alone in Previously Untreated Locally Advanced or Metastatic Non-Small-Cell Lung Cancer. *Journal of Clinical Oncology.* 2004;22(11):2184-2191.

[70] Hynes N. E., Stern D. F. The biology of erbB-2/neu/HER-2 and its role in cancer. *Biochem. Biophys. Acta.* 1994;1198:165-184.

[71] Overexpression of the c-erbB-2/neu-encoded P185 protein in primary lung cancer. *Mol. Carcinog.* 1992;5:213-218.

[72] Scheurle D., Jahanzeb M., Aronsohn R. S., Watzek L., Narayanan R. HER-2/neu expression in archival non-small cell lung carcinomas using FDA-approved HercepTest. *Anticancer Res.* 2000;20:2091-2096.

[73] Baselga J., Tripathy D., Mendelsohn J., Baughman S., Benz C. C., Dantis L., Sklarin N. T., Seidman A. D., Hudis C. A., Moore J., Rosen P. P., Twadell T., Henderson I. C., Norton L. Phase II study of weekly intravenous recombinant humanized anti-p185HER2 monoclonal antibody in patients with HER-2/neu-overexpressing metastatic breast cancer. *J. Clin. Oncol.* 1996;14:737-744).

[74] Krug LM, Miller VA, Patel J, Crapanzano J, Azzoli CG, Gomez J, Kris MG, Heelan RT, Pizzo B, Tyson L, Sheehan C, Ross JS, Venkatraman E. Randomized phase II study of weekly docetaxel plus trastuzumab versus weekly paclitaxel plus

trastuzumab in patients with previously untreated advanced nonsmall cell lung carcinoma. *Cancer.* 2005;104(10):2149-55.

[75] Gatzemeier U, Groth G, Butts C, et al: Randomized phase II trial of gemcitabine-cisplatin with or without trastuzumab in HER-2 positive non-small-cell lung cancer. *Ann. Oncol.* 2002;15:19-27.

[76] Johnson BE, Janne PA. Rationale for a phase II trial of pertuzumab, a HER-2 dimerization inhibitor, in patients with non-small cell lung cancer. *Clin. Cancer Res.* 2006;12(14 Pt 2):4436s-4440s.

In: Lung Cancer in Women
Editor: Varetta N. Torres, pp. 213-232

ISBN: 978-1-60021-659-6


*Chapter X*

# LUNG CANCER MOLECULAR PROFILE: DIFFERENCES BETWEEN SEXES

***Efi Nasothimiou, E. M. Karapanagiotou and K.N. Syrigos****

Oncology Unit, 3rd Department of Medicine, Athens Medical School, Sotiria General Hospital, Athens, Greece.

## ABSTRACT

The yearly number of new lung cancer cases in women is increasingly contrary to that of men. Women present an increased susceptibility in getting lung cancer, respond better to chemotherapy and biological therapies and live longer regardless of histology and stage. These statistical observations may be explained through molecular differences between the sexes.

K-ras gene mutations are three times more frequent in women, are associated mainly with adenocarcinoma and pose conflicting prognostic significance. CYP1A1 (P4501A1) overexpression alone or in combination with loss of expression of GSTM1 gene (glutathione S-transferase M1) is also correlated with the development of lung cancer in women. Decreased DNA repair capacity and increased levels of DNA adducts due to p53-pathway alterations or different bioavailability of phase I and phase II detoxifying enzymes correlate with the formation and progression of lung cancer in women. It is worthwhile noting that HER-2/neu is overexpressed in adenocarcinoma without overall survival improvement after the addition of monoclonal antibodies to standard chemotherapy. These basic molecular pathways in carcinogenesis as seen in women will be studied and analyzed with the hope of a better management.

* Address for Correspondence: Konstantinos N. Syrigos, MD, PhD; Assistant Professor of Oncology in Medicine; Athens University School of Medicine; Head, Oncology Unit, Third Department of Medicine; Building Z,

# INTRODUCTION

The yearly number of new lung cancer cases in women is increasingly contrary to that of men. Women present an increased susceptibility in getting lung cancer, develop mainly adenocarcinoma, respond better to chemotherapy or biological therapies and live longer regardless of stage. These statistical observations might be explained in part through molecular differences between the sexes. Genetic and epigenetic alterations of proto-oncogenes and tumor suppressor genes as well as an overexpression or aberrant expression of growth factors receptors present intriguing differences between the sexes. Moreover, decreased DNA repair capacity and increased levels of DNA adducts might correlate with the formation and progression of lung cancer in the female. These basic molecular pathways in carcinogenesis as seen in women will be studied and analyzed with the hope of a better management.

## CYP1AI (P4501A1)

CYP1A1 plays an important role in the metabolism of polycyclic aromatic hydrocarbons (PAHs), an important group of lung carcinogens. The human CYP1A1 gene codes for a central enzyme in the metabolic activation of PAHs, leading to the formation of highly reactive diol-epoxides that may bind to DNA. Polycyclic aromatic hydrocarbons (PAHs) and other tobacco-related carcinogens are oxidized by phase I enzymes into reactive metabolites that are then detoxified by phase II enzymes. Polymorphisms for genes encoding the metabolic enzymes cytochrome P450 1A1 (CYP 1A1) might contribute to the variability in individual susceptibility to lung cancer. The most important CYPs responsible for PAH activation in human lung are CYP1A1 and CYP1B1[1].

## Polymorphisms of CYP1A1 (P4501A1)

Two genetically linked polymorphisms of *CYP1A1*, *MspI* ($T^{3801}C$) and $Ile^{462}Val$, have been associated with increased risk of lung cancer. A one base substitution of thymine by cytosine in a noncoding region of the gene at position 3801 creates a *Msp*I recognition site (*CYP1A1*2A)*, which does not exist in the predominant genotype (*T/T)*. A one base substitution A:T→G:C at position 2455 in the heme-binding region of exon 7 induces an amino acid change of isoleucine to valine at codon 462 ($Ile^{462}Val$ polymorphism) This polymorphism is usually linked with the *MspI* polymorphism (*CYP1A1*2B)*. The presence of the $Ile^{462}Val$ polymorphism alone (*CYP1A1*2C*) is very rare in Caucasians. Another polymorphism in exon 7, i.e. a base substitution of cytosine by adenine at position 2453, leading to the $Thr^{461}Asn$ polymorphism (*CYP1A1*4*), has been also described [2]. The *CYP1A1* polymorphisms have been shown to increase microsomal catalytic activity for

Sotiria General Hospital; Mesogion 152; 115 27 Athens, Greece; Tel: +30 210 7475 034 / Fax: +30 210 7781 035; Email: knsyrigos@usa.net / ksyrigos@med.uoa.gr converting procarcinogens, including PAH and aromatic amines [3]. Positive associations of *CYP1A1* genetic polymorphisms and lung cancer risk were pointed out in an early Japanese study [4]. However, there is no consistent evidence of an association in other ethnic groups. A recent meta-analysis provided little support for an overall role of *CYP1A1* polymorphisms in lung cancer risk [5]. It is suggested that these inconsistencies might be due to the difference in allele frequencies in different populations. In a U.S. population study (more than 90% were Caucasians, (N = 343), women had a larger lung cancer risk than men (odds ratio 4.98 vs. 1.37) if they possessed the mutant type on exon 7 of *CYP1A1*, *CYP1A1*2C*. In this study, female patients with lung cancer were significantly more likely than female controls to have both the *CYP1A1* mutation and glutathione S-transferase (GST) M1 null genotype. The combined variant genotypes conferred an odds ratio of 6.54 for lung cancer in women versus 2.36 for men, independent of age or smoking history[5]. According to the data above, there was a meta-analysis of 11 studies, indicating that the *CYP1A1* exon 7 polymorphism may confer an increased risk of lung cancer. This association was stronger for squamous cell carcinoma (SCC) than adenocarcinoma, and appeared to be stronger in Caucasians than Asians (p: 0.03). Statistically significant interactions were also detected for smoking status and sex, with the effect of the polymorphism being stronger in never-smokers and in females[6].

## Overexpression of CYP1A1

Mollerup et al. *(1999)* reported the gender differences in lung CYP1A1 expression and DNA adduct levels among lung cancer patients[7]. By quantitative reverse transcription-PCR, female smokers exhibited a significantly higher expression level of lung *CYP1A1* (494 ± 334 CYP1A1 mRNA/$10^6$ glyceraldehyde-3-phophate dehydrogenase mRNA, $n$ = 15) compared with males (210 ± 208, $n$ = 12; $P$ = 0.016). In addition, a significantly positive correlation between *CYP1A1* expression and DNA adduct levels were found for both sexes($r$ = 0.50, $P$ = 0.009). Later, Mollerup et al (2006) reported in another study that CYP1A1 expression was significantly increased in smokers compared to ex-smokers and never-smokers. CYP1B1 expression showed a 40-fold variation between individuals and was also increased in smokers, although to a lesser extent than CYP1A1. For both sexes, however, there was no association between the number of cigarettes/day or pack years and the CYP1A1 expression level on an individual level. When analyzed in relation to sex, current smoking females had a 3.9-fold higher median level of CYP1A1 mRNA (smoking-induced CYP1A1 gene expression) compared to current smoking males ($p$ = 0.011). Median levels of CYP1A1 were similar among female and male ex-smokers and never-smokers, respectively, indicating similar "uninduced" CYP1A1 transcript levels in females and males. No indications of sex differences in CYP1B1 expression were found in any smoking category. Other studies on CYP1A1 gene expression in relation to smoking have come to similar conclusions[8;9]. CYP1A1 gene expression was found to correlate significantly with levels of PAH-DNA adducts irrespective of sex and smoking. The other genes analyzed (AHR and EPHX1) showed no relations to smoking or sex. Dresler et al. confirmed the risk of high CYP1A1 expression to the development of lung cancer in women versus men (OR, 4.98 vs.

1.37)[5]. These data are consistent with the hypothesis that CYP1A1 might play a significant role in lung cancer, through DNA adduct formation, and suggests that females may be particularly susceptible to the carcinogenic effect of PAH[10].

## POLYMORPHISMS AND EXPRESSION OF GLUTATHIONE S-TRANSFERASES (GST S)

GSTs, a major group of phase II enzymes, are involved in detoxification of tobacco-related carcinogenic PAHs, such as BaP- 7, 8-diol 9, 10-epoxide (BPDE)[11]. Genetic polymorphisms in GSTM1, GSTT1 and GSTP1 have been studied to find the etiology of lung cancer. Particularly, GST 0 has the highest expression in the lung and is one of the main detoxifiers of BPDE, the bioactivated form of BaP and a carcinogen of tobacco smoke[12]. In addition, GST 0 is encoded by a polymorphic gene, *GSTP1*. The polymorphism seen in *GSTP1* results from a single base pair substitution, A313G in exon 5, leading to Ile105Val. This substitution results in a lower enzymatic activity[13] and is associated with higher hydrophobic adduct levels in lung tissue[14] and higher levels of PAH-DNA adducts in human lymphocytes[15]. A Korean study has indicated that the presence of the mutant GSTP1 genotype and the mutant CYP1A1 exon 7 genotype enhanced the risk of adenocarcinoma and other lung cancers, including squamous cell carcinoma, respectively, in females. Involvement of the *GSTP1* genetic polymorphisms in lung cancer susceptibility is quite reasonable, based on characteristics of the GSTP1, which is locally expressed in the lung and has broad metabolic actions for xenobiotics[16]. However, the gender differences in the GSTP1 expression need further analysis. The expression of the glutathione S-transferase M1 (GSTM1) gene was also evaluated. GSTM1 has the ability to inactivate highly reactive intermediates that are carcinogenic; hence, reduced expression of this gene could lead to an increased risk for smoking-related cancers including lung cancer[17]. While non-expression (null phenotype) did not increase risk by itself, a null phenotype combined with high CYP1A1 expression raised the risk ratio for lung cancer in women as opposed to men (OR: 6.54 vs. 2.36), despite the fact that women in this study had a far less significant smoking history than men[5]. The GSTM1 null phenotype was also associated with an increased risk of lung cancer in non-smoking women with ETS. The OR was 2.6 for women with ETS exposure and GSTM1 null, compared to those expressing GSTM1. This risk increased with increasing exposure to ETS[18]. It is important to be cautious in interpreting and generalizing these findings beyond the study populations given the wide ethnic and racial differences in hepatic enzyme phenotypes[19]. Although the expression of *GSTM1* in lung is relatively low, loss of *GSTM1* enzyme activity (*GSTM1* null genotype) has been associated with host susceptibility in smoking-related lung cancer; however, its role in non-smoking-related lung cancer is still not established. Thus, is of great interest, a pooled analysis from 14 case–control studies on lung cancer with comparable information on genetic polymorphisms in nonsmokers suggest a possible role of *CYP1A1* $Ile^{462}Val$ polymorphisms in lung carcinogenesis among nonsmokers, particularly in combination with the *GSTM1* null genotype. The results for the *CYP1A1 MspI* polymorphism variants and *GSTM1* null genotype excluded an important effect of each of these polymorphisms alone on lung cancer risk. There was a combined effect of *CYP1A1 Ile*$^{462}$*Val* polymorphisms and the *GSTM1* null genotype observed in this analyses, in agreement with a biological hypothesis of a possible gene–gene interaction This stratified analysis on gender showed slightly different effects of genetic polymorphisms between males and females, however, the difference was not significant[19].

## K-*RAS* MUTATIONS AND OVEREXPRESSION

The K-*ras* gene encodes a protein that is known to be oncogenic when mutated or overexpressed[20]. Ras proteins are known to act as signalling switches that relay growth signals from the cell surface to the MAP kinase cascade[21]. As such, they are believed to contribute to hyperproliferative growth when they are mutated or overexpressed and may potentiate growth factor and hormone signalling. These proteins, however, are also involved in cell functions other than the MAP kinase cascade. Examples include interaction with the rho pathway[22;23] and integrin activation[24] suggesting that altered ras protein may affect the early metastatic potential of a neoplastic cell.

In lung cancer, K-*ras* mutations have been extensively studied. Typically, mutations in codons 12 or 13 are the predominant abnormality of *K-ras* observed in lung cancers, and mutations in codon 61 are so infrequent that they are ignored. These mutations are found in 15–35% of adenocarcinomas of the lung, with 80–90% of them occurring at codon 12 and consisting predominantly of G to T transversions[25;26]. On the other hand, some studies have showed that K-*ras* mutations are found in only 5–7% of lung tumors from non-smoking lung cancer patients[26;27]. These results suggested that K-*ras* mutations were induced primarily by tobacco-smoke carcinogens. The mutations occur in carcinogen-exposed cells during the misreplication of a bulky DNA adducts formed between a carcinogen(s), such as PAHs found in tobacco smoke, and guanine bases in the gene's sequence[10;28]. Nelson et al. reported there was a statistically significant association between female sex and K-*ras* codon 12 mutation after adjustment for carcinogen exposures (odds ratio = 3.3; 95% confidence interval [CI] = 1.3–7.9: N = 155), suggesting a possible role of estrogen exposure in either the initiation or the selection of K-*ras* mutant clones in adenocarcinoma[29]. A comparison of adenocarcinoma case patients with and without K-*ras* mutations in their tumors revealed a tendency for mutations to occur in former smokers and for those with mutations to have smoked for more pack-years and to have quit smoking for less time, although none of these associations were statistically significant. Among the patients with adenocarcinoma, 53.8% (95% CI = 46.8%-61.0%) were female. The prevalence of K-*ras* mutation was higher among women (26.2% [95% CI = 18.1%-35.6%]) than among men (17.4% [95% CI = 10.3%-26.7%]). When the spectrum of mutations in the K-*ras* gene at codon 12 was examined by sex, they observed that the majority of mutations were G→T and occurred at the second guanine, giving rise to a cysteine. When this change was compared with all other amino acid substitutions combined, there was an excess of cysteine mutations among women, which did not reach statistical significance (OR = 2.6; 95% CI = 0.73-9.1). They also observed that women were statistically significantly more likely to have mutations in codon 12 of the K-*ras* oncogene. There have been reports of a preponderance of K-*ras* mutations in males, but these were small studies, which primarily included only non-smoking women and none of the studies were in prospective design. Hence, the results of these other investigations either are not comparable or were subject to various selection biases[3,6,29].

At the same time, the increase in lung cancer incidence among women that has been consistently reported in recent years is clearly associated with an increase in adenocarcinoma incidence[30-37]. A mechanism for this increase might involve hormonally-mediated selection of K-*ras* mutant clones. The second event that is needed to negate the *ras*-induced senescence experimentally observed by Serrano et al.[38] might be related to hormonal effects on cells of an adenocarcinoma histology. It is known that the adenocarcinoma precursor cell can exhibit estrogen binding and express estrogen receptors [39]. Furthermore, Kato et al. have shown that the K-*ras* mutation can enhance the expression of estrogen receptors and induce cell transformation in NIH3T3 mouse embryo fibroblast cells[40].

## *p53* Mutation

The *p53* gene on chromosome 17p13.1 encodes a $M_r$ 53,000 nuclear phosphoprotein that is important in the control of the cell cycle and has been referred to as "the guardian of the human genome". In lung cancer, mutations of the *p53* gene have been reported to be present in 35–70% of cases [41,42]. Mutations in *p53* appear to be an early event in the formation of lung tumors because they have been observed in early bronchial neoplasia[43]. These changes, which occur almost exclusively within the highly conserved domains of the gene (exons 5–8), appear to have prognostic value. Several reports indicate that patients with tumors containing mutations in these regions have a significantly worse prognosis. Benzo[*a*]pyrene (BP), considered to be the most extensively studied carcinogen in cigarette smoke and has been known for a long time to be involved in the causation of lung cancer[44]. The distribution of adducts formed by BP within DNA[45;46] corresponds closely to the sites in the *p53* gene with the highest mutation frequencies in lung tumor tissue from smokers, but not in that from nonsmokers[47]. *In vitro* studies have shown that PAH adducts form preferentially at the mutational hotspots in the *p53* gene[48,49]. PAHs form guanine-adducts and preferentially induce G to T. Interestingly, the frequency of G to T transversions at *p53* has been found to be elevated in lung tumors from female smokers compared with male smokers[50]. Another study reported a higher frequency of G:C to T:A transversions among female smokers compared to female never-smokers. This was in contrast to the mutational spectra of male never-smokers and smokers, where no major differences were found[51]. This may indicate a specific role of tobacco smoke carcinogens (PAH) in generating this particular signature mutation in women.

Furthermore, a study in 1999 by Robert Gealy et al., compared the mutation in *p53* in 55 cases of lung carcinoma from smoking and non-smoking women. *P53* mutations were found in 10 of 30 long-term female smokers (33,3%) which was not significantly different from the 26,1% incidence in nonsmokers(P=0.764). However, the types of these mutations differed significantly from those found in nonsmokers. In nonsmokers, p53 mutations consisted of five transitions (including three C to T, one G to A, and one T to C) and one T to A transversion. In comparison, *p53* mutations identified in short- and long-term smokers, consisted of six transversions (four G to T, one A to T, and one G to C), one A to G transition, one C to T transition, and two deletions of one to four base pairs. Mutations in the *p53* gene found in nonsmokers also occurred in either different codons or different positions within a codon compared with those seen in long-term smokers. These results, according to this study, suggest the mutagen(s) and /or mechanisms of *p53* mutation in woman are different from those responsible for *p53* mutation in woman smokers, which are probably largely induced by tobacco mutagens[52].

## DNA Repair Capacity and Adducts

Carcinogens undergo metabolism which may lead either to detoxification and excretion or to activation to a more reactive form that can bind to DNA. Most carcinogens require metabolism for binding to DNA, although some will react directly. The epoxides, for example, can be further metabolized by microsomal epoxide hydrolase (EPHX1) and CYP-enzymes leading to the formation of highly reactive diol-epoxides that can react with DNA. Covalent binding to DNA results in production of "DNA adducts" in which the carcinogen metabolite is chemically bound to one of the DNA bases or to phosphate. This binding is critical to the carcinogenic process. There are cellular repair mechanisms which remove these adducts and return the DNA to its normal form, but, unfortunately, these are not always efficient. If the adducts persist during DNA replication, miscoding can occur leading to permanent mutations. If the mutations occur in critical genes such as oncogenes and tumor suppressor genes, loss of normal cellular growth control processes can result and, ultimately, cancer occurs[19].

The DNA adduct level in a given tissue is thought to reflect cumulative unrepaired DNA damage: the internal dose, the net effect of carcinogen exposure, metabolic activation/detoxification pathways and DNA repair capacity. It has been suggested that the DNA adduct level may be predictive of cancer risk[19].

Molecular studies have pointed to sex differences in PAH metabolism, DNA repair capacity and cell proliferation potential. There is little information on sex differences in DNA repair capacity. Wei et al. have shown that women have a significantly lower DNA repair capacity (DRC ) than men[53]. DRC was measured in the host-cell reactivation assay utilizing lymphocytes transfected with a reporter damaged by BaP. PAHs and tobacco-specific nitrosamines via tobacco smoke are major risk factors exerting their genotoxic effects through the formation of DNA adducts and mutations in transforming gene. DNA adduct levels have been shown to correlate with the level of AHH (arylhydrocarbon hydroxylase) activity[53], which again correlates with the level of cytochrome P450 (CYP)1A1 mRNA[54]. McLemore et al. reported the gender differences in lung CYP1A1 expression and DNA adduct levels among lung cancer patients[55]. Female smokers had a significantly higher levels of aromatic/hydrophobic DNA adducts in their non-tumor lung tissue ($15.39 \pm 9.47$ adducts/$10^8$nucleotides, $n = 29$) than male smokers ($12.08 \pm 8.14$, $n = 93$; $P = 0.047$), higher levels of adducts/pack-year (females $0.95 \pm 0.82$ adducts/pack-year and males $0.46 \pm 0.46$; $P = 0.0004$), and higher levels of adducts/cigarette/ day (females $1.48 \pm 1.29$ and males $0.89 \pm 0.74$, $P = 0.015$). These reports suggest that the susceptibility to PAH-induced DNA damage may be higher in women than men despite smoking significantly less[53,56]. It may be inferred from the study above that expression of CYP1A1 is an important determinant for DNA adduct levels in the human lung, and the sex differences in adducts and CYP1A1 expression are in support of an increased susceptibility to lung cancer among women. The mechanism(s) behind these sex differences is not known. An attractive hypothesis considers a possible interaction between AHR and estrogen receptor pathways[9,57]. However, the results of *in vitro* and animal studies do not support this hypothesis, at least not regarding the involvement of estrogens receptor-α [57]. The estrogen receptor-β is, in contrast to the α-receptor, ambiguously expressed in human lung tissue and primary epithelial cells at the RNA level[58]. Therefore, a role of this receptor in regulating CYP-gene expression in the lung cannot be excluded.

## Epidermal Growth Factor Receptor (EGFR) Mutation and Expression

The Erb B family of receptors tyrosine kinases (RTKs) consists of four structurally related members: Erb-1 (HER-1), Erb-2 (HER-2/Neu), Erb-3 (HER-3) and Erb-4 (HER-4)[59]. The EGFR is a cell-surface, 170-kDA protein that presents three main parts, one extracellular ligand-binding domain, one transmembrane region, and one intracellular domain with tyrosine kinase activity. Upon direct ligand stimulation through transforming growth factors (TGF-α) and epidermal growth factors (EGF) or indirect stimulation through lymphokines, cytokines, hormones and stress factors, the receptor forms homo/heterodimers which lead to activation of its intracellular kinase domain and autophosphorylation of tyrosine residues in the intracellular domain. Following the EGFR activation, a cascade of cytoplasmic and nuclear signalling pathways is emerging[60-63]. The Ras-Raf-MEK-ERK and the P13-PDK1-Akt kinase pathways are mainly activated resulting in gene transcription[64,65]. Biological effects of gene transcription on cell are proliferation, differentiation, adhesion and migration[66-69]. Moreover, overexpression or aberrant expression of EGFR seems to play a critical role in lung carcinogenesis referring to more aggressive disease and poorer prognosis. Ligand overexpression, heterodimerization with other ErbB members, in particular HER2, transactivation by heterologues signaling networks or mutations are some of other potential mechanisms which may induce aberrant EGFR kinase activity[66-68]. Although more than thirty different mutations which have been identified in the tyrosine kinase domain of EGFR, the vast majority of them could be categorized in three classes: in-frame deletion at exon 19, single-nucleotide substitution at exon 18 or 21 and in-frame duplication at exon 20[70-72]. Among these mutations, only L858R missense mutation in exon 21 and deletions in exon 19 seems to be activated mutations[10,70-72]. Mutations in EGFR have been largely studied due to the clinical observation that patients with mutant EGFR present better clinical responses when they receive the EGFR-TK inhibitors, erlotinib and gefinitib[73].

It is unknown if overexpression or aberrant expression of EGFR is more frequent in women than in men and if these molecular differences play a role in lung carcinogenesis, better therapy responses and longer survival of women. D'Amico et al. studied nine molecular markers inclusive EGFR-gene and proto-oncogene HER 2 in pathologic specimens from 408 consecutive patients with NSCLC stage I. They did not found overexpression of

EGFR in women compared to men. 54% of women's specimens that were examined expressed EGFR compared to 51% of men's specimens[74]. In the same way, Cappuzzo et al. evaluated EGFR status by fluorescence in situ hybridization (FISH), DNA sequencing, and immunohistochemistry in 102 NSCLC patients treated with gefinitib. Amplification or high polysomy of the EFGR gene by FISH were seen in 51% of the examined men and 48% of the examined women. EGFR protein overexpression by immunohistochemistry was presented in 64% and 36% of men and women, respectively. Finally, EGFR gene mutation by DNA sequencing was presented in 47% of the male population and in the 53% of the female population. There were no statistically significant differences in the EGFR expression between sexes in that study[75]. Contrary to that, Tsao et al. evaluated EGFR expression in a subanalysis of erlotinib versus placebo clinical trial for NSCLC patients. From a pool of 325 specimens evaluated immunohistochemically, 197 samples were analyzed for EGFR mutations and 221 samples were analyzed for EGFR genes. Mutant EGFRs were more frequently observed in female patients and even more so, these patients presented better responses[76]. Shigematsu et al. sequenced exons 18-21 of the EGFR TK domain from genomic DNA isolated from 617 non-small-cell lung cancers (NSCLCs) in Japan, Taiwan, the United States, and Australia. They detected a total of 134 EGFR TK domain mutations in 130 (21%) of the 617 NSCLCs. The mutations were more frequent in females than in males with a proportion of 42% versus 14%, respectively ($P < .001$)[77]. When Sasaki et al. examined EGFR status in 575 non-small cell lung cancer patients using polymerase chain reaction (PCR) and direct sequencing for EGFR genes, they found that from 117 patients who presented mutant EGFR status, seventy-five (75) were women. In this group, 40.3% of the examined women presented mutations in the tyrosine kinase part of the receptor. The females investigated had presented with a L858R mutation (arginine for leucine substitution at amino acid 858) in a proportion of 69.8% and deletion type 1 in a proportion of 55.6%. These percentages were statistically significantly higher than that of men. Moreover, in a multivariate analysis, L858R mutation was correlated with longer overall survival [78]. Sugio et al. examined somatically acquired mutations in the epidermal growth factor receptor (EGFR) gene in lung cancer. Of the 469 resected tumors of patients with lung cancer that were examined, the majority (322) were adenocarcinomas. Using PCR for the identification of any possible deletion in exon 19 and the amplification of any mutation in codon 858 of exon 21, it was found that there was an increased incidence of EGFR mutations in women ($p=0.0004$), in adenocarcinoma and well-differentiated tumors[79]. In a smaller study which was performed in a Japanese population, Tokumo et al. studied the relationship between EGFR mutation status and clinicopathological factors in surgically resected specimens of 120 NSCLC patients stage I-IV. Out of 83 males and 37 females, it was found that EGFR mutations were more frequent in women ($p=0,003$)[80].

In general, EGFR overexpression or aberrant expression are more often observed in female, never-smokers with adenocarcinoma and Asian origin. These patients responded better to biological therapies with EFGR-TK inhibitors erlotinib or gefinitib. However, there is no clear evidence for women who are not in this subgroup. We cannot draw safe conclusions for all women around the world due to the fact that the majority of trials have been performed on populations with Asian origin. Additional investigations must be done to ascertain whether these results are independent of potential confounding covariates.

Erb-B2 (HER-2/neu) is member of the type I growth factor gene family which has an established role in breast carcinogenesis and an apparent critical role in lung carcinogenesis Approximately 25-30% of invasive breast cancers overexpress HER-2/neu protein. This overexpression is correlated with a more aggressive disease and poorer outcome. Similarly, HER-2/neu is overexpressed in 20%-40% of patients with lung carcinoma and is correlated with poor prognosis in early and advanced-stage NSCLC[81-84]. When proto-oncogene erb-B2 was immunohistochemically studied in 408 surgically resected NSCLC stage I, it showed a predilection for men, and not for women, and it was correlated with a shorter overall survival[74]. Contrary to that, Vallbohmer et al. investigated the association between gene expression levels of HER-2/neu and prognosis in 90 patients with curable resected NSCLC. They found HER-2/neu mRNA overexpression in 68.9% of the patients. When they divided the patients into men and women with low or high expression levels, they found that women with a low expression level of HER-2/neu had a significantly longer survival time compared to women who had a high HER-2/neu expression levels (median survival time of≥94.7 months versus 26.4 months, respectively.)[85]. Despite these observations, treatment with monoclonal antibody to HER-2/neu in addition to standard chemotherapy failed to improve outcome[86]. In another study, mutation status of erb-B2 was examined in correlation to EGFR status in 95 surgically treated Japanese NSCLC patients. Erb-B2 mutation at exon 20 was found only in one never-smoker female patient [87].

## Gastrin-Releasing-Peptide

In the case of lung cancer, GRP has been well-documented as an autocrine growth factor for both small-cell lung cancer and non-small cell lung cancer (NSCLC). All forms of GRP are generated by processing a 125-amino acid prohormone; recent studies have indicated that C-terminal amidation of GRP18-27 is not essential for bioactivity, and that peptides derived from residues 31 to 125 of the prohormone are present in normal tissue and in tumors. GRP receptors can be divided into four classes, all of which belong to the 7 transmembrane domain family and bind GRP and/or GRP analogues with affinities in the nM range. Overexpression of GRP and its receptors has been demonstrated at both the mRNA and the protein level in many types of tumors including lung, prostate, breast, stomach, pancreas and colon [83]. A number of studies have shown that gastrin-releasing (GRP) plays a role in neoplasia by stimulating cell proliferation. In normal tissues, GRP stimulates the growth of bronchial epithelial cells and has been implicated as a regulator of human lung development. The effect of this peptide is mediated mainly through and interaction with the gastrin–releasing peptide receptor (GRPR). The gene for the GRP receptor is X linked, located on chromosome Xp 22, near a cluster of genes that escape X inactivation. Woman, therefore, can have 2 actively transcribed alleles of the GRPR gene compared with only one in men.

Shriver and colleagues reported that GRPR mRNA expression was noted in 55% of female nonsmokers but none were seen in male nonsmokers. In addition, 75% of woman, who were short-term smokers (1-25 pack-years), had GRPR mRNA expression compared with 20% of male short-term smokers[88].

Seigfried also demonstrated that the expression of GRPR mRNA in lung fibroblasts was elevated following exposure to nicotine and hypothesized that woman may be at increased risk to the carcinogenic effects of nicotine through the induction of GRPR expression. Shriver and colleagues have also shown increased expression of the GRPR gene when human airway cells were exposed to estrogen, suggesting that the GRPR gene could also be regulated by the hormone [84-88]. The gene for the gastrin-releasing peptide receptor, which has been implicated in human lung development, was found to be induced by smoking and to be expressed to a higher degree in females compared to males[89].

## Parathyroid Hormone-Related Protein (PTHrP)

The Parathyroid hormone-related protein (PTHrP) is commonly expressed in lung cancer and is very often responsible for hypercalcemia observed in these cancers. Expression of the protein might present implications in lung cancer development and progression because it regulates cancer cell growth, apoptosis, and angiogenesis [90]. When PTHrP immunohistochemical expression was examined in paraffin-embedded tumor samples from 407 patients with NSCLC and correlated to overall survival, it was found that women positive for PTHrP had a longer overall survival compared to women without PTHrP overexpression. This was translated as 55 versus 22 months, respectively, after adjustment for additional covariates. Median male overall survival was 38 months independent of PTHrP status[91].

## Estrogen Receptors

Recently, estrogen receptors have been identified in pulmonary adenocarcinomas in both men and women[92]. It is suggested that estrogens act as estrogen receptors ligands mediating cell proliferation through indirect actions on lung fibroblasts or through metabolic activation to reactive intermediates that can produce DNA adducts or cause oxidative damage[93]. However, the estrogen receptor expression in lung cancer cells and tissues does not clarify whether these receptors are involved in the estrogen-related carcinogenic effects on pulmonary tissues, even though it is known that estrogen can induce lung tissue differentiation and maturation. Two principal types of estrogen receptors have been described.

The *estrogen receptor-α* is a ligand-activated transcription factor that is associated with the development of estrogen-dependent cancers such as breast and endometrial cancers. Several studies have reported the immunohistochemically expression of estrogen receptors in human lung cancer in varying percentages [94-97].

The *estrogen receptor-β* was recently identified and found to be localized to chromosome 14. Relative higher quantities of estrogen receptor-β mRNA have been found in human granulose cells, endothelial cells, ovarian cells and even lung cells [98,99]. This type of receptor is expressed in both lung tumors as well as in normal tissues[100].

These two types of estrogen receptors present similarities in function and structure. Their important role in gene transcription could be explained through opposite mechanism of action. Estradiol-estrogen receptor-α complexes activate transcription, while estradiol-estrogen receptor-β complexes inhibit transcription. There are not enough clinical studies to explain the role of these receptors in lung carcinoma and their impact on female adenocarcinoma. Stabile and colleagues have shown that there is a relationship between b-estradiol and proliferation in NSCLC while the anti-estrogens could block this interaction [93]. Moreover, Taioli et al. showed an interaction between estrogens and the development of lung adenocarcinoma in women using case-control data[34,101].

## Conclusion

The incidence of lung cancer has increased sharply among women. Recently, conflicting data about lung carcinogenesis is that women may be at higher risk of smoking-associated lung cancer than men [34;102]. Several studies have reported the relative risk of lung cancer among females to exceed that of males by a factor of 1.5-2.5[34]. However, not all epidemiological studies have been able to confirm this increased risk [102,103]. Thus, the question regarding the increased susceptibility in females to lung cancer remains challenged.

The higher risk for women could not be explained by differences in baseline exposure, smoking history, or body size. Several investigators have reasoned that shifts in the histology of lung cancer are a reflection of changes in the composition of cigarettes, as well as alterations in smoking behavior. However, few molecular studies have indicated sex differences that may support this hypothesis [104-106]. More studies and further analyses are warranted. Furthermore, understanding these differences may help improve the therapeutic approach to this disease.

## References

[1] Syrigos KN, Nutting C, Roussos C, Tumors of the chest. Biology, Diagnosis and Management. Verlag, New York, May 2006.

[2] Cascorbi I, Brockmoller J, Roots I. A C4887A polymorphism in exon 7 of human CYP1A1: population frequency, mutation linkages, and impact on lung cancer susceptibility. *Cancer Res.* 1996;56:4965-9.

[3] Bartsch H, Nair U, Risch A, Rojas M, Wikman H, Alexandrov K. Genetic polymorphism of CYP genes, alone or in combination, as a risk modifier of tobacco-related cancers. *Cancer Epidemiol. Biomarkers Prev.* 2000;9:3-28.

[4] Kawajiri K, Nakachi K, Imai K, Yoshii A, Shinoda N, Watanabe J. Identification of genetically high risk individuals to lung cancer by DNA polymorphisms of the cytochrome P450IA1 gene. *FEBS Lett.* 1990;263:131-3.

[5] Dresler CM, Fratelli C, Babb J, Everley L, Evans AA, Clapper ML. Gender differences in genetic susceptibility for lung cancer. *Lung Cancer.* 2000;30:153-60.

[6] Le ML, Guo C, Benhamou S, Bouchardy C, Cascorbi I, Clapper ML et al. Pooled analysis of the CYP1A1 exon 7 polymorphism and lung cancer (United States). *Cancer Causes Control.* 2003;14:339-46.

[7] Mollerup S, Ryberg D, Hewer A, Phillips DH, Haugen A. Sex differences in lung CYP1A1 expression and DNA adduct levels among lung cancer patients. *Cancer Res.* 1999;59:3317-20.

[8] Mollerup S, Berge G, Baera R, Skaug V, Hewer A, Phillips DH et al. Sex differences in risk of lung cancer: Expression of genes in the PAH bioactivation pathway in relation to smoking and bulky DNA adducts. *Int. J. Cancer.* 2006;119:741-4.

[9] McLemore TL, Adelberg S, Liu MC, McMahon NA, Yu SJ, Hubbard WC et al. Expression of CYP1A1 gene in patients with lung cancer: evidence for cigarette smoke-induced gene expression in normal lung tissue and for altered gene regulation in primary pulmonary carcinomas. *J. Natl. Cancer Inst.* 1990;82:1333-9.

[10] Konstantinos N.Syrigos Christopher M.Nutting Charalambos Roussos (Eds.). *Tumors of the Chest Biology, Diagnosis and Management.* 2006.

[11] Landi S. Mammalian class theta GST and differential susceptibility to carcinogens: a review. *Mutat. Res.* 2000;463:247-83.

[12] Fields WR, Morrow CS, Doss AJ, Sundberg K, Jernstrom B, Townsend AJ. Overexpression of stably transfected human glutathione S-transferase P1-1 protects against DNA damage by benzo[a]pyrene diol-epoxide in human T47D cells. *Mol. Pharmacol.* 1998;54:298-304.

[13] Watson MA, Stewart RK, Smith GB, Massey TE, Bell DA. Human glutathione S-transferase P1 polymorphisms: relationship to lung tissue enzyme activity and population frequency distribution. *Carcinogenesis.* 1998;19:275-80.

[14] Ryberg D, Skaug V, Hewer A, Phillips DH, Harries LW, Wolf CR et al. Genotypes of glutathione transferase M1 and P1 and their significance for lung DNA adduct levels and cancer risk. *Carcinogenesis.* 1997;18:1285-9.

[15] Butkiewicz D, Grzybowska E, Phillips DH, Hemminki K, Chorazy M. Polymorphisms of the GSTP1 and GSTM1 genes and PAH-DNA adducts in human mononuclear white blood cells. *Environ. Mol. Mutagen.* 2000;35:99-105.

[16] Coles B, Yang M, Lang NP, Kadlubar FF. Expression of hGSTP1 alleles in human lung and catalytic activity of the native protein variants towards 1-chloro-2,4-dinitrobenzene, 4-vinylpyridine and (+)-anti benzo[a]pyrene-7,8-diol-9,10-oxide. *Cancer Lett.* 2000;156:167-75.

[17] Seidegard J, Pero RW, Markowitz MM, Roush G, Miller DG, Beattie EJ. Isoenzyme(s) of glutathione transferase (class Mu) as a marker for the susceptibility to lung cancer: a follow up study. *Carcinogenesis.* 1990;11:33-6.

[18] Bennett WP, Alavanja MC, Blomeke B, Vahakangas KH, Castren K, Welsh JA et al. Environmental tobacco smoke, genetic susceptibility, and risk of lung cancer in never-smoking women. *J. Natl. Cancer Inst.* 1999;91:2009-14.

[19] Kiyohara C, Otsu A, Shirakawa T, Fukuda S, Hopkin JM. Genetic polymorphisms and lung cancer susceptibility: a review. *Lung Cancer.* 2002;37:241-56.

[20] Barbacid M. ras genes. *Annu.Rev.Biochem.* 1987;56:779-827.:779-827.

[21] Bos JL. p21ras: an oncoprotein functioning in growth factor-induced signal transduction. *Eur. J. Cancer.* 1995;31A:1051-4.

[22] Khosravi-Far R, Solski PA, Clark GJ, Kinch MS, Der CJ. Activation of Rac1, RhoA, and mitogen-activated protein kinases is required for Ras transformation. *Mol. Cell Biol.* 1995;15:6443-53.

[23] Qiu RG, Chen J, Kirn D, McCormick F, Symons M. An essential role for Rac in Ras transformation. *Nature.* 1995;374:457-9.

[24] Hughes PE, Renshaw MW, Pfaff M, Forsyth J, Keivens VM, Schwartz MA et al. Suppression of integrin activation: a novel function of a Ras/Raf-initiated MAP kinase pathway. *Cell.* 1997;88:521-30.

[25] Siegfried JM, Gillespie AT, Mera R, Casey TJ, Keohavong P, Testa JR et al. Prognostic value of specific KRAS mutations in lung adenocarcinomas. *Cancer Epidemiol. Biomarkers Prev.* 1997;6:841-7.

[26] Gealy R, Zhang L, Siegfried JM, Luketich JD, Keohavong P. Comparison of mutations in the p53 and K-ras genes in lung carcinomas from smoking and nonsmoking women. *Cancer Epidemiol. Biomarkers Prev.* 1999;8:297-302.

[27] Rodenhuis S, Slebos RJ. Clinical significance of ras oncogene activation in human lung cancer. *Cancer Res.* 1992;52:2665s-9s.

[28] Greenblatt MS, Bennett WP, Hollstein M, Harris CC. Mutations in the p53 tumor suppressor gene: clues to cancer etiology and molecular pathogenesis. *Cancer Res.* 1994;54:4855-78.

[29] Nelson HH, Christiani DC, Mark EJ, Wiencke JK, Wain JC, Kelsey KT. Implications and prognostic value of K-ras mutation for early-stage lung cancer in women. *J. Natl. Cancer Inst.* 1999;91:2032-8.

[30] Lubin JH, Blot WJ. Assessment of lung cancer risk factors by histologic category. *J. Natl. Cancer Inst.* 1984;73:383-9.

[31] Wynder EL, Hoffmann D. Smoking and lung cancer: scientific challenges and opportunities. *Cancer Res.* 1994;54:5284-95.

[32] Peto R, Lopez AD, Boreham J, Thun M, Heath C, Jr., Doll R. Mortality from smoking worldwide. *Br. Med. Bull.* 1996;52:12-21.

[33] McDuffie HH, Klaassen DJ, Dosman JA. Female-male differences in patients with primary lung cancer. *Cancer.* 1987;59:1825-30.

[34] Risch HA, Howe GR, Jain M, Burch JD, Holowaty EJ, Miller AB. Are female smokers at higher risk for lung cancer than male smokers? A case-control analysis by histologic type. *Am. J. Epidemiol.* 1993;138:281-93.

[35] Alavanja MC, Brownson RC, Boice JD, Jr., Hock E. Preexisting lung disease and lung cancer among nonsmoking women. *Am. J. Epidemiol.* 1992;136:623-32.

[36] O'Neall MA, Brownson RC. Teaching evidence-based public health to public health practitioners. *Ann. Epidemiol.* 2005;15:540-4.

[37] Travis WD, Travis LB, Devesa SS. Lung cancer. *Cancer.* 1995;75:191-202.

[38] Serrano M, Lin AW, McCurrach ME, Beach D, Lowe SW. Oncogenic ras provokes premature cell senescence associated with accumulation of p53 and p16INK4a. *Cell.* 1997;88:593-602.

[39] Saunders PT, Maguire SM, Gaughan J, Millar MR. Expression of oestrogen receptor beta (ER beta) in multiple rat tissues visualised by immunohistochemistry. *J. Endocrinol.* 1997;154:R13-R16.

[40] Kato K, Ueoka Y, Kato K, Hachiya T, Nishida J, Wake N. Contribution of enhanced transcriptional activation by ER to [12Val] K-Ras mediated NIH3T3 cell transformation. *Oncogene.* 1997;15:3037-46.

[41] Vogelstein B, Kinzler KW. p53 function and dysfunction. *Cell.* 1992;70:523-6.

[42] Levine AJ, Momand J, Finlay CA. The p53 tumour suppressor gene. *Nature.* 1991;351:453-6.

[43] Nishio M, Koshikawa T, Yatabe Y, Kuroishi T, Suyama M, Nagatake M et al. Prognostic significance of cyclin D1 and retinoblastoma expression in combination with p53 abnormalities in primary, resected non-small cell lung cancers. *Clin. Cancer Res.* 1997;3:1051-8.

[44] Sozzi G, Miozzo M, Donghi R, Pilotti S, Cariani CT, Pastorino U et al. Deletions of 17p and p53 mutations in preneoplastic lesions of the lung. *Cancer Res.* 1992;52:6079-82.

[45] Vineis P, Bartsch H, Caporaso N, Harrington AM, Kadlubar FF, Landi MT et al. Genetically based N-acetyltransferase metabolic polymorphism and low-level environmental exposure to carcinogens. *Nature.* 1994;369:154-6.

[46] Vineis P. Molecular epidemiology: low-dose carcinogens and genetic susceptibility. *Int. J. Cancer.* 1997;71:1-3.

[47] Ambrosone CB, Freudenheim JL, Graham S, Marshall JR, Vena JE, Brasure JR et al. Cigarette smoking, N-acetyltransferase 2 genetic polymorphisms, and breast cancer risk. *JAMA.* 1996;276:1494-501.

[48] Smith LE, Denissenko MF, Bennett WP, Li H, Amin S, Tang M et al. Targeting of lung cancer mutational hotspots by polycyclic aromatic hydrocarbons. *J. Natl. Cancer Inst.* 2000;92:803-11.

[49] Kure EH, Ryberg D, Hewer A, Phillips DH, Skaug V, Baera R et al. p53 mutations in lung tumours: relationship to gender and lung DNA adduct levels. *Carcinogenesis.* 1996;17:2201-5.

[50] Guinee DG, Jr., Travis WD, Trivers GE, De B, V, Cawley H, Welsh JA et al. Gender comparisons in human lung cancer: analysis of p53 mutations, anti-p53 serum antibodies and C-erbB-2 expression. *Carcinogenesis.* 1995;16:993-1002.

[51] Toyooka S, Tsuda T, Gazdar AF. The TP53 gene, tobacco exposure, and lung cancer. *Hum. Mutat.* 2003;21:229-39.

[52] Vahakangas KH, Bennett WP, Castren K, Welsh JA, Khan MA, Blomeke B et al. p53 and K-ras mutations in lung cancers from former and never-smoking women. *Cancer Res.* 2001;61:4350-6.

[53] Wei Q, Cheng L, Amos CI, Wang LE, Guo Z, Hong WK et al. Repair of tobacco carcinogen-induced DNA adducts and lung cancer risk: a molecular epidemiologic study. *J. Natl. Cancer Inst.* 2000;92:1764-72.

[54] Alexandrov K, Rojas M, Geneste O, Castegnaro M, Camus AM, Petruzzelli S et al. An improved fluorometric assay for dosimetry of benzo(a)pyrene diol-epoxide-DNA adducts in smokers' lung: comparisons with total bulky adducts and aryl hydrocarbon hydroxylase activity. *Cancer Res.* 1992;52:6248-53.

[55] McLemore TL, Adelberg S, Liu MC, McMahon NA, Yu SJ, Hubbard WC et al. Expression of CYP1A1 gene in patients with lung cancer: evidence for cigarette smoke-induced gene expression in normal lung tissue and for altered gene regulation in primary pulmonary carcinomas. *J. Natl. Cancer Inst.* 1990;82:1333-9.

[56] Shigematsu H, Lin L, Takahashi T, Nomura M, Suzuki M, Wistuba II et al. Clinical and biological features associated with epidermal growth factor receptor gene mutations in lung cancers. *J. Natl. Cancer Inst.* 2005;97:339-46.

[57] Haugen A. Women who smoke: are women more susceptible to tobacco-induced lung cancer? *Carcinogenesis.* 2002;23:227-9.

[58] Mollerup S, Jorgensen K, Berge G, Haugen A. Expression of estrogen receptors alpha and beta in human lung tissue and cell lines. *Lung Cancer.* 2002;37:153-9.

[59] Yarden Y, Sliwkowski MX. Untangling the ErbB signalling network. *Nat. Rev. Mol. Cell Biol.* 2001;2:127-37.

[60] Carpenter G. Employment of the epidermal growth factor receptor in growth factor-independent signaling pathways. *J. Cell Biol.* 1999;146:697-702.

[61] Graus-Porta D, Beerli RR, Daly JM, Hynes NE. ErbB-2, the preferred heterodimerization partner of all ErbB receptors, is a mediator of lateral signaling. *EMBO J.* 1997;16:1647-55.

[62] Karunagaran D, Tzahar E, Beerli RR, Chen X, Graus-Porta D, Ratzkin BJ et al. ErbB-2 is a common auxiliary subunit of NDF and EGF receptors: implications for breast cancer. *EMBO J.* 1996;15:254-64.

[63] W Saif, A Zalonis KN Syrigos. The clinical significance of autoantibodies in gastrointestinal malignancies: an overview. Expert Opinion on Biological Therapies . 2006.
Ref Type: In Press

[64] Pinkas-Kramarski R, Soussan L, Waterman H, Levkowitz G, Alroy I, Klapper L et al. Diversification of Neu differentiation factor and epidermal growth factor signaling by combinatorial receptor interactions. *EMBO J.* 1996;15:2452-67.

[65] Riese DJ, van Raaij TM, Plowman GD, Andrews GC, Stern DF. The cellular response to neuregulins is governed by complex interactions of the erbB receptor family. *Mol. Cell Biol.* 1995;15:5770-6.

[66] Ozanne B, Richards CS, Hendler F, Burns D, Gusterson B. Over-expression of the EGF receptor is a hallmark of squamous cell carcinomas. *J. Pathol.* 1986;149:9-14.

[67] Tang CK, Gong XQ, Moscatello DK, Wong AJ, Lippman ME. Epidermal growth factor receptor vIII enhances tumorigenicity in human breast cancer. *Cancer Res.* 2000;60:3081-7.

[68] Woodburn JR. The epidermal growth factor receptor and its inhibition in cancer therapy. *Pharmacol. Ther.* 1999;82:241-50.

[69] Syrigos KN, Karayiannakis AJ. Adhesion molecules as targets for the treatment of neoplastic diseases. *Curr. Pharm. Des.* 2006;12:2849-61.

[70] Paez JG, Janne PA, Lee JC, Tracy S, Greulich H, Gabriel S et al. EGFR mutations in lung cancer: correlation with clinical response to gefitinib therapy. *Science.* 2004;304:1497-500.

[71] Lynch TJ, Bell DW, Sordella R, Gurubhagavatula S, Okimoto RA, Brannigan BW et al. Activating mutations in the epidermal growth factor receptor underlying responsiveness of non-small-cell lung cancer to gefitinib. *N. Engl. J. Med.* 2004;350:2129-39.

[72] Pao W, Miller V, Zakowski M, Doherty J, Politi K, Sarkaria I et al. EGF receptor gene mutations are common in lung cancers from "never smokers" and are associated with sensitivity of tumors to gefitinib and erlotinib. *Proc. Natl. Acad. Sci. U.S.A.* 2004;101:13306-11.

[73] G J Papaetis, C. Roussos K. N. Syrigos. Targeted therapy for Non-Small Cell Lung Cancer. *Current Pharmaceutical Design* . 2006. Ref Type: In Press

[74] D'Amico TA, Aloia TA, Moore MB, Herndon JE, Brooks KR, Lau CL et al. Molecular biologic substaging of stage I lung cancer according to gender and histology. *Ann. Thorac. Surg.* 2000;69:882-6.

[75] Cappuzzo F, Hirsch FR, Rossi E, Bartolini S, Ceresoli GL, Bemis L et al. Epidermal growth factor receptor gene and protein and gefitinib sensitivity in non-small-cell lung cancer. *J. Natl. Cancer Inst.* 2005;97:643-55.

[76] Tsao MS, Sakurada A, Cutz JC, Zhu CQ, Kamel-Reid S, Squire J et al. Erlotinib in lung cancer - molecular and clinical predictors of outcome. *N. Engl. J. Med.* 2005;353:133-44.

[77] Shigematsu H, Lin L, Takahashi T, Nomura M, Suzuki M, Wistuba II et al. Clinical and biological features associated with epidermal growth factor receptor gene mutations in lung cancers. *J. Natl. Cancer Inst.* 2005;97:339-46.

[78] Sasaki H, Endo K, Takada M, Kawahara M, Kitahara N, Tanaka H et al. L858R EGFR mutation status correlated with clinico-pathological features of Japanese lung cancer. *Lung Cancer.* 2006;54:103-8.

[79] Sugio K, Uramoto H, Ono K, Oyama T, Hanagiri T, Sugaya M et al. Mutations within the tyrosine kinase domain of EGFR gene specifically occur in lung adenocarcinoma patients with a low exposure of tobacco smoking. *Br. J. Cancer.* 2006;94:896-903.

[80] Tokumo M, Toyooka S, Kiura K, Shigematsu H, Tomii K, Aoe M et al. The relationship between epidermal growth factor receptor mutations and clinicopathologic features in non-small cell lung cancers. *Clin. Cancer Res.* 2005;11:1167-73.

[81] Shi D, He G, Cao S, Pan W, Zhang HZ, Yu D et al. Overexpression of the c-erbB-2/neu-encoded p185 protein in primary lung cancer. *Mol. Carcinog.* 1992;5:213-8.

[82] Harpole DH, Jr., Marks JR, Richards WG, Herndon JE, Sugarbaker DJ. Localized adenocarcinoma of the lung: oncogene expression of erbB-2 and p53 in 150 patients. *Clin. Cancer Res.* 1995;1:659-64.

[83] Micke P, Hengstler JG, Ros R, Bittinger F, Metz T, Gebhard S et al. c-erbB-2 expression in small-cell lung cancer is associated with poor prognosis. *Int. J. Cancer.* 2001;92:474-9.

[84] Brabender J, Danenberg KD, Metzger R, Schneider PM, Park J, Salonga D et al. Epidermal growth factor receptor and HER2-neu mRNA expression in non-small cell lung cancer Is correlated with survival. *Clin. Cancer Res.* 2001;7:1850-5.

[85] Vallbohmer D, Brabender J, Yang DY, Danenberg K, Schneider PM, Metzger R et al. Sex differences in the predictive power of the molecular prognostic factor HER2/neu in patients with non-small-cell lung cancer. *Clin. Lung Cancer.* 2006;7:332-7.

[86] Gatzemeier U, Groth G, Butts C, Van ZN, Shepherd F, Ardizzoni A et al. Randomized phase II trial of gemcitabine-cisplatin with or without trastuzumab in HER2-positive non-small-cell lung cancer. *Ann. Oncol.* 2004;15:19-27.

[87] Sasaki H, Shimizu S, Endo K, Takada M, Kawahara M, Tanaka H et al. EGFR and erbB2 mutation status in Japanese lung cancer patients. *Int. J. Cancer.* 2006;118:180-4.

[88] Shriver SP, Bourdeau HA, Gubish CT, Tirpak DL, Davis AL, Luketich JD et al. Sex-specific expression of gastrin-releasing peptide receptor: relationship to smoking history and risk of lung cancer. *J. Natl. Cancer Inst.* 2000;92:24-33.

[89] Patel O, Shulkes A, Baldwin GS. Gastrin-releasing peptide and cancer. *Biochim. Biophys. Acta.* 2006;1766:23-41.

[90] Hastings RH. Parathyroid hormone-related protein and lung biology. *Respir. Physiol. Neurobiol.* 2004;142:95-113.

[91] Hastings RH, Laux AM, Casillas A, Xu R, Lukas Z, Ernstrom K et al. Sex-specific survival advantage with parathyroid hormone-related protein in non-small cell lung carcinoma patients. *Clin. Cancer Res.* 2006;12:499-506.

[92] Dabbs DJ, Landreneau RJ, Liu Y, Raab SS, Maley RH, Tung MY et al. Detection of estrogen receptor by immunohistochemistry in pulmonary adenocarcinoma. *Ann. Thorac. Surg.* 2002;73:403-5.

[93] Stabile LP, Davis AL, Gubish CT, Hopkins TM, Luketich JD, Christie N et al. Human non-small cell lung tumors and cells derived from normal lung express both estrogen receptor alpha and beta and show biological responses to estrogen. *Cancer Res.* 2002;62:2141-50.

[94] Canver CC, Memoli VA, Vanderveer PL, Dingivan CA, Mentzer RM, Jr. Sex hormone receptors in non-small-cell lung cancer in human beings. *J. Thorac. Cardiovasc. Surg.* 1994;108:153-7.

[95] Cagle PT, Mody DR, Schwartz MR. Estrogen and progesterone receptors in bronchogenic carcinoma. *Cancer Res.* 1990;50:6632-5.

[96] Ollayos CW, Riordan GP, Rushin JM. Estrogen receptor detection in paraffin sections of adenocarcinoma of the colon, pancreas, and lung. *Arch. Pathol. Lab Med.* 1994;118:630-2.

[97] Beattie CW, Hansen NW, Thomas PA. Steroid receptors in human lung cancer. *Cancer Res.* 1985;45:4206-14.

[98] Enmark E, Pelto-Huikko M, Grandien K, Lagercrantz S, Lagercrantz J, Fried G et al. Human estrogen receptor beta-gene structure, chromosomal localization, and expression pattern. *J. Clin. Endocrinol. Metab.* 1997;82:4258-65.

[99] Kuiper GG, Carlsson B, Grandien K, Enmark E, Haggblad J, Nilsson S et al. Comparison of the ligand binding specificity and transcript tissue distribution of estrogen receptors alpha and beta. *Endocrinology.* 1997;138:863-70.

[100] Omoto Y, Kobayashi Y, Nishida K, Tsuchiya E, Eguchi H, Nakagawa K et al. Expression, function, and clinical implications of the estrogen receptor beta in human lung cancers. *Biochem. Biophys. Res. Commun.* 2001;285:340-7.

[101] Taioli E, Wynder EL. Re: Endocrine factors and adenocarcinoma of the lung in women. *J. Natl. Cancer Inst.* 1994;86:869-70.

[102] Kreuzer M, Boffetta P, Whitley E, Ahrens W, Gaborieau V, Heinrich J et al. Gender differences in lung cancer risk by smoking: a multicentre case-control study in Germany and Italy. *Br. J. Cancer.* 2000;82:227-33.

[103] Henschke CI, Miettinen OS. Women's susceptibility to tobacco carcinogens. *Lung Cancer.* 2004;43:1-5.

[104] Thun MJ, Lally CA, Flannery JT, Calle EE, Flanders WD, Heath CW, Jr. Cigarette smoking and changes in the histopathology of lung cancer. *J. Natl. Cancer Inst.* 1997;89:1580-6.

[105] Zang EA, Wynder EL. Differences in lung cancer risk between men and women: examination of the evidence. *J. Natl. Cancer Inst.* 1996;88:183-92.

[106] Zang EA, Wynder EL. Cumulative tar exposure. A new index for estimating lung cancer risk among cigarette smokers. *Cancer.* 1992;70:69-76.

In: Lung Cancer in Women
Editor: Varetta N. Torres, pp. 233-245
ISBN: 978-1-60021-659-6


*Chapter XI*

# INCIDENCE AND TRENDS IN LUNG CANCER IN WOMEN: ALBERT CALMETTE HOSPITAL EXPERIENCE IN 15 YEARS

***Demosthenes Makris*[*], *Andreiy Bondarief, Arnaud Schepereel, Xavier Dallouin, Guillame Colin, Charles-Hugo Marquette, Jean-Jaques Lafitte***
Clinique des Maladies Respiratoires, Service de Pneumologie
et d'Oncologie Thoracique, CHRU, Lille

## ABSTRACT

### Background

Lung cancer is the leading cause of cancer-related mortality in both men and women. Emerging data demonstrate sex-specific differences in lung cancer incidence and trends.

### Aim

To estimate lung cancer incidence and trends in women and to find whether there are significant differences in treatment modalities and survival between men and women.

[*] Correspondance: Demosthenes MAKRIS ; Clinique des Maladies Respiratoires ; Hôpital Albert Calmette ; Centre Hospitalier Régional Universitaire de Lille ; 59037 Lille cedex ;e-mail: appollon7@hotmail.com

### Subjects and Methods

This retrospective analysis included all cases with bronchopulmonary cancer registered in the Thoracic Oncology Department database in Albert Calmette University Hospital in Lille, France, between 1990 and 2005. Lung cancer histologic pattern and staging, main treatment modalities and survival data were analyzed by gender and by two different time periods, 1990-1999 and 2000-2005.

### Results

The proportion of new lung cancer cases in women significantly increased over the last five-year period compared to the last decade (18.8% vs 9.6%, p=0.001). Adenocarcinoma was the histologic type of cancer which predominated in women (51%). A change in the histologic pattern in men, from squamous cell towards lung adenocarcinoma, was observed. Women presented less often complications to chemotherapy than men, especially in the period between 1990 and 1999 (p=0.001). The overall median survival time was better in women than men (p=0.01) although there were no significant gender differences in median survival time when each treatment modality was considered separately.

### Conclusion

In view of the increased number of new lung cancer cases in women, tobacco control and early detection screening programs for lung cancer with reference to gender should be high priorities for health care services.

**Key words**: lung cancer; incidence; female; smoking.

## INTRODUCTION

Lung cancer is still a leading cause of cancer mortality with an overall 5-year survival of less than 20% in Europe and in the United States of America [1]. The main reason of low survival rates and treatment failure is late diagnosis of extensive disease [2]. Although the prevalence of lung cancer has started to decrease among men in countries like the United States, it is the most common tumor and it is clearly advancing in both men and women in France as it was shown by recent mortality rates [3][4][5][6]. In 2000 lung cancer was responsible for about 150000 deaths, representing more than a quarter of total mortality in France. In men, lung cancer ranked as the first cause of death from neoplastic diseases while it ranked as fourth cause in women [7]. However, this patterns may change as the number of female smokers increases and because there is evidence that women may be in greater risk to develop the disease than men [8][9]. The male/female incidence ratio narrowed dramatically, from 3.65 in 1975 to 1.65 in 1999, while the incidence rate in women continued to rise slowly [10]. Notably, although lung cancer predominates in men, it ranks now as the first cause of death from neoplastic diseases among women in the United States of America [11].

It has been suggested that there are distinct differences between women and men in respect of lung cancer histopathology, response to treatment and prognosis [12][13][14]. Women may be more susceptible to lung cancer than men. Molecular and genetic epidemiology studies are underway to prove this hypothesis. However, women are still underrepresented in cancer trials and definitive conclusion can not be derived from existing data [15][16]. Thus, there is a need for wide-ranging studies to compare differences between males and females in respect of incidence, susceptibility and treatment outcome.

It has been reported that in north France (Nord – Pas de Calais region) lung cancer incidence rate in women was lower compared to the mean rate for women in France (figure 1) [17]. In contrast, the regional incidence rate in men was higher than the national mean rate. In our institution, we observed an increase in rates of hospitalization of women with lung cancer during the last years. We therefore conducted this investigation to monitor trends in lung cancer in women to find whether there are significant differences in treatment modalities and survival between men and women. Monitoring cancer incidence and mortality time trends is essential for setting prevention measures, for evaluating mass screening, for planning treatment resources and for setting public health policy. We analyzed retrospectively collected data from all lung cancer cases diagnosed between 1990 and 2005 in this tertiary health centre which serves a population of about 4.000.000 inhabitants.

**Incidence rates of lung cancer in France**

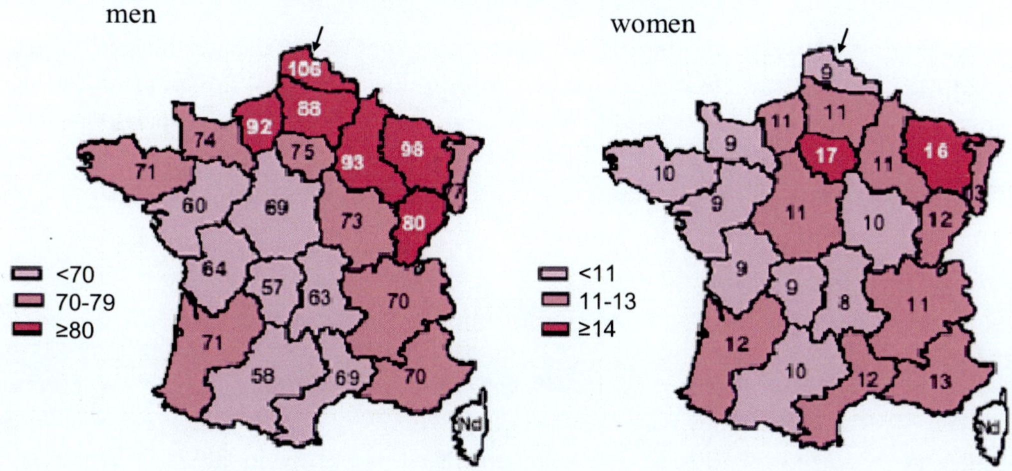


Arrows indicate the Nord-Pas de Calais region;
Figure modified from reference 17.

Figure 1. Lung cancer incidence rates in the year 2000 in France (new cases per 100.000 inhabitants).

## Material and Methods

This analysis included all lung cancer cases registered in the Thoracic Oncology Department database in Albert Calmette University Hospital in Lille, France, between 1$^{st}$ January 1990 and the 31$^{st}$ December 2005. This database includes all cases with bronchopulmonary cancer diagnosed and treated in this hospital. For all lung cancer cases presented here, therapeutic planning and decision have been discussed systematically in weekly multidisciplinary meeting in this tertiary hospital. In the present study the following rules were applied in data collection and analysis: i) only primary lung tumours were included; ii) mesothelioma cases were excluded; iii) survival was calculated as the time between the start of treatment for each case until time death occurred or time of data analysis; iv) only the main initial treatment modality was included in analysis; v) data were analyzed by gender and vi) by dividing the whole 15-year period in two shorter periods, 1990 to 1999 and 2000 to 2005. Karnofski performance score (KPS) has was used as a global indicator of the functional status of patients; KPS ranges between 100 (best) and 0 [18]. In addition to the quality checks made at the registry level, others were carried out secondarily. Each record in error was returned to the registry for correction to be included in analysis.

## Statistical Analysis

Results are presented as mean (SE) values for continuous data or as percentage for categorical data. Survival data are presented as median (25$^{th}$ -75$^{th}$ percentile) values. Continuous data were compared with the Mann- Whitney U test. Comparisons between groups on categorical data were done using chi-square or Fisher's exact test. The statistical package SPSS 13.0 (Chicago.IL; USA) was used for the entire analysis.

## Results

A total of 3942 cases were studied. There were 2411 new lung cancer cases between 1990 and 1999 and 1531 new cases between 2000 and 2005. Lung cancer cases, histologic pattern and the stage of disease at time of diagnosis are presented in table 1. The percentage of male lung cancer patients was consistently higher than women in the whole studied period. Although, the number of new cases diagnosed annually in men remained relatively stable, a steady increase was evident in women (figure 2). Two hundred forty five new lung cancer cases in women were registered between 2000 and 2005 (18.8% of lung cancer cases in this period) while less cases were found during the past ten years (233 cases, 9.6% of lung cancer cases in that period) (p=0.001). In men, there were 2178 new lung cancer cases between 1990 and 1999 (93.4% of total cases in this period), and 1287 (81.2%) cases between 2000 and 2005. No significant difference was found between sexes in respect of the age of patients at time of lung cancer diagnosis. Median (25$^{th}$ -75$^{th}$ percentile) ages at diagnosis were 61 (49-71) and 59 (48-69) for men and women respectively (p=0.15). No significant gender differences were found in smoking trends or in Karnofski performance score. The proportion of women with co-morbidities was lower than that of men but the difference did not reach statistical significance (23.2% vs 28.5%, p=0.4).

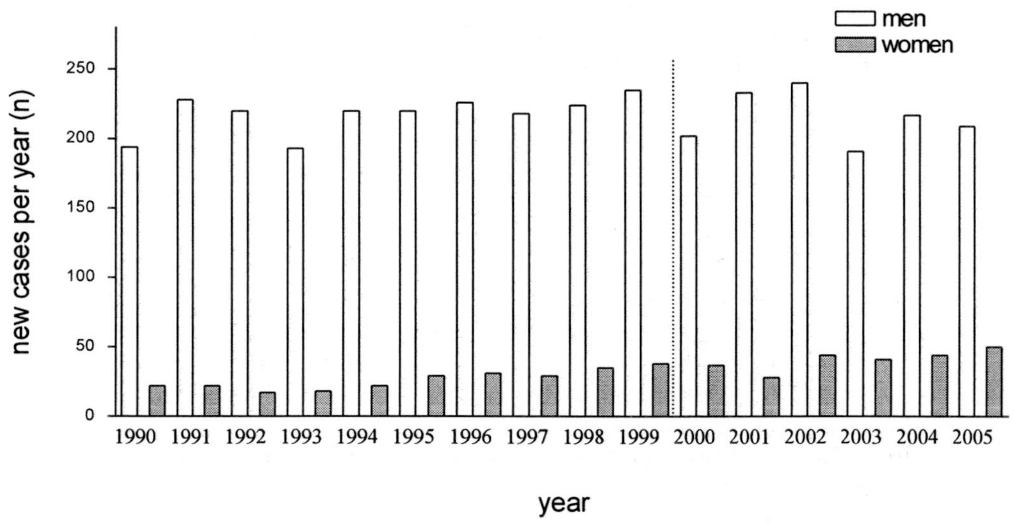


Figure 2. New lung cancer cases in the period 1990-2005 in men and women.

**Table 1. Characteristics of new lung cancer cases in women between 1990 and 2005**

| | 1990 – 1999n=233 | 2000 -2005 n=244 |
|---|---|---|
| % of total lung cancer cases | 9.6 | 18.8* |
| age at diagnosis | 58.7 (49-71) | 59.6 (47-69) |
| age started smoking | 17 (14 – 19) | 18 (16-20) |
| age stopped smoking | 56 (46-43) | 48.5 (41 -54) |
| cigarettes per day | 15 (10-20) | 10 (5- 20) |
| Karnofski performance score | 80 (70-90) | 90 (70-90) |
| histologic type | | |
| squamous | 46 (19.7) | 39 (18.4) |
| adenocarcinoma | 118 (51.5) | 108 (51) |
| small cell lung cancer | 38 (16.3) | 27 (12.7) |
| giant cell | 1 (0.4) | - |
| miscellaneous types | 3 (1.3) | - |
| non differentiate | 27 (11.6) | 38 (17.9) |
| disease staging | | |
| stage I | 18 (9.7) | 30 (13.8) |
| stage II | 14 (7.5 ) | 12 (5.5) |
| stage III | 32 (17 ) | 34 (15.5) |
| stage IV | 122 (65.5) | 144 (65) |

Data are presented as n (% of cases in each category), age and smoking trends are presented as median ($25^{th}$ – $75^{th}$) values; *difference between time periods, p=0.001.

The most common histologic type of cancer in women was adenocarcinoma (51% of types). The histologic pattern in women did not change over the studied period. A significant decrease in the rate of squamous cell carcinoma was noted while the rate of adenocarcinoma rised significantly in male population (figure 3). Lung cancer was already in an advanced stage at the time of diagnosis. Sixty five per cent of diagnosed cases in women were of stage IV at the time of diagnosis.

Chemotherapy was the most common option of treatment in women (33.5%) over the 15-year period. In men palliative treatment was more common than other type of treatment (31%) in this period. Table 2 shows the main initial modalities of treatment in men and women. Complications of chemotherapy included haematologic disorders, infection, electrolytic disturbances, renal impairment and gastrenterologic disorders. In women a significantly lower percentage of complications was observed compared to men; this difference was statistically significant in the period between 1990 and 1999 ($p=0.001$).

The median ($25^{th}$ –$75^{th}$ percentile) overall survival time for the period 1990-1999 was 295 (95-606) and 220 (71-485) days for women and men respectively ($p=0.01$). Median survival for small cell lung cancer (SCLC) was 270 (95-565) and 217 (70-502) days for women and men respectively ($p=0.01$). Median survival was also better in women with non-small cell lung cancer (NSCLC) than in men with the same type of cancer, 301 (47-600) vs 220 (71-485) days respectively ($p=0.005$). Survival rates although better in women were not significantly different when each treatment modality was studied separately.

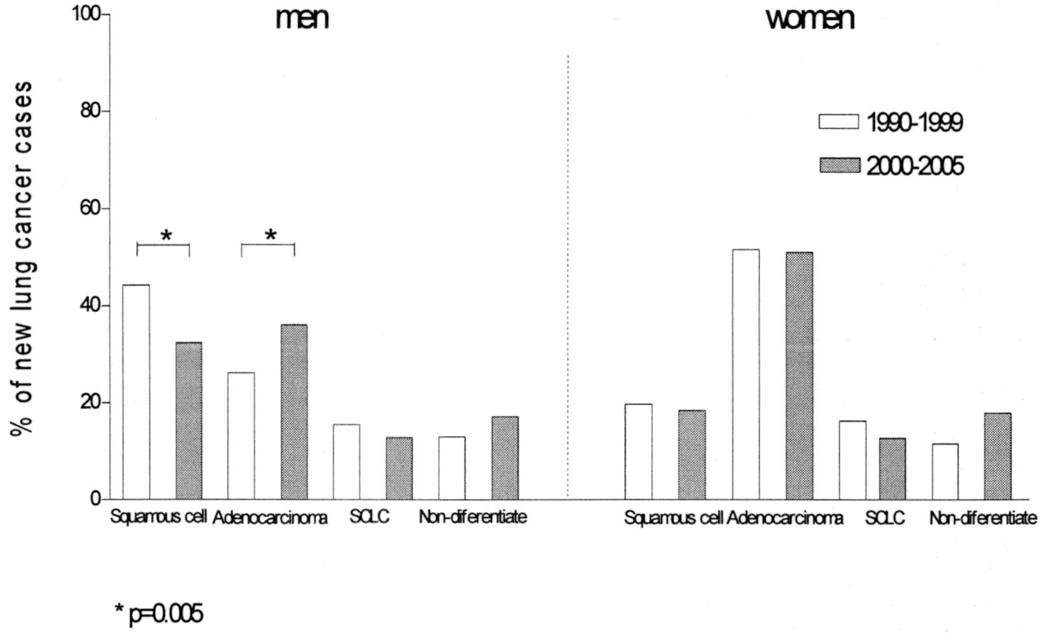


Figure 3. Histologic pattern of lung cancer in men and women, in the period 1990-1999 and 2000-2005.

**Table 2. Main initial treatment modalities for lung cancer and complications related to treatment in men and women**

| | 1990-1999 | | 2000-2005 | |
|---|---|---|---|---|
| | females n=233 | males n=2178 | females n=244 | males n=1287 |
| treatment | | | | |
| Chemotherapy | 94 (40.1)* | 693 (31.8) | 68 (27.8) | 321 (24.9) |
| Curative Surgery | 46 (19.7) | 383 (17.5) | 30 (12.8) | 173 (8.7) |
| Radiotherapy | 21 (9) | 307 (15) | 16 (6.5) | 97 (7.5) |
| Palliative medical care | 50 (21.5) | 573 (26) | 90 (36.8) | 460 (35.7) |
| Palliative intervention† | 22 (9.5) | 222 (10.2) | 40 (16.4) | 236 (18.3 ) |
| complications during treatment | | | | |
| Chemotherapy | 40 (25)* | 481 (44.7) | 22.5 (33) | 155 (48) |
| radiotherapy | - | 7 (0.6) | - | - |
| surgical | 3 (6.5) | 33 (8.6) | 2 (6.5) | 26 (15) |

Data are presented as n (% of treated cases) in each category; † minor palliative surgical procedure, endobronchial airway debulking or airway stent placement ;*differences between men and women, $p<0.01$

# Discussion

In the year 2000, lung cancer represented 10.0% of all incident cancers and was responsible for 18.1% of deaths from cancer in France [7]. During the two decades before 2000, the incidence of lung cancer increased from 47.4 to 52.2 per hundred thousand in French men. In the same period, the incidence in women was doubled from 3.7 to 8.6 per hundred thousand [17][19][20]. Especially, the risk of developing lung cancer was increased considerably (+451%) between the generation of women born in 1953 and those born in 1913 [21]. In the present survey, we found that the new lung cancer cases diagnosed during the last five years in a reference centre in North France exceeded the number of lung cancer cases of the previous decade. Our results confirm the findings of recent analyses which have detected a clear trend toward a higher incidence in women in France and elsewhere [11][12][17] and provide useful information considering that lung cancer incidence in women in North France is considered to be one of the lowest in France.

Our findings may be skewed due to the retrospective nature of our investigation because of lost or unavailable data, particularly in these cases where patients were transferred to other hospitals or health care regions. In addition, this is one-centre study. However, our institution is the main tertiary health centre in North France serving a large population and useful information can be provided by studying lung cancer incidence in such a long time period. In addition, our results are consistent with the rates reported elsewhere in the literature regarding trends in lung cancer in women [11][14]. Moreover, figures gathered systematically by other authors or for certain areas based on similar case finding methods and yielded similar trends and annual incidence rates [22][23][24]. In this respect our findings deserve consideration.

The rate of female lung cancer patients in North France has been always less than 15% and less than men [7]. Female lung cancer incidence in this region of France was one of the lowest in the country [17]. However, our results suggest a significant increase in the number of lung cancer cases in women. Furthermore the age of patients at the time of diagnosis of lung cancer was lower than other series which have reported to be around 63 to 67 years [25][26]. In addition, cigarette smoking is the main culprit for lung cancer epidemic. A significant proportion of women in this region of France remain active smokers according to recent data [7]. The overall prevalence of current smoking among women of this region is estimated as 25% [7][27]. The percentage of active smokers among is about 30% thirty per cent for those women who were born between 1951 and 1960 and around 35% for those who were born between 1961 and 1970. The percentage of active smokers for those women who will be 50-60 years between 2010 and 2020 is alarmingly high. Furthermore, according to estimations regarding smoking trends in other countries smoking rates among women are expected to surpass those among men in the next years [28]. Although overall smoking rates have declined during the last decades we must still expect the incidence and mortality rates to continue rising for at least a decade due to the latency time between a fall in the rate of smoking and the start of a reduction in the incidence of lung cancer. Only after that, and if the prevalence of smoking addiction falls, a reduction in the incidence of lung cancer will be expected. On this basis, the increase of new lung cancer cases that was found in this study may be an early indication that lung cancer has the potential to reach epidemic proportions in women in this region affecting significantly mortality rates and expectancy of life.

The distribution of histologic types of lung cancer differed consistently among men and women. The most common histologic type was consistently adenocarcinoma among women. Squamous cell carcinoma was the most common type among men during the past decade. A trend towards an increase in the rate of adenocarcinoma was observed in the last five years of the studied period in men whereas the rate of small cell lung cancer was lower compared to the last decade in this study. This new trend has already been confirmed in the United States [29][30]. Several explanations have been proposed for the distribution of the histologic types of lung cancer. First, the decline in smoking observed in the past decades may lead to a decrease in certain type of cancers. Although, smoking is a risk factor for all histologic types of lung cancer, the association is much stronger for squamous cell, small cell, and large cell carcinomas than for adenocarcinomas. Second, the systematic use of low-nicotine and filtered cigarettes may also be a plausible explanation. Smokers try to achieve high nicotine levels by deeper inhalation of tobacco and as a consequence, carcinogenic substances can reach deeper areas of the lung. This pattern may favor malignancies which are more prevalent in lung parenchyma than in central bronchial tree, such as adenocarcinoma. However, these hypotheses do not fully explain the observed differences. Men smokers have similar risk for the development of squamous cell and small cell carcinomas, whereas women smokers appear to have a much higher risk for the development of small cell compared to squamous cell carcinoma [3][32][33][34]. Thus, gender differences in the distribution of histologic types of lung cancer may also be due to basic differences in the etiology of lung cancer in male and female patients.

In the present investigation the vast majority of patients had already advanced lung at the time that treatment was started. Especially, the percentage of patients with stage IV disease was alarmingly high to that reported in the literature. Unfortunately, lung cancer is asymptomatic in its early stages. Only 18% of cases are still confined to the primary site at diagnosis (local disease) while almost 40% are diagnosed after the cancer has already spread to other parts of the body [11]. This affects significantly survival rates (5 year survival rates are 51.3% for localized and 2.1% for metastatic disease) [2][34]. Therefore, attempts at early detection of lung cancer should be pursued. Unfortunately, the role of screening programs (chest radiography, low radiation computed tomography) is not yet clear [35][36]. However, in respect of the poor prognosis of lung cancer patients with metastatic disease, the evaluation of early detection screening programs with specific reference to gender should be a priority.

In the analysis for survival we did not include the period 2000-2005 since follow up data of this period are not yet available. In the period between 1990 and 1999, the overall survival in women was better compared to men. An explanation for this finding cannot be derived from the current study. There were no significant gender differences in terms of smoking history, age or co-morbidities that could affect significantly survival after treatment. Survival according to different types of treatment was not significantly better in women compared to men although it was consistently better in women. Gender differences found in treatment modalities and complications during treatment cannot explain sufficiently why median survival was superior in women. We speculate that basic gender differences may the difference in the outcome of lung cancer in men and women. Data from previous studies support this hypothesis. It has been shown that women with non-small cell lung cancer have a better survival than men when treated with surgery, radiation therapy with or without chemotherapy, and trimodality therapy, (chemotherapy, radiation therapy, and surgery) [37][38][39]. The same applies also in small cell lung cancer [40]. These data underline the fact that gender should be addressed as a specific research variable and that women should be actively recruited for inclusion from lung cancer clinical trials, in contrast to what has been done to a large degree in the past [41].

In summary, the overall message conveyed by our data is that the passing years have seen a gradual increase in the number of female patients diagnosed with lung cancer. Adenocarcinoma was the histologic type of cancer which predominated in women while a change in the histologic pattern in men, from squamous cell towards lung adenocarcinoma, was observed. The data suggested that women presented less often complication to chemotherapy than men, especially in the period between 1990 and 1999. The overall median survival time was better in women than in men in the same period. In view of the increased number of new lung cancer cases in women and the advanced stage of cancer at time of diagnosis findings, not only tobacco control but also early detection screening for lung cancer with reference to gender should be high priorities of the health care services.

**Table 3. Median survival in men and women by stage and treatment modalities in non small cell lung cancer and small cell lung cancer, in the period 1990-1999**

| | *non small cell lung cancer* | | *small cell lung cancer* | |
|---|---|---|---|---|
| | *Women* | *Men* | *Women* | *Men* |
| *all stages* | *270 (95-565)** | *217 (70-502)* | *301 (47-600)*** | *220 (71-485)* |
| *local disease* | *465 (190-785)* | *424 (218 - 946)* | *364 (275-607)* | *344 (158 – 474)* |
| *metastatic disease* | *265 (117-458)** | *191 (67-350)* | *247 (35-593)* | *208 (33 – 349)* |
| *Chemotherapy* | *250 (84-504)* | *233 (115-420)* | *364 (70-617)* | *277 (163-450)* |
| *Curative Surgery* | *568 (262-1138)* | *549 (210-1281)* | - | *235 (93 -555)* |
| *Radiotherapy* | *286 (94 -595)* | *298 (135-562)* | - | *155 (42-294)* |
| *Palliative medical care* | *96 (26-260)* | *46 (14-192)* | *36 (9-53)* | *35 (10-47)* |
| *Palliative intervention†* | *275 (19-613)* | *114 (49-380)* | - | *69 (22-432)* |

Data are presented as median ($25^{th}$ – $75^{th}$ percentile) values; † ie. minor palliative surgical procedure, endobronchial airway debulking, airway stent placement; *difference between men and women with non- small cell lung cancer, p=0.01; **difference between men and women with small cell lung cancer, p=0.001.

## REFERENCES


[1] Smith, RA, Glynn, TJ. Epidemiology of lung cancer. *Radiol. Clin. North Am.* 2000; 38:453-470.

[2] Henschke CI, Yankelevitz DF, Miettinen OS. International Early Lung Cancer Action Program Investigators. Computed tomographic screening for lung cancer: the relationship of disease stage to tumor size. *Arch. Intern. Med.* 2006; 166:321-5.

[3] Imbernon E. Estimation du nombre de cas de certains cancers attribuables à des facteurs professionnels en France. Institut de veille sanitaire, 2003 ; http://www.invs.sante.fr/publications/2003/cancers_pro/rapport_cancer_pro.pdf. [accessed December 20, 2006]

[4] Janssen-Heijnen ML, Coebergh JW. The changing epidemiology of lung cancer in Europe. *Lung Cancer.* 2003; 41 (3): 245-258.

[5] Menegoz F, Cherie-Challine L. Le cancer en France : Incidence et Mortalité. Situation en 1995. Evolution entre 1975 et 1995. Réseau FRANCIM, Ministère de l'Emploi et de la Solidarité, La documentation Française, 1998: 25-69.

[6] De Zelicourt M. et al, Epidémiologie et coûts du cancer du poumon en France. *Bull. Cancer.* 2001; 88 (8): 753-758.

[7] Institut National de la Statistique et des Études Économiques. Regards sur la parité. Cancers; 2006. http://www.insee.fr/fr/insee_regions/Nord-Pas-de-calais/zoom/6_2.htm [accessed December 20, 2006]

[8] Gorlova OY, Zhang Y, Schabath MB, Lei L, Zhang Q, Amos CI, et al. Never smokers and lung cancer risk: a case-control study of epidemiological factors. *Int. J. Cancer.* 2006; 118:1798-804.

[9] Environmental protection agency (EPA). Respiratory health effects of passive smoking: lung cancer and other disorders; 1992. http://cfpub.epa.gov/ncea/cfm/ets/etsindex.cfm [accessed December 20, 2006].

[10] Fu JB, Kau TY, Severson RK, Kalemkerian GP. Lung cancer in women: analysis of the national surveillance, epidemiology, and end results database. *Chest.* 2005; 127:768-77.

[11] Jemal A, Murray T, Ward E, Samuels A, Tiwari RC, Ghafoor Ac.Cancer statistics, 2005. *CA Cancer J. Clin.* 2005; 55:10-30.

[12] Liu Y, Inoue M, Sobue T, Tsugane S. Reproductive factors, hormoneuse and the risk of lung cancer among middle-aged never-smoking Japanese women: a large-scale population based cohort study. *Int. J. Cancer.* 2005;117:662-6.

[13] Schwartz AG, Ruckdeschel JC. Familial lung cancer: genetic susceptibility and relationship to chronic obstructive pulmonary disease. *Am. J. Respir. Crit. Care Med.* 2006; 173:16-22.

[14] International Early Lung Cancer Action Program Investigators- Henschke CI, Yip R, Miettinen OS. Women's susceptibility to tobacco carcinogens and survival after diagnosis of lung cancer. *JAMA.* 2006; 296:180-4.

[15] Du W, Gadgeel SM, Simon MS. Predictors of enrollment in lung cancer clinical trials. *Cancer.* 2006; 106:420-5.

[16] Murthy VH, Krumholz HM, Gross CP. Participation in cancer clinical trials: race-, sex-, and age-based disparities. *JAMA.* 2004; 291:2720-6.

[17] Salem G, Rican S, Jougla E. Géographie d'une épidémie silencieuse: le cancer du poumon féminin en France (1973-1999). *Oncologie.* 2004; 6(8): 535-539

[18] Yates JW, Chalmer B, McKegney FP. Evaluation of patients with advanced cancer using the Karnofsky performance status. *Cancer.* 1980; 45(8):2220-4.

[19] Parkin DM. Global Cancer Statistics in the year 2000. *The Lancet Oncology.* 2002; 2: 533-43.

[20] Howe HL, Wingo PA, Thun MJ, et al. Annual report to the nation on the status of cancer (1973 through 1998), featuring cancers with recent increasing trends. *J. Natl. Cancer Inst.* 2001; 93: 824-42.

[21] Molinie F, Velten M, Remontet L, Bercelli P, Reseau Francim. The progression of lung cancer incidence in France (1978-2000). *Rev. Mal. Respir.* 2006; 23(2 ):127-34.

[22] Hernández Hernández JR, Tapias del Pozo JA, Moreno Canelo P, Rodríguez Puebla A, Paniagua Tejo S, Sánchez Marcos JC. Incidencia del cáncer de pulmón en la provincia de Ávila. Año 2002 y tendencias en una década. *Arch. Bronconeumol.* 2004; 40:304-10is

[23] Mäkitaro R, Pääkkö P, Huhti E, Bloigu R, Kinnula VL.. An epidemiological study of lung cancer: history and histological types in a general population in northern Finland. *Eur. Respir. J.* 1999; 13:436-40is.

[24] Andrews JL, Bloom S, Balogh K, et al. Lung cancer in women—Lahey Clinic experience, 1957-1980. *Cancer.* 1985; 55:2894-98

[25] Sánchez de Cos Escuín J, Miravet Sorribes L, Núñez Ares A, Hernández Hernández J, Abal Arca J, Montero Martínez C, et al. Lung cancer in Spain. Last epidemiological trends concerning age, gender, smoking prevalence and histological types. Proceedings of the 11th World Conference on Lung Cancer; 2003, Barcelona, Spain.

[26] Stabile LP, Siegfried JM. Sex and gender differences in lung cancer. *J. Gend. Specif. Med.* 2003; 6:37—48.

[27] Aliaga C. Le tabac : vingt ans d'usage et de consommation. Institut National de la Statistique et des Études Économiques (Insee). Première n°808: 2001. p 1-4..

[28] Pierce JP, Fiore MC, Novotny TE, et al. Trends in cigarette smoking in the United States: projections to the year 2000. *JAMA.* 1989; 26:61-65

[29] Beckles MA, Spiro SG, Colice GL, Rudd RM. Initial evaluation of the patient with lung cancer. *Chest.* 2003; 123:97S-104S.

[30] Spiro SG.. Clinical features and assessment of lung cancer. In: Gibson GJ, Geddes DM, Dostabel U, Sterk PJ, Corrib B, editors. Respiratory medicine. 3rd ed. London: Elsevier; 2003. p. 1828-49.

[31] Schoenberg JB, Wilcox HB, Mason TJ, et al. Variation in smoking-related lung cancer risk among New Jersey women. *Am. J. Epidemiol.* 1989; 130:688-95.

[32] Osann KE. Lung cancer in women: the importance of smoking, family history of cancer, and medical history of respiratory disease. *Cancer Res.* 1991; 51:4893-97.

[33] Osann KE, Anton-Culver H, Kuosaki T, et al. Sex differences in lung-cancer risk associated with cigarette smoking. *Int. J. Cancer.* 1993; 54:44-48.

[34] Surveillance, epidemiology and end results (SEER) data base Fast Stats: lung and bronchus cancer. http://seer.cancer.gov/ [accessed Decemcer 20, 2006].

[35] Strauss GM, Gleason RE, Sugarbaker DJ. Chest x-ray screening improves outcome in lung cancer: a reappraisal of randomized trials on lung cancer screening. *Chest.* 1995; 107: 270S-79S.

[36] Weiss W, Boucot KR. The Philadelphia Pulmonary Neoplasm Research Project: early roentgenographic appearance of bronchogenic carcinoma. *Arch. Intern. Med.* 1974; 134:306-11.

[37] Mitsudomi T, Tateishi M, Oka T, et al. Longer survival after resection of non-small cell lung cancer in Japanese women. *Ann. Thorac. Surg.* 1989; 48:639-42.

[38] Graham MV, Purdy JA, Emami B, et al. Preliminary results of a prospective trial using three dimensional radiotherapy for lung cancer. *Int. J. Radiat. Oncol. Biol. Phys.* 1995; 33:993-1000.

[39] Albain KS, Rusch VW, Crowley JJ, et al. Concurrent cisplatin/etoposide plus chest radiotherapy followed by surgery for stages IIIA(N2) and IIIB non-small cell lung

cancer: mature results of Southwest Oncology Group phase II study 8805. *J. Clin. Oncol.* 1995; 13:1880-1992.

[40] Skarin AT. Analysis of long-term survivors with small-cell lung cancer. *Chest.* 1993; 103:440S-44S.

[41] Patterson WB, Emanuel EJ. The eligibility of women for clinical research trials. *J. Clin. Oncol.* 1995; 13:293-99.

In: Lung Cancer in Women
Editor: Varetta N. Torres, pp. 247-277
ISBN: 978-1-60021-659-6


*Chapter XII*

# OUTDOOR AIR POLLUTION AND LUNG CANCER: ARE WOMEN AT A HIGHER RISK?

***Stefano Parodi**** 
Epidemiology and Biostatics Section, Scientific Directorate, G.Gaslini Children's Hospital, L.go G. Gaslini, 5, 16147 Genoa, Italy

## ABSTRACT

Lung cancer accounts for more than 1 million deaths worldwide per year. Even if most of them are caused by tobacco smoking, the role of environmental causes, including outdoor air pollution, is now generally recognized.

Early evidence for a higher risk of developing lung cancer for populations residing in highly polluted areas came from ecological studies published in the '60s. Such evidence was repeatedly confirmed by many other ecological and semi-ecological investigations, including migrant studies and point source analyses. However, the more compelling evidence came from analytical investigations (case-control and cohort studies), which allow a more strict control for potential confounding. In particular, population-based cohort studies made in the USA and, more recently, in Northern Europe, have definitively demonstrated the role of air pollution as a risk factor for lung cancer.

In many recent investigations, expecially case-control studies, females have been found to have a higher susceptibility than males to tobacco smoking, which contains many known or alleged carcinogens also present in urban and industrial air pollution (*e.g.*, benzene, polycyclic aromatic hydrocarbons, thin particulate matter and formaldehyde). Moreover, such a finding was confirmed by a recent large screening survey and supported by results from many genetic and biochemical investigations, even if some recent cohorts studies have reported similar rates between female and male smokers. The difficulty of assessing the individual past exposure both to air pollution and to possible confounding factors has hampered the production of reliable estimates of the excess risk due to the exposure to air pollutants. As a consequence, comparisons between

* Stefano Parodi: Tel 0039 010 5636 301; fax 0039 010 377 6590; e-mail stefanoparodi@ospedale-gaslini.ge.it.

risks in males and in females are often lacking, while studies reporting estimates of the impact of air pollution separately in the two sexes have provided conflicting results. However, some recent investigations, especially ecological comparisons and point source analyses, have occasionally shown a higher risk for the female gender. Uncontrolled smoking habits, including passive smoking, indoor exposures to other pollutants, occupational exposures, chronic pulmonary diseases, dietary habits and socio-economic status are all factors that may account for most of differences in the risks observed by gender, but the hypothesis of a higher susceptibility of women cannot be completely ruled out. This chapter reviews the evidence both in favour of and against this hypothesis, using the more relevant epidemiological literature from the last 20 years.

## INTRODUCTION

Lung cancer is the most frequent neoplasia occurring in the world, accounting for about 1.2 million incidence cases in 2000, with more than 50% in developed countries. It is the most common cancer in men and the fifth most common cancer in females. In women the worldwide incidence rate, expressed as number of new cases per 100,000 persons per year, has been estimated to be 11.1, while in men the corresponding figure is 34.9 (Ginsberg, 2005).

In most western countries, incidence is increasing in women, even if it has recently shown a tendency to reach a plateau in the USA and in many European countries, while in men incidence and mortality rates are now decreasing, according to changes in the pattern of smoking habits in the last decades (Ginsberg, 2005; Levi *et al*, 2006). In many less developed countries, where smoking in women is generally rare, there is little change in risk (Parkin, 2002). Incidence of histologic subtypes in general differs by gender; in particular, small cell carcinoma and adenocarcinoma are more common in women than in men (Ginsberg, 2005).

Worldwide mortality figures indicate that approximately 1.1 million deaths were attributed to lung cancer in 2000 (Whitrow *et al*, 2003; Parkin *et al*, 2000). In fact, in spite of advances in theurapeutical regimes, lung cancer remains a highly lethal disease, being the first cause of death from cancer in males in most of the developed countries. In the USA lung cancer in females is now the first cause of death from cancer, even passing breast cancer since 1987, and accounts for about 32% and 25% of all cancer deaths in males and females, respectively (Patel *et al*, 2004; Ginsberg, 2005). In Europe, in 2002 it became the second main cause of death from cancer in women after breast cancer, passing colo-rectal cancer (Levi *et al*, 2006). Time trend of mortality rates is consistent with that observed for incidence, due to the high lethality of this disease.

Tobacco smoke has been recognized to be by far the main risk factor for lung cancer, accounting for about 85-90% of the total incidence burden (Doll *et al*, 1994; Thomas *et al*, 2005; Thun *et al*, 2006). However, due to the high incidence and mortality of such a disease, the burden of lung cancer not related to tobacco smoking cannot be considered as negligible. In fact, if the impact of the exposure to tobacco smoking is eliminated, lung cancer will remain the sixth cause of death from cancer in the USA (Thun *et al*, 2006). Apart from passive exposure to tobacco smoking and to other indoor air pollutants, in particular residential radon, which have been recognized as important risk factors in nonsmokers in numerous studies (Boffetta, 2004), many other environmental factors have been found to be associated with the risk of developing this disease, including chronic nonmalignant lung diseases, occupational exposures, diet, and outdoor air pollutants.

The carcinogenic effect of outdoor air pollution was proposed since the early 1960s in studies comparing incidence and mortality in urban and in rural areas, and, in the following decades, by many other ecologic and case-control studies comparing areas of higher *vs.* lower pollution. However, compelling evidence of an effect of outdoor air pollutants was obtained only after the publication of 3 important cohort studies in the USA in the 1990s (Dockery *et al*, 1993; Pope *et al*, 1995; Beeson *et al*, 1998), and further confirmed by many other more recent investigations.

In spite of this increasing amount of evidence, the difficulty to assess previous exposure to an individual level, the presence of different mixtures of carcinogenic pollutants at different areas and other limitations of observational epidemiological studies (including statistical power and residual confounding) made estimates of the association between air pollutants and lung cancer risk rather unsettled. In light of such uncertainty, different risks occasionally observed by gender are difficult to interpret and the possibility of a higher susceptibility for females has not been explicitly addressed in most of such investigations. However, many studies, in particular those analyzing exposure to cigarette smoking, have suggested that females might be more susceptible to the effect of inhaled carcinogenic compounds, despite some conflicting evidence (Blot and McLaughlin, 2004; Risch and Miller, 2004). Furthermore, recent results from molecular biological studies suggest that a different susceptibility to carcinogenic air pollutants in the two sexes cannot be completely excluded.

This chapter reviews the main evidence in the scientific literature about the impact of outdoor air pollutants on the risk of developing lung cancer, comparing risk estimates in females and males from analytical epidemiological studies published in the last 20 years. Due to their relevance, cohort studies will be described in more detail.

## Risk Factors for Lung Cancer

Cigarette smoking is recognised to be the most important risk factor in the development of lung cancer, accounting for approximately 85 to 90% of the whole incidence of this disease (Thomas *et al*, 2005). There are at least two ways that smoking is associated with lung cancer. Polycyclic aromatic hydrocarbons (PAH), mainly released by the combustion process, may induce mutations in the p53 gene, especially G to T transversions (Stellman *et al*, 1997). p53 is the most frequently mutated gene in most of the human cancer sites, including the lung (Alberg *et al*, 2005). It encodes for a 53-kd nuclear phosphoprotein that induces cell cycle arrest or alternatively may cause apoptosis, acting as a tumor suppressor. Agents causing mutations in p53 facilitate the accumulation of DNA damage in target cells and, preventing apoptosis, may eventually lead to malignant transformation (Sun, 2006).

Moreover, tobacco contains many other substances, including several N-nitroso compounds that are recognized cancerogens and whose presence is sufficient to explain the induction of cancer in human beings (IARC, 1986; Stellman *et al*, 1997). Finally, many molecular changes have been recently reported in the different steps of lung cancerogenesis induced by cigarette smoking, including allelic loss in 3p chromosomal regions, epigenetic changes in many tumor suppressor genes, mutation of the K-ras oncogene and overexpression of MYCN (Alberg *et al*, 2005). Smoking is more related to squamous and small cell carcinoma than adenocarcinoma. However, in the past few decades, the incidence of adenocarcinoma increased more rapidly than that of the other types. Such a change seemed to be related to the decrease in tar contents in modern cigarettes and to the increase of nitrosamines (Stellman *et al*, 1997).

Occupational exposure accounts for about 2-4% of the total cancer burden, but it is responsible for more than 20% of cancer risk in exposed workers (Doll and Peto, 1981; Boffetta *et al*, 1995). Regarding lung cancer, many known or probable carcinogens have been identified in the occupational setting, including asbestos, arsenic, bis(chloromethyl)ether, chromium, nickel, vinyl chloride, PAH, cadmium, accrylonitrile and formaldehyde (Williams and Sandler, 2001; Boffetta, 2004). The impact of such substances is difficult to evaluate in occupationally exposed individuals, due to the difficulty to control for residual confounding by smoking habit, which is more present in blue collar workers, and for the possibility of interaction with tobacco smoke (Williams and Sandler, 2001). Investigations restricting the analyses to nonsmoker workers are rather rare and often lack statistical power. A recent multicenter case-control study in Europe, which included 223 lung cancer cases and 1039 controls, suggested a rather limited effect of occupational exposures on lung cancer risk in nonsmokers, but confirmed the independent carcinogenic effect of nonferrous metal dust and fumes, and silica. Interestingly, a higher risk was observed among females (Zeka *et al*, 2006).

Chronic lung diseases may predispose to lung cancer. In particular, pulmonary fibrosis, asthma, emphysema, tuberculosis, chronic bronchitis and pneumonia have been reported to be associated with lung cancer risk in nonsmokers, causing an excess risk of about 50% (Williams and Sandler, 2001; Wu *et al*, 1995). Other diseases suspected to be associated with the risk of developing lung cancer are a previous lung cancer, HIV infection (Parker *et al*, 1998; Bower *et al*, 2003; Thompson *et al*, 1996) and breast cancer treated with irradiation, these latter in smoking women, thus providing evidence of a possible interaction (Ford *et al*, 2003; Deutsch *et al*, 2003).

A high intake of fruits and vegetables have been consistently reported to have a protective effect against lung cancer, but most principles involved in such action remain to be elucidated (Miller *et al*, 2004). The hypothesis of a protective role of beta-carotene, alpha-tocopherol and retinol was seriously questioned by the negative results of a large chemo-preventive trial in the USA, which showed a higher risk of lung cancer for smokers receiving supplements of such nutrients in their diet, eventually causing the investigation to be stopped before completion (Omenn *et al*, 1996). However, recent epidemiological and molecular studies indicate that an anti-oxidant protective effect of beta-carotene is likely to exist at low doses, while at high concentrations or in the presence of chronic oxidative stress, *e.g.*, due to smoking habits, it may act as a prooxidant, propagating free radical-induced reactions and favouring DNA mutations and cancer (Palozza, 2005).

Recently, some studies have investigated the role of phytoestrogens, like flavonoids contained in soya beans, in inhibiting tumorigenesis promoted by steroid hormones and in reducing the effect of oxidative stress. Furthermore, other studies have indicated a protective role of isothiocyanates by the induction of phase II detoxification enzymes, providing a molecular basis for the protective effect of a regular consumption of cruciferous vegetables (cabbages, broccoli, brussels sprouts) (Alberg *et al*, 2005). The protective effect of such nutrients seems to be mediated by different genotypes of GSTM1 and GSTT1 genes, which are implicated in the elimination of isothiocyanates (Alberg *et al*, 2005; Brennan *et al*, 2005).

High levels of alcohol consumption have been consistently associated with an increased risk of lung cancer (Korte *et al*, 2002), but a possible influence of residual confounding by smoking habits cannot be completely excluded (Alberg *et al*, 2005).

Genetic predisposition to lung cancer have been consistently reported by many studies on cancer clusters in families (Williams and Sandler, 2001; Bilello *et al*, 2002). In particular, a large case-control study on 945 patients with lung cancer in Germany revealed an excess risk to have a close relative with lung cancer (Odds Ratio, OR = 1.67). OR is an estimator of relative risk and it increased to 4.75 when the analysis was restricted to patients aged less than 51 years (Bromen *et al*, 2000). This finding was recently confirmed by a case-control study in Liverpool (UK), including 579 incident cases and 1157 controls, which estimated an OR = 4.89 for subjects with a diagnosis of lung cancer before 60 years to have a first-degree relative with cancer in the same age group (Cassidy *et al*, 2006). Such findings strongly point out a genetic component in lung cancer risk, especially in young and middle aged adults.

Further studies have been addressed to identify molecular mechanisms responsible for genetic susceptibility to lung cancer. In particular, such investigations tried to identify mechanisms of interaction between carcinogenic compounds, especially from tobacco smoking, and probability of DNA damage (Novello and Baldini, 2006). Among such investigations, many studies were focused to the difference, if any, between male and female susceptibility to inhaled carcinogenic compounds, and they may be particularly important in addressing the question of a higher susceptibility of women to outdoor air pollutants. For such reason results from such investigations will be reviewed in a dedicated paragraph.

Indoor air pollution is another recognized cause of lung cancer and women are in general more exposed than men (Pauk *et al*, 2005). Four components of indoor air pollution have been recognised, *i.e.*: radon, combustion products, chemicals, and biological agents (Lissowska *et al*, 2005).

Radon is the main contributor to lung cancer risk from indoor air pollution, and it was considered the second cause of lung cancer deaths in the USA (Pawel and Puskin, 2004).

Combustion products from heating and cooking and fumes from frying oils have been studied especially in developing countries, where they have been found to be associated with the risk of developing lung cancer (Gupta *et al*, 2001; Kleinemann *et al*, 2002, Boffetta *et al*, 2004). Moreover, a recent large case-control study (Lissowska *et al*, 2005) in six Eastern Central European countries and in the UK reported a moderate but statistically significant excess risk for the use of solid fuel for cooking and/or for heating (ORs ranged between 1.2 and 1.4), confirming previous evidence also in more developed areas. Among combustion products, environmental tobacco smoke is another recognized cause of lung cancer. In fact, in nonsmokers who lived with smokers a significant excess risk of 24% was estimated, with an evidence of a dose-response trend (Hackshaw *et al*, 1997).

The carcinogenic effect of outdoor air pollution was repeatedly proposed in the 1960s by studies (most ecologic) comparing lung cancer mortality or incidence in urban *vs.* rural areas

(Katsouyanni and Pershagen, 1997). Ecologic studies are considered as merely descriptive, due to their inability in assessing previous exposures, in controlling for many possible confounders and due to the availability of exposure at an aggregate level only, that may generate false evidence of an effect, a phenomenon known as "ecological fallacy" (Kleinbaum *et al*, 1987). However, in the following years such evidence was confirmed by many ecologic and semi-ecologic investigations (including point source analyses around industrial sites) and by many case-control studies, which allow a better control for the confounding effect from personal exposures, including smoking habits and occupation (Breslow and Day, 1980). However, evidence of the impact of air pollution remained somewhat controversial. Moreover, case-control studies may be prone to some biases in particular related to the anamnestic source of information about exposure and about many possible confounders. For instance, cases may have a different ability than controls in remembering the occurrence or the intensity of some exposures, a phenomenon known as recall bias (Breslow and Day, 1980). Such a bias may be even more insidious when information about exposure is obtained by interview from the next-of-kin of deceased subjects, which frequently occurs when very lethal diseases are considered or when the selection of cases and controls is based on mortality records. Moreover, selection bias may occur during the recruitment of cases or, more frequently, of controls (Breslow and Day, 1980). Results from prospective cohort studies are considered as more reliable, in that the measure of the exposure precedes the onset of the disease (Kleinbaum *et al*, 1987; Vineis *et al*, 2004). Compelling evidence of an effect of outdoor air pollutants was obtained only after the publication of 3 important cohort studies in the USA in the 1990s, and further confirmed by many other recent investigations (Vineis *et al*, 2004; Dockery *et al*, 1993; Pope *et al*, 1995; Beeson *et al*, 1998). Evidence of a carcinogenic effect of air pollution is consistent, but the corresponding relative risks (RRs) between exposed and unexposed populations are small, ranging up to about 1.5 (Katsouyanni and Pershagen, 1997). The low attributable risk of air pollution exposure and the presence of many possible confounders hampered observational epidemiological studies and made problematic both precise risk assessment than (as a consequence) comparisons of risks measures between males and females. These issues will be discussed further in this chapter at the light of results from analytical epidemiological investigations (case-control and cohort studies) carried out in the last 20 years.

## OUTDOOR AIR POLLUTION: MAIN SOURCES AND DIFFERENT POLLUTANTS

Main sources of outdoor carcinogens are: industrial plants, power plants, motor vehicles and house heating systems.

Known carcinogens commonly found in urban air are particulates, photochemical compounds, including ozone ($O_3$), carbon monoxide (CO), sulfur oxides ($SO_2$ and $SO_3$), nitrogen oxides ($NO_2$, $NO_3$ and $NO_X$), and heavy metals (Cohen, 2000; Curtis *et al*, 2006). In the last few decades the level of many such air pollutants has decreased in most urban settings in developed countries, including $PM_{10}$, sulfur oxides, carbon monoxide and benzo[a]pyrene (Cohen, 2000; Curtis *et al*, 2006). However, high concentrations of $O_3$ are still observed, especially in summer, because their reduction in outdoor air is very difficult and costly (Weschler, 2006).

Particulates include a large range of different molecules, whose toxicity strongly depends on their size. In fact particulates less than 10 μm (inhalable particles, $PM_{10}$) may penetrate in lower respiratory tract and particulate less than 2.5 μm (fine particles, $PM_{2.5}$) may penetrate very deeply and remain in the lung causing many respiratory and cardiovascular diseases, ranging from inflammation to death (Cohen *et al*, 2005). Moreover, as illustrated in the following paragraphs, evidence from epidemiological studies has linked exposure to $PM_{2.5}$ to the risk of developing lung cancer. Particulates may include arsenic, asbestos, chromium and nickel, radionuclides, benzene, polycyclic aromatic hydrocarbons (PAH) and nitro-PAH (IARC, 1987). Moreover, inhalable and fine particles may adsorb other air pollutants enhancing their toxic effect, probably including carcinogenic ones.

Carcinogenic effect of PAH and benzene is well recognized. Major sources of these pollutants are combustion of fossil fuels from motor vehicles and coal or oil-fired power plants, and some other industrial activities, including coke production (Cohen, 2000; Curtis et al, 2006; Lambert *et al*, 2004; Parodi *et al*, 2005). Among PAH, benzo[a]pyrene has been used as a marker for combustion sources of air pollution, because its cancerogenicity has been well assessed (Cohen, 2000).

Ozone is an important component of photochemical air pollution, which is produced by complex atmospheric reactions catalyzed by sunlight, especially in summer. High $O_3$ concentrations are associated with many respiratory symptoms and disease and with acute mortality episodes for respiratory and cardiovascular diseases (Weschler, 2006). Evidence of a carcinogenic effect of $O_3$, even if suggested by results from a population based cohort study (Beeson *et al*, 1998), remains undemonstrated.

Carbon monoxide (CO) in the outdooor environment is produced by incomplete combustion, especially from vehicles, heating systems and power plants and it is a well known cause of severe acute poisoning in indoor environments (Mannaioni *et al*, 2006). No carcinogenic effect of exposure to outdoor concentration of CO is demonstrated.

Sulfur dioxide is mainly produced by vehicle emissions, burning coal and from refineries, coke ovens and some other industries, while $NO_2$ is largely produced by industrial or vehicle combustion. Even though they partly share the same sources, $SO_2$ is often used as a marker of air pollution from house heating, while $NO_2$ is considered as a marker of traffic related pollutants (Nyberg *et al*, 2000). Evidence of their association with lung cancer risk emerged from both case-control and cohort studies, that will be reviewed in a later paragraph.

Many toxic metals, including suspected or recognized carcinogens like cadmium (Cd) and arsenic (As), are released in outdoor air especially from waste incinerators (Franchini *et al*, 2004) and from many industrial processes including metal mining, smelting (Curtis *et al*, 2006) and coke production (Lambert *et al*, 2004; Parodi *et al*, 2005).

Outdoor air pollutants are present as components of complex mixtures whose effects, including carcinogenic activity, are in general difficult to separate.

# Evidence of a Different Susceptibility of Females Exposed to Carcinogenic Compounds

Most studies addressing the hypothesis of a higher susceptibility of females exposed to carcinogenic compounds, in comparison with males, are investigations about the effect of tobacco smoking, but the results are still controversial.

Early studies on lung cancer in smoking women tended to report a lower risk than in male smokers, due to the lower average cigarettes smoked per day (Blot and McLaughlin, 2004). In the 1980s the hypothesis of an equal or even highest susceptibility for females started to be reported, supported by the association between hormonal and reproductive factors and risk of lung cancer, especially adenocarcinoma (Blot and McLaughlin, 2004). In the 1990s, the evidence of a higher susceptibility of females exposed to tobacco smoking came mainly from many case-control studies (Brownson *et al*, 1992; McDuffie *et al*, 1987; Harris *et al*, 1993; Risch *et al*, 1993; Osann *et al*, 1993; Zang and Wynder, 1996), even if some other investigations provided conflicting results (IELCAP, 2006). Among positive studies, Risch *et al* (1993) in a large matched case-control investigation including 442 female and 403 male lung cancer patients, reported a RR=27.9 in women and a RR=9.6 in men exposed to a lifelong exposure of 40 pack-years, compared to nonsmokers. Difference was more evident for small cell lung cancer and adenocarcinoma. Such studies confirmed a previous finding from another large case-control study in Canada, involving nearly 1,900 cancer cases, which estimated a relative risk of 1.5 of developing lung cancer in females compared with males (Zang and Wynder, 1996). Furthermore, a recent paper (IELCAP, 2006) reports on the results of two screening campaigns carried out in the USA on 16,925 current or former smokers (7,498 women and 9,427 men), which found a near double risk of detectable asymptomatic lung cancer in women (OR = 1.9, 95%CI: 1.5;2.5). Results were consistent in both series after adjusting by age and smoking intensity (pack-years). Interestingly, after adjusting for smoking intensity, disease stage, tumor cell type and resection, females remained at a better prognosis (hazard ratio, HR = 0.48, 95%CI: 0.25;0.89) suggesting that lung cancer in females might be considered as a different entity. However, the effect of some selection bias cannot be completely excluded (Neugut and Jacobson, 2006).

In spite of such evidence, the hypothesis of a higher susceptibility of lung cancer for females is not substantiated by results from cohort studies, which are considered as the most important investigations to assess causality in observational epidemiology (Kleinbaum, 1987). In particular, Bain *et al* (2004) reports on the results from two large cohorts (121,700 females and 51,529 males, recruited among nurses and male professionals, respectively). Information about smoking habits and other possible confounders was assessed and followed up by the administration of a structured questionnaire every two years. Lung cancer rates were similar among men and women, thus not supporting the hypothesis of a higher susceptibility for females. Moreover, this finding was consistent with the results of 6 prospective studies about lung cancer incidence and mortality (Bach *et al*, 2003; Prescott *et al*, 1998; Thun *et al*, 1995, Friedman *et al*, 1997; Nilsson *et al*, 2001; Marang-van de Mheen *et al*, 2001), reviewed in the same paper. Discrepancy between such investigations may be due to the fact that baseline risks (*i.e.*, lung cancer rates in non smokers) were not considered in the analysis of cohort studies (Risch and Miller, 2004). However, case-control studies are more prone to biases, especially recall bias and selection bias of controls (Bain *et al*, 2004).

Other evidence of a different susceptibility to carcinogenic compounds came from molecular and genetic studies, which were supported by the finding of estrogen receptors in lung cancer tissues. A recent paper found that an activating mutation of the tyrosine kinase domain of the Epidermal Growth Factor Receptor (EGFR), which is more likely to occur in nonsmoking females than males with adenocarcinoma, correlates with the radiological response to Tyrosine-kinase inhibitors such as gefitinib and erlotinib (Janne *et al*, 2005). Furthermore, many investigations showed that women may be more predisposed to molecular aberrations caused by the carcinogenic effect of tobacco smoke (Novello and Baldini, 2006), even if with some exceptions. For instance, Kure *et al* (1996) reported a higher G:C to T:A mutation in the p53 gene. On the contrary, a recent case-control investigation (Marrogi *et al*, 2005) on 303 lung cancer cases (102 women and 201 men) reported a similar pattern of TP53 mutation between males and females. Shriver *et al* (2000) showed that GRPR gene (gastric-releasing peptide) is associated with a not inactivated cluster on the X chromosome. As a consequence, such a gene tends to be more expressed in women than in men. GRPR stimulates cell proliferation and it has been found to be more expressed in female than in male smokers. Furthermore, its activation occurs early in females in response to stimulation by tobacco smoke, indirectly suggesting that females might be at higher risk of developing lung cancer. Moreover, females seem to have a lower DNA repair capacity and more K-ras mutations in non small cell lung cancer among smokers (Nelson *et al*, 1999). Mollerup *et al* (2006) analyzed the expression of many genes involved in the PAH bioactivation in relation to sex, smoking habits and bulky DNA adducts, and reported an elevated expression of CYP1A1 and CYP1B1 among current smokers compared to former and never smokers. Levels of CYP1A1, but not of CYP1B1 were significantly higher in female smokers than in male smokers (median ratio = 3.9, p = 0.011). Moreover, lung DNA adducts were highly significantly associated with CYP1A1 expression, thus supporting the hypothesis of a higher susceptibility of females to lung cancer. Finally, an association between HPV infection and lung cancer has been occasionally reported in women, but it does not seem to be causal (Thomas et al, 2005).

Annesi-Maesano *et al* (2003) reviewed the evidence of different susceptibility by gender in studies analyzing risks from air pollution exposures of both acute and chronic diseases. A higher excess risk of lung cancer for females than males exposed to outdoor air pollution did not clearly emerge from the review of three USA cohort studies (Dockery *et al*, 1993; Pope *et al*, 1995; Abbey *et al*, 1999). Results from such investigations and from other more recent case-control and cohort studies will be discussed in more detail further in this chapter. However, as regards nonmalignant respiratory diseases, the authors reported a higher rate of respiratory symptoms in young females than young males (including children) and a diminished level of lung function, that have been found to be associated with a risk of developing lung cancer later in life (Williams and Sandler, 2001). Similar difference in susceptibility was also reported for the adults, even if with some conflicting results (Annesi-Maesano *et al*, 2003).

# EVIDENCE OF DIFFERENT RISK OF LUNG CANCER BY GENDER IN POPULATIONS EXPOSED TO OUTDOOR AIR POLLUTION

A different risk by gender in populations exposed to outdoor air pollution has been occasionally observed, especially in ecologic studies. In particular, an investigation in the Teesside (Northern England) found a higher risk for females than males residing in an industrial area, including a coke oven, compared with two less polluted zones, selected as referents (Pless-Mulloli *et al*, 1999). In Italy a point source investigation around a coke oven located close to an urban area highlighted a higher risk for females residing near the plant, while in males no trend of risk was found around the plant after adjusting for age and deprivation (Parodi *et al*, 2005). Finally, an ecologic investigation in another industrial area in Northern Italy found an excess risk for females residing in heavily polluted zones in comparison with the remaining female population of the same province, after controlling for urbanization, age and deprivation, while no excess risk emerged for the exposed males (Parodi *et al*, 2004). Most of the excess risk observed in females in the Teesside area was probably due to the uncontrolled confounding effect of smoking habits and socio-economic factors, as indicated by a recent case-control study on the same area, including 204 female cancer cases and 339 controls (Edward *et al*, 2006). However, an excess risk for residents in the more polluted area still remained (OR = 1.38) even if statistical significance was not reached. Unfortunately, the study was restricted to the female gender, thus comparison of risks by sex was not available. Considering the results from the two above cited Italian studies, the absence of an excess risk in males exposed to industrial air pollution may be due to the confounding effect of occupational exposures and smoking habits. In Italian females occupational exposures to carcinogenic substances were unlikely. Furthermore, until recently tobacco smoking in Italy was rare in females (La Vecchia, 1986). Finally, due to the high proportion of housewives in Italy, women were likely to reside in the polluted area for more time than men, thus undergoing a more intense exposure.

As mentioned above, evidence from observational analytical investigations (*i.e.*, case-control and cohort studies) may be considered as probative, provided that an adequate control for confounding and for other possible biases (*i.e.*, selection and information biases) is made (Kleinbaum *et al*, 1987). However, they have rarely addressed the issue of a different susceptibility of the female gender exposed to outdoor air pollutants (Annesi-Maesano *et al*, 2003).

The main characteristics and the more relevant results from case-control studies published in the last two decades (1985 to 2006) are resumed in Table 1. All studies reported estimates of the impact of air pollution adjusted for smoking habit and for other possible confounders, except for the investigation by Yang *et al* (1999) and by Chiu et al (2006), that analyzed the same female population with a low proportion of smokers (less than 10%). Exposure assessment was made in different ways, depending on the different availability of pollution measures and the main aim of the study (Table 1A). In spite of such heterogeneity, relative risks between more and less exposed populations, estimated by the ORs, ranged between 1.3 and 2.0 in most of such investigations (Table 1B). Such findings are consistent with many previous observations by ecologic studies and with results from large cohort investigations (Katsouyanni and Pershagen, 1997). Unfortunately, comparisons between female and male Odds Ratios (ORs) in such studies were rare also in recent investigations. In fact, among the 14 studies reviewed, 4 included only men (publications n. 1, 5, 7, and 8, Table 1A), 4 recruited only females (publications n. 3, 6, 12 and 14), one restricted the analyses to males only (publication n. 4) and 3 reported results only for the total population as a whole (publications n. 10, 11 and 13). The two investigations reporting a comparison by gender (publications n. 2 and 9) showed a higher excess risk for males than females, but the corresponding 95% confidence intervals (95%CI) largely overlapped.

Table 2 resumes the main characteristics and the more relevant results from cohort studies on outdoor air pollution and lung cancer. As mentioned above, the first three investigations (publications n. 1, 2 and 3, table 2A) were USA cohort studies and they had a strong impact on the scientific community, providing a compelling evidence of the effect of urban air pollution both on cancer risk (especially lung cancer) and on cardiovascular diseases. Publication of such findings led to the adoption of new air quality standard in the USA and many other countries (Pope *et al*, 2002). The first investigation (Dockery *et al*, 1993), commonly referred to in scientific literature as the Harvard Six Cities (HSC) study, was based on a cohort of 8,111 individuals of both sexes 25-74 years old, randomly selected from six USA communities. In particular, this investigation highlighted the importance of the impact of fine particulate matter ($PM_{2.5}$) on the risk of mortality including lung cancer. The second study (Pope *et al*, 1995), represents today the largest prospective cohort study specifically addressing the issue of the chronic effect of outdoor air pollution on human health. More than 550,000 individuals residing in 151 metropolitan areas were recruited in the framework of the Cancer Prevention Study II (CPS II) by the American Cancer Society. Results from this study, from its reanalysis (Krewski *et al*, 2000) and from an update of the follow-up on the same cohort (Pope *et al*, 2002, publication n. 5) provided the most exhaustive evidence of the effect of air pollution on cardiovascular mortality and on lung cancer. Finally, the third investigation (Beeson *et al*, 1998) was based on an extension of the follow-up of a previous cohort study (Mills *et al*, 1991) that enrolled 6,338 non-Hispanic Seventh Day Adventist adult (age 27-95 years) residents in Basins of San Francisco, South Coast and San Diego in California, and it is generally cited in the scientific literature as the AHSMOG (Adventist Health Study on Smog). It represents the first attempt in a cohort study to assess exposure at a fine level (*i.e.*, the home address of each individual) using a model based on an interpolation of environmental data recorded by fixed monitoring stations. Moreover, it was based on incidence data, which are more reliable than mortality data. An effect of many air pollutants, including ozone, was observed. The three USA cohort studies did not find an excess risk for females esposed to air pollution (Table 2B). In particular, the HSC study reported only on estimates for the two sexes combined, while the CPS II study showed slightly higher relative risks (RR) for males than females, but such a difference was not statistically significant. The AHSMOG study showed a stronger association between air pollutant concentrations and risk of lung cancer in males than in females. Moreover, RRs for males were higher than those generally observed in the other cohort investigations (Table 2B), but such a finding was based on 36 lung cancer cases only. A further analysis of the AHSMOG study (Abbey *et al*, 1999) confirmed the effect of $PM_{10}$ and $O_3$ in males only. Unfortunately, data about fine particulate matter ($PM_{2.5}$), which were indicated as a major health concern in the HSC study, were not available.

**Table 1A. Characteristics of case-control studies on outdoor air pollution and lung cancer risk**

| Publication | Exposure groups (details) | Area |
|---|---|---|
| 1) Pershagen, 1985 | Living within 20 Km from a copper smelter | Ronnskarsverken, Sweden |
| 2) Jedrychowski *et al*, 1990 a) | residence in highly polluted areas ($TSP>150\ \mu g/m^3$ and $SO_2>104\ \mu g/m^3$) | Cracow, Poland |
| b) | non smokers resident in highly polluted areas ($TSP>150\ \mu g/m^3$ and $SO_2>104\ \mu g/m^3$) | Cracow, Poland |
| 3) Katsouyanni *et al*, 1991 | non smokers resident in highly polluted areas (daily smoke values > 400 $\mu g/m^3$) vs. low polluted areas (less than 100 $\mu g/m^3$) | Athens, Greece |
| 4) Jockel *et al*, 1992 a) | semi-quantitative air pollution index based on BaP, TSP, SO2 | 5 cities in Germany |
| b) | semi-quantitative air pollution index based on BaP, TSP, SO2 and latency more than 20 years | 5 cities in Germany |
| 5) Barbone *et al*, 1995 | residence in areas with high levels of particle deposition (>0.298 vs. < 0.175 $g/m^2$/day) | Trieste, Italy |
| 6) Yang *et al*, 1999 | residence in highly polluted areas | Taiwan |
| 7) Nyberg *et al*, 2000 a) | long term exposure to $NO_2$ ($\geq 30.6$ *vs* $< 15.2\ \mu g/m^3$) | Stockholm, Sweden |
| b) | 10-year exposure to $NO_2$, lagged 20 years ($\geq 29.3$ *vs* $< 12.8\ \mu g/m^3$) | Stockholm, Sweden |
| c) | long term exposure to $SO_2$ ($\geq 78.2$ *vs* $<41.3\ \mu g/m^3$) | Stockholm, Sweden |
| d) | 10-year exposure to $SO_2$, lagged 20 years ($\geq 129.1$ *vs* $<66.2\ \mu g/m^3$) | Stockholm, Sweden |
| 8) Petrauskaite *et al*, 2002 | living within 5 Km from an industrial site with high levels of sulfuric acid | Kedainiai, Lithuania |
| 9) Besso *et al*, 2003 | Living near a copper smelter | Ronnskarsverken, Sweden |
| 10) Belli *et al*, 2004 | residence within 2 Km from a petrochemical plant | Brindisi, Italy |
| 11) Fano *et al*, 2004 | residence in a highly trafficked zone (southern outskirt) | Civitavecchia, Italy |
| 12) Edwards *et al*, 2006 | residence in an industrial highly polluted area for more than 25 years | Teesside, England |
| 13) Vineis *et al*, 2006 a) | residing nearby heavily trafficked roads | 10 European countries |
| b) | $NO_2 > 30\ \mu g/m^3$ | 10 European countries |
| 14) Chiu et al,, 2006 | air pollution index based on $PM_{10}$, $O_3$, CO, $NO_2$ and $SO_2$ concentrations and adjusted for urbanization level | Taiwan |

**Table 1B. Number of subjects and relative risk estimates (OR) associated with air pollution in case-control studies on outdoor air pollution and lung cancer risk**

| | Exposure | Males | | Females | | Total | |
|---|---|---|---|---|---|---|---|
| | | Cases/<br>Controls | OR<br>(95% CI) | Cases/<br>Controls | OR<br>(95% CI) | Cases/<br>Controls | OR<br>(95% CI) |
| 1) | industrial site<br>(copper smelter) | 212<br>386 | 2.0<br>(1.2-3.4) | n.e.<br>n.e. | n.e. | n.e.<br>n.e. | n.e. |
| 2) a) | TSP and $SO_2$ | 901<br>875 | 1.46<br>(1.06-1.99) | 198<br>198 | 1.17<br>(0.70-1.96) | 1099<br>1073 | n.e. |
| b) | TSP and SO2 in non smokers | 49<br>221 | 1.45<br>(0.74-2.87) | 79<br>166 | 1.16<br>(0.48-2.80) | 128<br>387 | n.e. |
| 3) | daily smoke concentration | n.e.<br>n.e. | n.e. | 101<br>89 | 1.09<br>($p>0.05$) | n.e.<br>n.e. | n.e. |
| 4) a) | air pollution index | 80<br>160 | 1.16<br>(0.64-2.13) | 48<br>96 | n.e. | n.e.<br>n.e. | n.e. |
| b) | air pollution index<br>(adjusted for latency) | 80<br>160 | 1.82<br>(0.61-5.41) | 48<br>96 | n.e. | n.e.<br>n.e. | n.e. |
| 5) | particle deposition | 755<br>755 | 1.4<br>(1.1-1.8) | n.e.<br>n.e. | n.e. | n.e.<br>n.e. | n.e. |
| 6) | highly polluted areas | n.e.<br>n.e. | n.e. | 399<br>399 | 1.66<br>(1.05-2.61) | n.e.<br>n.e. | n.e. |
| 7) a) | $NO_2$ (last vs. first quartile) | 1,042<br>2,364 | 1.28<br>(0.87-1.88) | n.e.<br>n.e. | n.e. | n.e.<br>n.e. | n.e. |
| b) | $NO_2$ (last vs. first quartile, adjusting for latency) | 1,042<br>2,364 | 1.60<br>(1.07-2.39) | n.e.<br>n.e. | n.e. | n.e.<br>n.e. | n.e. |
| c) | $SO_2$ (last vs. first quartile) | 1,042<br>2,364 | 0.92<br>(0.63-1.34) | n.e.<br>n.e. | n.e. | n.e.<br>n.e. | n.e. |
| d) | $SO_2$ (last vs. first quartile, adjusting for latency) | 1,042<br>2,364 | 0.95<br>(0.64-1.39) | n.e.<br>n.e. | n.e. | n.e.<br>n.e. | n.e. |

**Table 1B. (Continued).**

| | Exposure | Males | | Females | | Total | |
|---|---|---|---|---|---|---|---|
| | | Cases/ Controls | OR (95% CI) | Cases/ Controls | OR (95% CI) | Cases/ Controls | OR (95% CI) |
| 8) | residing in an industrial site (high $SO_2$ levels) | 181<br>727 | 1.03 (0.76-1.39) | n.e.<br>n.e. | n.e. | n.e.<br>n.e. | n.e. |
| 9) | residing in an industrial site (copper smelter) | 209<br>518 | 1.38 (0.89-2.14) | 107<br>209 | 0.88 (0.48-1.62) | 316<br>727 | n.e. |
| 10) | residing in an industrial site (petrochemical plant) | 121<br>127 | n.e. | 23<br>49 | n.e. | 144<br>176 | 3.1 (0.83-12) |
| 11) | residence in a highly trafficked zone | 201<br>626 | n.e. | 33<br>103 | n.e. | 234<br>729 | 1.51 (1.04-2.18) |
| 12) | residence in an industrial site (many sources) | n.e.<br>n.e. | n.e. | 204<br>339 | 1.83 (0.82-4.08) | n.e.<br>n.e. | n.e. |
| 13) a) | residence close to heavily trafficked roads | n.e.<br>n.e. | n.e. | n.e.<br>n.e. | n.e. | 152<br>432 | 1.46 (0.89-2.40) |
| b) | $NO_2$ | n.e.<br>n.e. | n.e. | n.e.<br>n.e. | n.e. | 122<br>352 | 1.30 (1.02-1.66) |
| 14) | higher *vs.* lower value of air pollution index | n.e.<br>n.e. | n.e. | 972<br>972 | 1.28 (1.02-1.61) | n.e.<br>n.e. | n.e. |

*n.e.* = not evaluated or not reported

**Table 2A. Characteristics of cohort studies on outdoor air pollution and lung cancer risk**

| Publication | Exposure groups (details) | Area (Follow-up period) |
|---|---|---|
| 1) Dockery *et al*, 1993 | PM2.5 29.6 vs. 11.0 μg/m$^3$ (highest polluted city, i.e., Steubenville vs. lowest polluted city, i.e., Portage). | 6 cities in USA (1974-1991) |
| 2) Pope *et al*, 1995 a) | increment in sulfate particulate of 19.9 μg/m$^3$ | 151 US cities (1982-1989) |
| b) | increment in PM2.5 of 24.5 μg/m$^3$ | 151 US cities (1982-1989) |
| 3) Beeson *et al*, 1998 a) | $O_3$ increment based on the interquartile range (556 hr/year increment) | 3 large areas in California (1977- 1992) |
| b) | $PM_{10}$ increment based on the interquartile range (24 μg/m$^3$) | 3 large areas in California (1977- 1992) |
| c) | SO2 increment based on the interquartile range (3.7 ppb) | 3 large areas in California (1977- 1992) |
| d) | $NO_2$ increment based on the interquartile range (1.98 ppb) | 3 large areas in California (1977- 1992) |
| 4) Pope *et al*, 2002 | 10 μg/m$^3$ increase in in $PM_{2.5}$. | 151 US cities (1982-1998) |
| 5) Hoek *et al*, 2002 a) | Black smoke in urban background and from local sources (trafficked streets) | 204 municipalities in The Netherlands (1986-1994) |
| b) | NO2 in urban background and from local sources (trafficked streets) | 204 municipalities in The Netherlands (1986-1994) |
| 6) Nafstad *et al*, 2003 a) | 10 μg/m$^3$ increase in NOx | Olso, Norway (1974-1998) |
| b) | 10 μg/m$^3$ increase in $SO_2$ | Olso, Norway (1974-1998) |
| 7) Filleul *et al*, 2005 a) | Increase in 10 μg/m$^3$ $NO_2$ | 24 areas in 7 towns, France (1974-1998) |
| b) | Increase in 10 μg/m$^3$ $NO_2$ | 18 areas in France with low $NO_2$/NO ratio (1974-1998) |

**Table 2A. (Continued).**

| Publication | Exposure groups (details) | Area (Follow-up period) |
|---|---|---|
| 8) Naess *et al*, 2006 a) | $NO_2$ quartile increase (51-70 years old) | 470 neighborhoods in Oslo, Norway (1992-1998) |
| b) | $NO_2$ quartile increase (71-90 years old) | 470 neighborhoods in Oslo, Norway (1992-1998) |
| c) | $PM_{10}$ quartile increase (51-70 years old) | 470 neighborhoods in Oslo, Norway (1992-1998) |
| d) | $PM_{10}$ quartile increase (71-90 years old) | 470 neighborhoods in Oslo, Norway (1992-1998) |
| e) | $PM_{2.5}$ quartile increase (51-70 years old) | 470 neighborhoods in Oslo, Norway (1992-1998) |
| f) | $PM_{2.5}$ quartile increase (71-90 years old) | 470 neighborhoods in Oslo, Norway (1992-1998) |
| 9) Nawrot *et al*, 2006 | residing in an area contaminated by Cd from 3 zinc smelters vs. not contaminated area | 3 areas contaminated by Cd in Belgium (1985-2004) |

**Table 2B. Number of subjects and relative risk estimates (RR) associated with air pollution in cohort studies on outdoor air pollution and lung cancer risk**

| | | Males | | Females | | Total | |
|---|---|---|---|---|---|---|---|
| | Exposure | Subjects/ events | RR (95%CI) | Subjects/ events | RR (95%CI) | Subjects/ events | RR (95%CI) |
| 1) | PM2.5 > 18.6 µg/m$^3$ vs. ? | n.e. | n.e. | n.e. | n.e. | 8,111<br>n.e. | 1.37<br>(0.81-2.31) |
| 2) a) | increment in sulfate particulate of 19.9 µg/m$^3$ | n.e. | 1.43<br>(1.13-1.81) | n.e. | 1.17<br>(0.80-1.72) | 552,138<br>n.e. | 1.36<br>(1.11-1.66) |
| b) | increment in $PM_{2.5}$ of 24.5 µg/m$^3$ | n.e. | 1.10<br>(0.81-1.47) | n.e. | 0.90<br>(0.55-1.44) | 552,138 | 1.03<br>(0.80-1337) |
| 3) a) | Interquartile range of $O_3$ | 4,060<br>16 | 3.56<br>(1.35-9.42) | 2,278<br>20 | 0.94<br>(0.41-2.16) | 6,338<br>36 | n.e. |
| b) | Interquartile range of $PM_{10}$ | 4,060<br>16 | 5.21<br>(1.94-14.0) | 2,278<br>20 | n.e. # | 6,338<br>36 | n.e. |
| c) | Interquartile range of $SO_2$ | 4,060<br>16 | 2.66<br>(1.62-4.39) | 2,278<br>20 | n.e. # | 6,338<br>36 | n.e. |
| d) | Interquartile range of $NO_2$ | 4,060<br>16 | 1.45<br>(0.67-3.14) | 2,278<br>20 | n.e. | 6,338<br>36 | n.e. |
| 4) | 10 µg/m$^3$ increase in in $PM_{2.5}$ | n.e. | n.e.§ | n.e. | n.e.§ | 1.2 million<br>10,749 | 1.14<br>(1.04-1.23) |
| 5) a) | Black smoke in urban background vs. local sources | n.e. | n.e. | n.e. | n.e. | 4492<br>60 | 1.06<br>(0.43;2.63) |
| b) | NO2 in urban background vs. local sources | n.e. | n.e. | n.e. | n.e. | 4492<br>60 | 1.25<br>(0.42-3.72) |
| 6) a) | 10 µg/m$^3$ increase in NOx | 16,209<br>418 | 1.12<br>(1.05-1.20) | n.e. | n.e. | n.e. | n.e. |
| b) | 10 µg/m$^3$ increase in $SO_2$ | 16,209<br>418 | 1.01<br>(0.94-1.08) | n.e. | n.e. | n.e. | n.e. |

**Table 2B. (Continued).**

| | | Males | | Females | | Total | |
|---|---|---|---|---|---|---|---|
| | Exposure | Subjects/ events | RR (95%CI) | Subjects/ events | RR (95%CI) | Subjects/ events | RR (95%CI) |
| 7) a) | Changes in 10 $\mu g/m^3$ $NO_2$ | 6802<br>153 | n.e. | 7482<br>25 | n.e. | 14,284<br>178 | 0.97<br>(0.85-1.10) |
| b) | Changes in 10 $\mu g/m^3$ $NO_2$, (restriction to 18 sub-areas) | n.e.<br>n.e. | n.e. | n.e.<br>n.e. | n.e. | n.e.<br>n.e. | 1.48<br>(1.05-2.06) |
| 8) a) | $NO_2$ quartile increase (in 51-70 years old persons) | n.e.<br>449 | 1.07<br>(0.97-1.18) | n.e.<br>424 | 1.23<br>(1.10-1.38) | n.e.<br>873 | n.e. |
| b) | $NO_2$ quartile increase (in 71-90 years old persons) | n.e.<br>295 | 1.09<br>(0.98-1.20) | n.e.<br>285 | 1.12<br>(0.98-1.27) | n.e.<br>580 | n.e. |
| c) | $PM_{10}$ quartile increase (in 51-70 years old persons) | n.e.<br>449 | 1.07<br>(0.97-1.18) | n.e.<br>424 | 1.27<br>(1.13-1.43) | n.e.<br>873 | n.e. |
| d) | $PM_{10}$ quartile increase (in 71-90 years old persons) | n.e.<br>295 | 1.08<br>(0.98-1.20) | n.e.<br>285 | 1.17<br>(1.03-1.33) | n.e.<br>580 | n.e. |
| e) | $PM_{2.5}$ quartile increase (in 51-70 years old persons) | n.e.<br>449 | 1.07<br>(0.97-1.18) | n.e.<br>424 | 1.27<br>(1.13-1.43) | n.e.<br>873 | n.e. |
| f) | $PM_{2.5}$ quartile increase (in 71-90 years old persons) | n.e.<br>295 | 1.07<br>(0.97-1.18) | n.e.<br>285 | 1.16<br>(1.02-1.32) | n.e.<br>580 | n.e. |
| 9) | residing in an area contaminated by Cadmium | 471<br>12 | n.e. | 523<br>7 | n.e. | 994<br>19 | 4.17<br>(1.21-14.4) |

*n.e.* = not evaluated or not reported; events = lung cancer cases or deaths.

§ Estimates of RR and related 95%CI reported in Figure 3 of the original paper, but not in the text or in the tables. No significant differences emerged between males and females. # RR > 1, but statistically significance not reached (corresponding figures not available in the original paper).

In 2002 Pope *et al* published the results of the extended follow-up of the CPS II cohort (publication n. 4, Table 2), including other possible confounding factors (diet, more occupational data, copollutants other than $PM_{2.5}$) and using a more sophisticated method of statistical analysis (*i.e.*, Cox regression model with random spatial effects), which took into account the possible spatial correlation of the observed events. The study confirmed the association between outdoor air pollution and mortality for some causes, including lung cancer. Moreover, an effect of $PM_{2.5}$ emerged even if at a lower extent than in the HSC study (RR=1.14, table 2B). No significant differences by sex were observed (corresponding RRs estimates and their 95% CI were not shown in the tables of the paper, then they cannot be reported in Table 2B).

Two cohort studies carried out in Northern Europe were published almost at the same time as the extended follow up analysis of the CPS II cohort (publications n. 5 and 6, Table 2). The first one (Hoek *et al*, 2002) was performed in The Netherlands, selecting 5,000 individuals among the Netherland cohort study on diet and cancer (NLCS cohort). Due to the quite homogenous distribution of some pollutants (in particular $O_3$) on the area under study, only traffic-related pollutants were considered, and exposure was estimated by a GIS model, using regional background pollution, urban sources, local sources (nearby streets), and data about black smoke and $NO_2$ concentrations. Statistical power was too small to allow the evaluation of the risk of lung cancer and, as a consequence, comparisons by gender were not available. However, RR estimates were consistent with that reported by the two first USA studies (HSC and CPS II, Table 2B). The other North European cohort study was carried out in Norway (Nafstad *et al*, 2003, publication n. 6 in Table 2). The study included more than 16,000 individuals, thus resulting in the largest cohort study after CPS II. Moreover, it was based on incidence data and exposure was assessed estimating the outdoor concentration for each air pollutant at the home address, using historical concentrations from monitoring stations and emissions and meteorological and topographical observations. The study confirmed the impact of $NO_X$, but not of $SO_2$ on the risk of developing lung cancer. Unfortunately, the cohort was made by males only, thus preventing any comparison between RR estimates by gender.

Results from three other cohort studies carried out in Western Europe have been recently published (publications n. 7, 8 and 9, Table 2). The PAARC (Pollution Atmosphérique et Affection Respiratoires Chroniques) cohort study was performed in France (Filleul *et al*, 2005, publication n. 7 in Table 2) to investigate the effect of air pollution on chronic respiratory diseases. The cohort included 14,284 individuals of both sexes. $SO_2$, acidimetric method, TSP (total suspended particulate), black smoke, $NO_2$ and NO were available by fixed monitoring stations in 24 areas located in 7 towns. An effect of $NO_2$ on lung cancer mortality was observed only after restricting the analysis to the 18 areas with a $NO_2$/NO ratio lower than 3 ppb (table 2B), that corresponded to the exclusion of areas with monitoring stations located too close to trafficked street, whose measures were likely to have been biased. Unfortunately, separated analyses by gender were not reported for mortality from specific causes of death, including lung cancer.

Another study (Naess *et al*, 2006) was carried out in 470 neighborhoods in Oslo (Norway), where the main sources of air pollution were car traffic, road dust, wood burning and transport by trucks (this latter mainly for $PM_{2.5}$ and $PM_{10}$). For each neighborhood, air pollution concentration was estimated by an air dispersion model (called "AirQUIS" model). A statistically significant effect was observed for $NO_2$, $PM_{10}$ and $PM_{2.5}$, which was slightly more pronounced in the female gender (Table 2B). However, data available in this study did not allow a direct control for smoking habit, which was indirectly accounted for using socio-economic variables (*i.e.*, occupation and education). A survey previously carried out on the same area suggested that prevalence of smoking habit was similar between the differently polluted zones (Sogaard *et al*, 2004), but residual confounding cannot be completely ruled out.

The last cohort study reported in Table 2 (Nawrot *et al*, 2006, publication n. 9) represents the only prospective cohort investigation, at least to my knowledge, aimed at assessing the impact of industrial air pollution on the residing population. The studied area involved six districts of the municipalities of Balen, Lommel and Overpelt in Belgium where more than 3 mg/Kg of cadmium was present in soil, due to the presence of 3 zinc smelters. In areas with historically contaminated soils, house dust is a persistent potential source of exposure. The lung is the main route of entrance and a potential target. The heavily exposed area included 9,840 residents, whose 521 were recruited in the cohort. A reference area with a low contamination level of Cd was identified in 4 districts of the villages Hechtel and Eksel, with 9,390 inhabitants (473 included in the cohort). Data about previous and current exposures and possible confounders were obtained by a validated questionnaire. Moreover, urine samples were collected at the house of each participant at the beginning of the study and 1 week later; on that occasion also a blood sample was collected. Exposure to environmental Cd was associated with the risk of lung cancer. The RR, estimated by the Hazard Ratio, for living in the higher exposure areas was 4.17 (95%CI: 1.21-14.4, Table 2B). Furthermore, RR of 1.70 (95%CI: 1.13-2.57) and 1.57 (95%CI: 1.11-2.24) were found for doubling urinary cadmium concentration or cadmium concentration in the soil. Unfortunately, separated RR for males and females were not estimated, probably due to the small number of observed events.

## Discussion

Evidence of a higher susceptibility to develop lung cancer for females exposed to carcinogenic compounds was mainly provided by a study on tobacco smoking, but the results between case-control and cohort investigations were conflicting, the latter indicating a similar risk in male and female smokers. Even if results from cohort studies are in general considered more reliable than those from case-control investigations, the possibility that the higher susceptibility of females observed in the latter might be entirely due to residual confounding or to recall or selection bias, seems quite unlikely. One reason for the discrepancy may be a lower rate in unexposed (*i.e.*, not smoker) females than in males and to the presence of similar rates in similarly exposed subjects (*i.e.*, in ex and in current smokers). Such a pattern might have caused similar RRs to be estimated in cohort studies by the ratio of incidence or mortality rates in male and female smokers, and to different ORs observed by sex in case-control investigations (Blot and McLaughlin, 2004). The evaluation of a different susceptibility in the two sexes corresponds to assessing an interaction between exposure to tobacco smoking and gender, which should be performed by including in the model the baseline rates, *i.e.*, considering also the unexposed population (Risch and Miller, 2004). However, as noted by Blot and McLaughlin (2004), baseline rates are quite variable, reflecting the effects of uncontrolled exposures. This statement implicitly considers the effects of such factors and, probably, their interaction with genetic characteristics, as negligible in the comparison of risk estimates in male and female smokers, an assumption which remains undemonstrated. Nevertheless, it is known that smokers differ from never smokers in many characteristics, which are hardly accounted for even in well conducted analytical investigations (Leffondre *et al*, 2002). As a consequence, statistical models including interaction terms between exposure to tobacco smoking (or to other risk factors for lung cancer) and gender might provide unreliable results, and investigations aimed at assessing a different susceptibility by gender should also be addressed to explain the large variability of risk estimates in nonsmoker populations.

Evidence of different susceptibility by gender from genetic and molecular studies is more compelling (Thomas *et al*, 2005), but some results remain partly controversial. The presence of receptors for estrogen and progesterone in lung cancer tissues is an intriguing finding, which should be further investigated (Novello and Baldini, 2006).

Females might be at a different risk, especially in childhood and adolescence, of developing chronic nonmalignant lung diseases in response to exposure to air pollutants (Annesi-Maesano *et al*, 2003), which could predispose to lung cancer and, perhaps, rise their susceptibility to air pollution. Reasons for such a difference by gender relies on genetic and biological mechanisms, including a smaller lung and airways calibre in young females and a higher level of bronchial hyperresponsiveness (Annesi-Maesano *et al*, 2003).

If a higher risk for smoking females were demonstrated, it would not necessarily indicate a higher risk also for outdoor air pollutants, which are generally present in much lower concentrations than in tobacco smoking. However, molecular studies, especially about the efficiency of detoxification enzymes and DNA repair in the two sexes, will help in assessing the impact of inhaled carcinogens from both sources and to highlight differences in risk, if any, by gender.

As regards epidemiological studies on air pollution and lung cancer, they have not yet provided evidence of a higher risk for exposed females than males. However, as mentioned above, observational investigations are prone to many biases. Ecologic studies cannot be considered as probative, mainly due to ecological fallacy and uncontrolled confounding (Kleinbaum *et al*, 1987). Case-control studies may be affected by several limitations (Breslow and Day, 1980), the most commonly considered, as stated above, being recall bias and selection bias of controls. Moreover, some investigations based on mortality included among the control group some individuals that could be deceased by causes indirectly related to air pollution exposure, like cardio-vascular diseases, probably causing a bias toward null. Furthermore, as highlighted by Whitrow (2004), another insidious bias may be due to a higher compliance of controls living in exposed areas in participating in the investigation, thus masking the excess risk, if any, in exposed populations. This phenomenon could also explain the reverse bias (*i.e.* the false evidence of a protective effect of the exposure to outdoor air pollutants) occasionally encountered in some case-control studies (*e.g.*, Pawlega *et al*, 1997; Gupta *et al*, 2001; Whitrow, 2004).

Finally, as illustrated above in detail, most case-control studies reported only risk estimates for either males or females, or for both sexes combined, preventing any comparison by sex to be performed. Cohort studies are considered more reliable, but they are also prone to some biases, in particular information bias about exposure, especially when the risk factors and the possible confounders are measured only at the beginning of the follow up period. Moreover, the power required to identify small effect is hard to achieve (Whitrow *et al*, 2003). Furthermore, air pollution is a mixture of different compounds whose singular effects are hardly separable. In such a context, and in light of the low attributable risk of outdoor air pollutants at the commonly observed concentrations in urban air, even if females were more susceptible than males to some specific agents, significant different risks might not emerge.

Another limit deriving from the available sources of air pollution is the difficulty to assess exposure concentrations at an individual level, which may cause a misclassification bias of the exposure. A not differential (*i.e.*, a completely random) misclassification is likely to induce a bias toward null, also hampering comparison of relative risks by gender. However, results from the reanalyses of the HSC and CPS II cohorts (Krewski *et al*, 2000) found an interaction between exposure and socio-economic condition, indicating that such a bias could be, at least in part, not differential, because highly educated people could have experienced a lower individual exposure than lower educated ones. Very interesting, the only study reporting precise measures of individual cumulative exposures (Pawlega *et al*, 2006, publication n. 9 in Table 2), even if based on a rather small cohort with relatively few events, showed the highest RR. This finding suggests that indirect measures of personal exposure in the other studies might have caused the corresponding risks to be underestimated. Consequences of such biases on the comparison between male and female RRs are difficult to evaluate.

Finally, in the absence of individual measures of exposure, confounded by indoor air pollution, which is more likely to impact on females (especially housewives), cannot be excluded. Some studies have reported a high correlation between outdoor and indoor air pollutants, especially particulate matter (Brunekreef, 1999; Janssen *et al*, 1998). Concentration of some pollutants may be lower in indoor than in outdoor environments. For instance, ozone concentrations tend to be reduced in domestic environments, even if they may generate other toxic compounds by an oxidative mechanism (Weschler, 2006). Finally, other toxic substances, in particular benzene, may be more concentrated in indoor than in outdoor air. As highlighted by a survey by Cocheo *et al* (1999), carried out in 6 European towns, correlation between indoor and outdoor concentrations may depend on the different pollutants considered and by climatic and meteorological factors. In particular, as regards benzene, the association between indoor and outdoor pollution strongly varied with the latitude, probably due to a role of the different adsorbent surfaces on walls and floors (carpets, linoleum, wood, especially used in Northern countries, and tiling, marble and bare, prevalent in Southern Europe). In light of such a finding, most studies aimed at assessing the relationship between outdoor air pollution and risk of developing disease (including lung cancer) may be influenced by the confounding role of indoor air pollution even in the absence of active or passive smoking. Such a bias might also partly account for the heterogenity in lung cancer risk in nonsmoker women reported in many studies in different geographical areas.

## CONCLUSION

The hypothesis of a higher susceptibility of women to air-pollution-related lung cancer is not substantiated by epidemiological evidence, but most studies have not specifically addressed this issue. Moreover, a higher susceptibility to carcinogenic compounds is supported by many biological and genetic studies, even if with some conflicting results, thus such a hypothesis cannot be ruled out. However, the excess risk, if any, for females exposed to outdoor air pollution is expected to barely exceed the corresponding risk in males. Apart from the possibility of a higher susceptibility, in some situations females might be at a higher risk than males of developing lung cancer due to a more intense exposure. In particular, housewives living close to industrial sources of air pollution, contaminated areas or heavily trafficked streets could experience a higher cumulative exposure to air pollution and eventually a higher risk of developing lung cancer. Furthermore, indoor produced air pollutants, like radon and, especially in less developed countries, chemicals from heating and cooking combustion processes, passive smoking and asbestos, might enhance the impact of pollutants from outdoor sources. As a consequence, in some instances, females might be at a higher risk than males not occupationally exposed and with similar smoking habits.

Appropriate study designs are needed to investigate the presence of different susceptibility or different individual levels of exposure. Such research should be based on a prospective cohort design, should stratify (rather than adjust) for gender, take into account comparable exposure between males and females, and analyze the biological differences between males and females when exposed to air pollution (Annesi-Maesano *et al*, 2003). However, studies designated to specifically address these issues are expected to be very expensive, and the limited availability of funding might prevent them from being carried out. As suggested by Cohen (2003), a good option may be identifying existing cohorts, especially those with large numbers of non-smokers and for whom biological samples have been stored. However, since the impact of air pollution on human health is not limited to lung cancer, an integrated approach including many disciplines (environmental chemistry, epidemiology, molecular biology, genetics and clinical medicine) may help to design appropriate studies with the aim of further investigating the effect of outdoor air pollutants on human health. In such a framework, the issue of the identification of subpopulations at different levels of susceptibility might be addressed, including analysis restricted to lung cancer risk. In this context, the use of GIS models based on fixed monitoring station records (Bellander *et al*, 2001) and on climatic and meteorological values may integrate measures from individual and house specific indoor and outdoor samplers, which cannot be extensively used for long time periods, due to their high cost.

Investigations aimed at identifying subpopulations with characteristics that predispose them to the adverse effects of air pollutants, including carcinogenic ones, may have a strong impact on the scientific community, public opinion and public health providers. As suggested by Annesi-Maesano *et al* (2003), exploring the specific role of each pollutant and its mechanism of effect will also provide a basis for public health interventions.

# REFERENCES

Alberg AJ, Brock MV, Samet JM. Epidemiology of lung cancer: looking to the future. *J. Clin. Oncol.* 2005;23:3175-85.

Abbey DE, Nishino N, McDonnell WF, Burchette RJ, Knutsen SF, Beeson WL, Yang JX. Long-term inhalable particles and other air pollutants related to mortality in nonsmokers. *Am. J. Respir. Crit. Care Med.* 1999;159:373-82.

Annesi-Maesano I, Agabiti N, Pistelli R, Couilliot MF, Forastiere F. Subpopulations at increased risk of adverse health outcomes from air pollution. *Eur. Respir. J.* 2003; Suppl.40:57s-63s.

Bach PB, Kattan MW, Thornquist MD, Kris MG, Tate RC, Barnett MJ, Hsieh LJ, Begg CB. Variations in lung cancer risk among smokers. *J. Natl. Cancer Inst.* 2003;95:470-8.

Bain C, Feskanich D, Speizer FE, Thun M, Hertzmark E, Rosner BA, Colditz GA. Lung cancer rates in men and women with comparable histories of smoking. *J. Natl. Cancer Inst.* 2004;96:826-34.

Barbone F, Bovenzi M, Cavallieri F, Stanta G. Air pollution and lung cancer in Trieste, Italy. *Am. J. Epidemiol.* 1995;141:1161-9.

Beeson WL, Abbey DE, Knutsen SF. Long-term concentrations of ambient air pollutants and incident lung cancer in California adults: results from the AHSMOG study.Adventist Health Study on Smog. *Environ. Health Perspect.* 1998;106:813-23.

Bellander T, Berglind N, Gustavsson P, Jonson T, Nyberg F, Pershagen G, Jarup L. Using geographic information systems to assess individual historical exposure to air pollution from traffic and house heating in Stockholm. *Environ. Health Perspect.* 2001;109:633-9.

Belli S, Benedetti M, Comba P, Lagravinese D, Martucci V, Martuzzi M, Morleo D, Trinca S, Viviano G. Case-control study on cancer risk associated to residence in the neighbourhood of a petrochemical plant. *Eur. J. Epidemiol.* 2004;19:49-54.

Besso A, Nyberg F, Pershagen G. Air pollution and lung cancer mortality in the vicinity of a nonferrous metal smelter in Sweden. *Int. J. Cancer.* 2003;107:448-52.

Bilello KS, Murin S, Matthay RA. Epidemiology, etiology, and prevention of lung cancer. *Clin. Chest. Med.* 2002;23:1-25.

Blot WJ, McLaughlin JK. Are women more susceptible to lung cancer? *J. Natl. Cancer Inst.* 2004;96:812-13.

Boffetta P, Kogevinas M, Simonato L, Wilbourn J, Saracci R. Current Perspectives on Occupational Cancer Risks. *Int. J. Occup. Environ. Health.* 1995;1:315-325.

Boffetta P, Jourenkova N, Gustavsson P. Cancer risk from occupational and environmental exposure to polycyclic aromatic hydrocarbons. *Cancer Cause Control.* 1997;8:444-472.

Boffetta P. Epidemiology of environmental and occupational cancer. *Oncogene.* 2004;23:6392-6403.

Bower M, Powles T, Nelson M, Shah P, Cox S, Mandelia S, Gazzard B. HIV-related lung cancer in the era of highly active antiretroviral therapy. *AIDS.* 2003;17:371-375.

Brennan P, Hsu CC, Moullan N, Szeszenia-Dabrowska N, Lissowska J, Zaridze D, Rudnai P, Fabianova E, Mates D, Bencko V, Foretova L, Janout V, Gemignani F, Chabrier A, Hall J, Hung RJ, Boffetta P, Canzian F. Effect of cruciferous vegetables on lung cancer in patients stratified by genetic status: a mendelian randomisation approach. *Lancet.* 2005 ;366:1558-60.

Breslow N.E., and Day N.E.. Statistical Methods in Cancer Research – Volume 1 – The analysis of case-control studies. IARC Scientific Publications N. 32, Lyon, 1980.

Bromen K, Pohlabeln H, Jahn I, Ahrens W, Jockel KH. Aggregation of lung cancer in families: results from a population-based case-control study in Germany. *Am. J. Epidemiol.* 2000;152:497-505.

Brownson RC, Chang JC, Davis JR. Gender and histologic type variations in smoking-related risk of lung cancer. *Epidemiology.* 1992;3:61-64.

Brunekreef B. All but quiet on the particulate front. *Am. J. Respir. Crit. Care Med.* 1999;159:354-6.

Cassidy A, Myles JP, Duffy SW, Liloglou T, Field JK. Family history and risk of lung cancer: age-at-diagnosis in cases and first-degree relatives. *Br. J. Cancer.* 2006;95:1288-90.

Chiu HF, Cheng MH, Tsai SS, Wu TN, Kuo HW, Yang CY. Outdoor air pollution and female lung cancer in Tiwan. *Inhal Toxicol.* 2006;18:1025-31.

Cohen AJ. Outdoor air pollution and lung cancer. *Environ. Health Perspect.* 2000;108 Suppl 4:743-50.

Cohen AJ. Air pollution and lung cancer: what more do we need to know? *Thorax.* 2003;58:1010-1012.

Cohen AJ, Ross Anderson H, Ostro B, Pandey KD, Krzyzanowski M, Kunzli N, Gutschmidt K, Pope A, Romieu I, Samet JM, Smith K. The global burden of disease due to outdoor air pollution. *J. Toxicol. Environ. Health. A* 2005;68:1301-7.

Cocheo V, Sacco P, Boaretto C, De Saeger E, Ballesta PP, Skov H, Goelen E, Gonzalez N, Caracena AB. Urban benzene and population exposure. *Nature.* 2000;404:141-142.

Curtis L, Rea W, Smith-Willis P, Fenyves E, Pan Y. Adverse health effects of outdoor air pollutants. *Environ. Int.* 2006;32:815-30.

Deutsch M, Land SR, Begovic M, Wieand HS, Wolmark N, Fisher B. The incidence of lung carcinoma after surgery for breast carcinoma with and without postoperative radiotherapy. Results of National Surgical Adjuvant Breast and Bowel Project (NSABP) clinical trials B-04 and B-06. *Cancer.* 2003;98:1362-1368.

Dockery DW, Pope CA 3rd, Xu X, Spengler JD, Ware JH, Fay ME, Ferris BG Jr,Speizer FE. An association between air pollution and mortality in six U.S. cities. *N. Engl. J. Med.* 1993;329:1753-9.

Doll R, Peto R, Wheatley K, Gray R, Sutherland I. Mortality in relation to smoking: 40 years' observations on male British doctors. *BMJ.* 1994;309:901-11.

Doll R, Peto R. The causes of cancer: quantitative estimates of avoidable risks of cancer in the United States today. *J. Natl. Cancer Inst.* 1981;66:1191-1308.

Edwards R, Pless-Mulloli T, Howel D, Chadwick T, Bhopal R, Harrison R, Gribbin H. Does living near heavy industry cause lung cancer in women? A case-control study using life grid interviews. *Thorax.* 2006;61:1076-82.

Fano V, Michelozzi P, Ancona C, Capon A, Forastiere F, Perucci CA. Occupational and environmental exposures and lung cancer in an industrialised area in Italy. *Occup. Environ. Med.* 2004;61:757-63.

Filleul L, Rondeau V, Vandentorren S, Le Moual N, Cantagrel A, Annesi-Maesano I, Charpin D, Declercq C, Neukirch F, Paris C, Vervloet D, Brochard P, Tessier JF, Kauffmann F, Baldi I. Twenty five year mortality and air pollution: results from the French PAARC survey. *Occup. Environ. Med.* 2005;62:453-60.

Ford MB, Sigurdson AJ, Petrulis ES, Ng CS, Kemp B, Cooksley C, McNeese M, Selwyn BJ, Spitz MR, Bondy ML. Effects of smoking and radiotherapy on lung carcinoma in breast cancer survivors. *Cancer.* 2003;98:1457-1464.

Franchini M, Rial M, Buiatti E, Bianchi F. Health effect of exposure to waste incinerator emissions: a review of epidemiological studies. *Ann. Ist. Super Sanità.* 2004;40:101-115.

Friedman GD, Tekawa I, Sadler M, Sidney S. Chapter 6. Smoking and mortality; the Kaiser-Permanente experience. In: Burns DM, Garfinkel L, Samet J, editors. Smoking and Tobacco Control Monograph No. 8: Changes in cigarette-related disease risks and their implication for prevention and control. Bethesda (MD): U.S. Department of Health and Human Service, National Institute of Health, National Cancer Institute: 1997. p. 477-99. NIH Publ No. 97-4213.

Ginsberg MS. Epidemiology of lung cancer. *Semin. Roentgenol.* 2005;40:83-9.

Gupta D, Boffetta P, Gaborieau V, Jindal SK. Risk factors of lung cancer in Chandigarh, India. *Indian J. Med. Res.* 2001;113: 142–50.

Hackshaw AK, Law MR, Wald NJ. The accumulated evidence on lung cancer and environmental tobacco smoke. *BMJ.* 1997;315:980-988.

Harris RE, Zang EA, Anderson HI, Wynder EI. Race and sex differences in lung cancer risk associated with cigarette smoking. *Int. J. Epidemiol.* 1993;22:592-599.

Hoek G, Brunekreef B, Goldbohm S, Fischer P, van den Brandt PA. Association between mortality and indicators of traffic-related air pollution in the Netherlands: a cohort study. *Lancet.* 2002;360:1203-9.

IARC. Tobacco smoke. *IARC Monogr. Eval. Carcinog. Risk. Chem. Hum,* 1986;38:83 – 126.

IARC. IARC Monographs on the evaluation of carcinogenic risks to humans. Supplement 7: overall evaluations of carcinogenity, an updating of IARC Monographs. Lyon: International Agency for Research on Cancer, 1987.

IELCAP: International Early Lung Cancer Action Program Investigators; Henschke CI, Yip R, Miettinen OS. Women's susceptibility to tobacco carcinogens and survival after diagnosis of lung cancer. *JAMA.* 2006;296:180-4.

Janne PA, Engelman JA, Johnson BE. Epidermal growth factor receptor mutations in non-small-cell lung cancer: implications for treatment and tumor biology. *J. Clin. Oncol.* 2005;23:3227-34.

Janssen NAH, Hoek G, Brunekreef B, Harssema H, Mensink I, Zuidhof A. Personal sampling of PM10 among adults: relation between personal, indoor and outdoor concentrations. *Am. J. Epidemiol.* 1998;147:537–547.

Jedrychowski W, Becher H, Wahrendorf J, Basa-Cierpialek Z. A case-control study of lung cancer with special reference to the effect of air pollution in Poland. *J. Epidemiol. Community Health.* 1990;44:114-20.

Jockel KH, Ahrens W, Wichmann HE, Becher H, Bolm-Audorff U, Jahn I, Molik B, Greiser E, Timm J. Occupational and environmental hazards associated with lung cancer. *Int. J. Epidemiol.* 1992;21:202-13.

Katsouyanni K, Trichopoulos D, Kalandidi A, Tomos P, Riboli E. A case-control study of air pollution and tobacco smoking in lung cancer among women in Athens. *Prev. Med.* 1991;20:271-8.

Katsouyanni K, Pershagen G. Ambient air pollution exposure and cancer. *Cancer Causes Control.* 1997;8:284-91.

Kleinbaum DG, Kupper LL, Muller KE. Maximum Likelihood method: theory and applications. In: Applied Regression Analysis and Other Multivariable Methods, PWS-Kent Publishing Company, Boston (USA) 1987: 483-518.

Kleinerman RA, Wang Z, Wang L, Metayer C, Zhang S, Brenner AV, Zhang S, Xia Y, Shang B, Lubin JH. Lung cancer and indoor exposure to coal and biomass in rural China. *J. Occup. Environ. Med.* 2002;44:338–44.

Korte JE, Brennan P, Henley SJ, Boffetta P. Dose-specific meta-analysis and sensitivity analysis of the relation between alcohol consumption and lung cancer risk. *Am. J. Epidemiol.* 2003;157:569-70.

Krewski D, Burnett RT, Goldberg MS, Hoover K, Siemiatycki J, Jerrett M, Abrahamovitz M, White WH. Reanalysis of the Harvard Six Cities study and the American Cancer Society study of particulate air pollution and mortality. A special report of the Institute's Particle Epidemiology Reanalysis Project. Cambridge MA, Health Effects Institute, 2000.

Kure EH, Ryberg D, Hewer A, Phillips DH, Skaug V, Baera R, Haugen A. p53 mutations in lung tumours: relationship to gender and lung DNA adduct levels. *Carcinogenesis.* 1996;17:2201-5.

La Vecchia C. Smoking in Italy, 1949-1983. *Prev. Med.* 1986;15:274—81.

Lambert TW, Lane S. Lead, arsenic and polycyclic aromatic hydrocarbons in soil and house dust in the communities surrounding the Sydney, Nova Scotia, Tar Ponds. *Environ. Health Perspect.* 2004;112:35—41.

Leffondre K, Abrahamowicz M, Siemiatycki J, Rachet B. Modeling smoking history: a comparison of different approaches. *Am. J. Epidemiol.* 2002;156:813-23.

Levi F, Lucchini F, Negri E, La Vecchia C. Continuing declines in cancer mortality in the European Union. *Ann. Oncol.* 2006 Dec 12; [Epub ahead of print]

Lissowska J, Bardin-Mikolajczak A, Fletcher T, Zaridze D, Szeszenia-Dabrowska N, Rudnai P, Fabianova E, Cassidy A, Mates D, Holcatova I, Vitova V, Janout V, Mannetje A, Brennan P, Boffetta P. Lung cancer and indoor pollution from heating and cooking with solid fuels: the IARC international multicentre case-control study in Eastern/Central Europe and the United Kingdom. *Am. J. Epidemiol.* 2005;162:326-33.

Mannaioni PF, Vannacci A, Masini E. Carbon monoxide: the bad and the good side of the coin, from neural death to anti-inflammatory activity. *Inflamm. Res.* 2006;55:261-273.

Marang-van de Mheen PJ, Smith GD, Hart CL, Hole DJ. Are women more sensitive to smoking than men? Findings from the Renfrew and Paisley study. *Int. J. Epidemiol.* 2001;30:787-92.

Marrogi AJ, Mechanic LE, Welsh JA, Bowman ED, Khan MA, Enewold L, Shields PG, Harris CC. TP53 mutation spectrum in lung cancer is not different in women and men. *Cancer Epidemiol. Biomarkers Prev.* 2005;14:1031-3.

McDuffie HH, Klaassen DJ, Dosman JA. Female-male differences in patients with primary lung cancer. *Cancer.* 1987;59:1825-1830.

Miller AB, Altenburg HP, Bueno-de-Mesquita B, Boshuizen HC, Agudo A, Berrino F, Gram IT, Janson L, Linseisen J, Overvad K, Rasmuson T, Vineis P, Lukanova A, Allen N, Amiano P, Barricarte A, Berglund G, Boeing H, Clavel-Chapelon F, Day NE, Hallmans G, Lund E, Martinez C, Navarro C, Palli D, Panico S, Peeters PH, Quiros JR, Tjonneland A, Tumino R, Trichopoulou A, Trichopoulos D, Slimani N, Riboli E. Fruits and vegetables and lung cancer: Findings from the European Prospective Investigation into Cancer and Nutrition. *Int. J. Cancer.* 2004;108:269-76.

Mills PK, Abbey D, Beeson WL, Petersen F. Ambient air pollution and cancer in California Seventh-day Adventists. *Arch. Environ. Health.* 1991;46:271-80

Mollerup S, Berge G, Baera R, Skaug V, Hewer A, Phillips DH, Stangeland L,Haugen A. Sex differences in risk of lung cancer: Expression of genes in the PAH bioactivation pathway in relation to smoking and bulky DNA adducts. *Int. J. Cancer.* 2006;119:741-4.

Nafstad P, Haheim LL, Oftedal B, Gram F, Holme I, Hjermann I, Leren P. Lung cancer and air pollution: a 27 year follow up of 16 209 Norwegian men. *Thorax.* 2003;58:1071-6.

Naess O, Nafstad P, Aamodt G, Claussen B, Rosland P. Relation between Concentration of Air Pollution and Cause-Specific Mortality: Four-Year Exposures to Nitrogen Dioxide and Particulate Matter Pollutants in 470 Neighborhoods in Oslo, Norway. *Am. J. Epidemiol.* 2006 Nov 29; [Epub ahead of print]

Nawrot T, Plusquin M, Hogervorst J, Roels HA, Celis H, Thijs L, Vangronsveld J, Van Hecke E, Staessen JA. Environmental exposure to cadmium and risk of cancer: a prospective population-based study. *Lancet Oncol.* 2006;7:119-26.

Nelson HH, Christiani DC, Mark EJ, Wiencke JK, Wain JC, Kelsey KT. Implications and prognostic value of K-ras mutation for early-stage lung cancer in women. *J. Natl. Cancer. Inst.* 1999;91:2032-8.

Neugut AI, Jacobson JS. Women and lung cancer: gender equality at a crossroad? *JAMA.* 2006;296:218-9.

Nilsson S, Carstensen JM, Pershagen G. Mortality among male and female smokers in Sweden: a 33 year follow up. *J. Epidemiol. Community Health.* 2001;55:825-30.

Novello S, Baldini E. Women and lung cancer. *Ann. Oncol.* 2006;17 Suppl 2:ii79-82.

Nyberg F, Gustavsson P, Jarup L, Bellander T, Berglind N, Jakobsson R, Pershagen G. Urban air pollution and lung cancer in Stockholm. *Epidemiology.* 2000;11:487-95.

Omenn GS, Goodman G, Thornquist M, Barnhart S, Balmes J, Cherniack M, Cullen M, Glass A, Keogh J, Liu D, Meyskens F Jr, Perloff M, Valanis B, Williams J Jr. Chemoprevention of lung cancer: the beta-Carotene and Retinol Efficacy Trial (CARET) in high-risk smokers and asbestos-exposed workers. *IARC Sci. Publ.* 1996;(136):67-85.

Osann KE, Anton-Culver H, Kurosaki R, Taylor T. Sex differences in lung cancer risk associated with cigarette smoking. *Int. J. Cancer.* 1993;54:44-48.

Palozza P. Can beta-carotene regulate cell growth by a redox mechanism? An answer from cultured cells. *Biochim. Biophys. Acta.* 2005;1740:215-21.

Patel JD, Bach PB, Kris MG. Lung cancer in US women a contemporary epidemic. *JAMA.* 2004;291:1763-1768.

Parodi S, Baldi R, Benco C, Franchini M, Garrone E, Vercelli M, Pensa F, Puntoni R, Fontana V. Lung cancer mortality in a district of La Spezia (Italy) exposed to air pollution from industrial plants. *Tumori.* 2004;90:181-5.

Parodi S, Stagnaro E, Casella C, Puppo A, Daminelli E, Fontana V, Valerio F, Vercelli M. Lung cancer in an urban area in Northern Italy near a coke oven plant. *Lung Cancer.* 2005;47:155-64.

Parker MS, Leveno DM, Campbel TJ, Worrell JA, Carozza SE. AIDS-related bronchogenic carcinoma. Fact or fiction? *Chest.* 1998;113:154-161.

Parkin DM, Bray F, Ferlay J, Pisani P. Estimating the worls cancer burden: GLOBOCAN 2000. *Int. J. Cancer,* 2001;94:153-156.

Parkin DM. Global cancer statistics in the year 2000. *Lancet Oncol.* 2002;2:533-543.

Pauk N, Kubik A, Zatloukal P, Krepela E. Lung cancer in women. *Lung Cancer* 2005;48:1-9.

Pawel DJ, Puskin JS. The U.S. Environmental Protection Agency's assessment of risks from indoor radon. *Health Phys.* 2004;87:68-74.

Pawlega J, Rachtan J, Dyba T. Evaluation of certain risk factors for lung cancer in Cracow (Poland) – a case-control study. *Acta Oncol.* 1997;36:471-6.

Pershagen G. Lung cancer mortality among men living near an arsenic-emitting smelter. *Am. J. Epidemiol.* 1985;122:684-94.

Petrauskaite R, Pershagen G, Gurevicius R. Lung cancer near an industrial site in Lithuania with major emissions of airway irritants. *Int. J. Cancer.* 2002;99:106-11.

Pless-Mulloli T, Phillimore P, Moffatt S, Bhopal R, Foy C, Dunn C, Tate J. Lung cancer, proximity to industry, and poverty in northeast England. *Environ. Health Perspect.* 1998;106:189-96.

Pope CA 3rd, Thun MJ, Namboodiri MM, Dockery DW, Evans JS, Speizer FE, Heath CW Jr. Particulate air pollution as a predictor of mortality in a prospective study of U.S. adults. *Am. J. Respir. Crit. Care Med.* 1995;151(3 Pt 1):669-74.

Pope CA 3rd, Burnett RT, Thun MJ, Calle EE, Krewski D, Ito K, Thurston GD. Lung cancer, cardiopulmonary mortality, and long-term exposure to fine particulate air pollution. *JAMA.* 2002;287:1132-41.

Prescott E, Osler M, Hein HO, Borch-Johnsen K, Lange P, Schnohr P, Vestbo J. Gender and smoking-related risk of lung cancer. The Copenhagen Center for Prospective Population Studies. *Epidemiology.* 1998 ;9:79-83.

Radzikowska E, Glaz P, Roszkowski K. Lung cancer in women: age, smoking, histology, performance status, stage, initial treatment and survival. Population-based study of 20 561 cases. *Ann. Oncol.* 2002;13(7):1087-93.

Risch HA, Howe GR, Jain M, Burch JD, Holowaty EJ, Miller AB. Are female smokers at higher risk for lung cancer than male smokers? a case-control analysis by histologic type. *Am. J. Epidemiol.* 1993;138:281-293.

Risch HA, Miller AB. Re: Are women more susceptible to lung cancer? *J. Natl. Cancer Inst.* 2004;96:1560

Sogaard AJ, Selmer R, Bjertness E, et al. The Oslo Health Study: the impact of self-selection in a large, population-based survey. *Int. J. Equity Health.* 2004;3:3.

Sun Y. p53 and its downstream proteins as molecular targets of cancer. *Mol. Carcinog.* 2006;45:409-15.

Shriver SP, Bourdeau HA, Gubish CT, Tirpak DL, Davis AL, Luketich JD, Siegfried JM. Sex-specific expression of gastrin-releasing peptide receptor: relationship to smoking history and risk of lung cancer. *J. Natl. Cancer Inst.* 2000;92:24-33.

Stellman SD, Muscat JE, Thompson S, Hoffmann D, Wynder EL. Risk of squamous cell carcinoma and adenocarcinoma of the lung in relation to lifetime filter cigarette smoking. *Cancer.* 1997;80:382-8.

Thomas L, Doyle LA, Edelman MJ. Lung cancer in women: emerging differences in epidemiology, biology, and therapy. *Chest.* 2005;128:370-81.

Thompson SC, Nanni C, Levine A. The stressors and stress of being HIV-positive. *AIDS Care.* 1996;8:5-14.

Thun MJ, Day-Lally CA, Calle EE, Flanders WD, Heath CW Jr. Excess mortality among cigarette smokers: changes in a 20-year interval. *Am. J. Public Health.* 1995;85(9):1223-30.

Thun MJ, Henley SJ, Burns D, Jemal A, Shanks TG, Calle EE. Lung cancer death rates in lifelong nonsmokers. *J. Natl. Cancer Inst.* 2006;98:691-9.

Vineis P, Alavanja M, Buffler P, Fontham E, Franceschi S, Gao YT, Gupta PC, Hackshaw A, Matos E, Samet J, Sitas F, Smith J, Stayner L, Straif K, Thun MJ, Wichmann HE, Wu AH, Zaridze D, Peto R, Doll R. Tobacco and cancer: recent epidemiological evidence. *J. Natl. Cancer Inst.* 2004;96:99-106.

Vineis P, Hoek G, Krzyzanowski M, Vigna-Taglianti F, Veglia F, Airoldi L, Autrup H, Dunning A, Garte S, Hainaut P, Malaveille C, Matullo G, Overvad K, Raaschou-Nielsen O, Clavel-Chapelon F, Linseisen J, Boeing H, Trichopoulou A, Palli D, Peluso M, Krogh V, Tumino R, Panico S, Bueno-De-Mesquita HB, Peeters PH, Lund EE, Gonzalez CA, Martinez C, Dorronsoro M, Barricarte A, Cirera L, Quiros JR, Berglund G, Forsberg B, Day NE, Key TJ, Saracci R, Kaaks R, Riboli E. Air pollution and risk of lung cancer in a prospective study in Europe. *Int. J. Cancer.* 2006;119:169-74.

Weschler CJ. Ozone's impact on public health: contributions from indoor exposures to ozone and products of ozone-initiated chemistry. *Environ Health Perspect* 2006;114:1489-96

Whitrow MJ, Smith BJ, Pilotto LS, Pisaniello D, and Nitschke M. Environmental exposure to carcinogens causing lung cancer:evidence from the medical literature. *Respirology.* 2003;8:513-521.

Whitrow MJ. The association between air pollution and lung cancer in the NOrth West of Adelaide: a case control study and air quality monitoring. PhD Thesis, 2004, available at the web address: http://thesis.library.adelaide.edu.au, last access December, 2006.

Williams MD, Sandler AB. The epidemiology of lung cancer. *Cancer Treat. Res.* 2001;105:31-52.

Wu AH, Fontham ET, Reynolds P, Greenberg RS, Buffler P, Liff J, Boyd P, Henderson BE, Correa P. Previous lung disease and risk of lung cancer among lifetime nonsmoking women in the United States. *Am. J. Epidemiol.* 1995;141:1023-32.

Yang CY, Cheng MF, Chiu JF, Tsai SS. Female lung cancer and petrochemical air pollution in Taiwan. *Arch. Environ. Health.* 1999;54:180-5.

Zang EA, Wynder EL. Differences in lung cancer risk between men and women: examination of the evidence. *J. Natl. Cancer Inst.* 1996;88:183-92.

Zeka A, Mannetje A, Zaridze D, Szeszenia-Dabrowska N, Rudnai P, Lissowska J, Fabianova E, Mates D, Bencko V, Navratilova M, Cassidy A, Janout V, Travier N, Fevotte J, Fletcher T, Brennan P, Boffetta P. Lung cancer and occupation in nonsmokers: a multicenter case-control study in Europe. *Epidemiology.* 2006;17:615-23.

In: Lung Cancer in Women
Editor: Varetta N. Torres, pp. 279-307

ISBN: 978-1-60021-659-6


*Chapter XIII*

# Functional Imaging in the Management of Lung Cancer

***Ehab M. Kamel**, *Sabine Schmidt*, *Pierre Schnyder* and *Francesco Doenz***

Department of Diagnostic and Interventional Radiology and Division of Nuclear Medicine, Lausanne University Hospital (CHUV), 1011-Lausanne, Switzerland

## Abstract

Despite the remarkable reduction in the incidence of lung cancer among men in many developed countries, there has been a fourfold increase in lung cancer in women over the past 30 years associated with a rising trend in female lung cancer related mortality. Early diagnosis and appropriate treatment of lung cancer are two important determinants of prognosis and overall disease outcome. Functional imaging has recently gained a prominent role in the management of numerous pulmonary malignancies. The successful introduction of $^{18}$F-fluorodeoxyglucose ($^{18}$F-FDG) along with PET/CT image fusion has revolutionized diagnostic imaging in lung cancer. Currently, $^{18}$F-FDG PET/CT is considered the most precise diagnostic test for a wide range of pulmonary malignancies. This is primarily attributed to its unique ability to assess the global metabolic state of each individual tumor. In fact, the high sensitivity and the whole body mode of data acquisition are two critical advantages that favor $^{18}$F-FDG PET/CT over other cross sectional imaging modalities like CT and MRI. Noteworthy, however, is the complementary role of dynamic contrast enhanced CT in characterizing indeterminate pulmonary nodules and adrenal lesions. Besides its distinguished diagnostic potentials, especially in unmasking occult tumor foci, $^{18}$F-FDG PET/CT can precisely delineate the locoregional tumor burden for an accurate radiotherapy treatment planning. Furthermore,

* Correspondence to: Ehab M. Kamel, M.D. Department of Diagnostic and Interventional Radiology and Division of Nuclear Medicine, Lausanne University Hospital (CHUV), 1011-Lausanne, Switzerland. Tel; 0041 21 314 45 69; Fax; 0041 21 314 44 43; E-mail; Mohamed-ehab.kamel@chuv.ch

PET can offer reliable prognostic information since the avidity of both de novo and previously treated cancerous lesions to $^{18}$F-FDG has been shown to correlate with the overall disease outcome and patient survival. In the near future, further brilliant horizons are expected since the development trials of other radiotracers that target tumor proliferation, apoptosis, and hypoxia are emerging.

## INTRODUCTION

Lung cancer is the leading cause of cancer mortality around the world. In the United States, the disease now accounts for 29 percent of deaths from cancer [1]. Among women, there has been a 600 percent increase in the incidence of lung cancer during the past 80 years, and rates of death among women with lung cancer in the United States are the highest of any elsewhere [2]. In fact, lung cancer deaths in women have surpassed those of breast, ovarian and uterine cancers combined, accounting for 26 percent of all cancer deaths among females in the United States [1-3]. The increase of incidence of lung cancer in women is primarily attributed to an increase in their tobacco use [3]. Furthermore, several case control studies have argued that women are more susceptible to the carcinogenic effect of cigarette smoke than men with a significantly higher risk for developing lung cancer [4, 5]. For instance, the lower DNA repair capacity along with the tobacco-related p53 mutations are more common in female lung cancer patients than in their male counterparts, suggesting that women may be more vulnerable to the carcinogenic effect of tobacco smoke than men [6, 7]. Another potential contributing factor is the role of female steroid sex hormones in inducing lung carcinogenesis. In fact, *ß*-Estradiol, through its proliferative effect on lung cancer cell lines, is believed to mediate cell division in lung neoplasm, an effect that can be blocked by antiestrogens [8]. This argument can be strengthened by the well established interaction between oestrogen replacement therapy, smoking and the development of lung cancer [9]. Some other residential factors like indoor Radon and indoor fumes from cooking and heating stoves are possible lung carcinogens to which women could be selectively exposed [10].

Lung cancer histologies include squamous cell carcinoma, adenocarcinoma, large cell carcinoma and small cell carcinoma. The former 3 histological subtypes, which accounts for approximately 85 percent of lung cancer, constitute non-small cell lung cancer (NSCLC). Cigarette smoking is linked to all 4 histological subtypes of lung cancer especially squamous-cell and small-cell carcinomas, whereas, the proportion of non-smokers is highest in those who present with adenocarcinoma [7, 11]. Despite uniform staging and treatment, the 5-year survival rate of women with stage I-III NSCLC is better than men overall and at each stage. Women are more likely to have adenocarcinoma, to present with earlier stage disease, and to show better response to neoadjuvant chemotherapy [12].

## THE SOLITARY PULMONARY NODULE

Continuous efforts have been devoted to detect lung cancer at an early stage. However, since both chest radiography and cytologic analysis of sputum, which were the mainstay of most screening programs, were not proven to significantly reduce mortality from lung cancer, high-resolution CT screening has emerged as an efficient tool for early detection of lung cancer [13]. Preliminary outcome data has revealed a significant reduction in mortality of patients with lung cancer detected by CT screening with an overall five-year survival rate of 84 percent in comparison with 49 percent for those who have been screened by chest radiography [13]. Despite the high sensitivity of high-resolution CT, 25 to 39 percent of malignant nodules are misclassified as benign after radiologic assessment of morphologic characteristics and about half of the biopsied indeterminate pulmonary nodules turn out to be benign lesions [14-16]. Accordingly, improving the specificity of CT in characterizing indeterminate pulmonary nodules would be of great clinical value.

Characterizing indeterminate pulmonary nodules or mass lesions has matured dramatically with the advent of new technologies in imaging and follow-up. Some authors have advocated CT volumetric measurements follow-up for non calcified nodules that measure less than 1 cm in diameter (figures 1 and 2). In this radiologic analysis, an increase in the measured volume of the entire nodule or of the solid component of a partially solid nodule by more than 25 percent within the usual 2-year surveillance is considered an alarming sign for an underlying malignancy, whereas size stability over the same period is a strong indicator of benignity [17, 18]. For low-risk patients (i.e., those with minimal or absent history of smoking and of other known risk factors), recently published guidelines for the management of small pulmonary nodules have recommended no CT follow-up for nodules ≤4 mm, whereas, for nodules >4-6 mm and >6-8 mm, follow-up at 12 months, and 6-12 months must be considered, respectively. On the other hand, for high risk patients (i.e., those with a history of smoking or of other known risk factors), follow-up CT at 12 months is recommended for nodules ≤4 mm, whereas, for those >4-6 mm and >6-8 mm, follow-up must be considered at 6-12 months and 3-6 months, respectively [19, 20]. Among persons who are referred for needle biopsy on the basis of nodule growth, the rate of diagnosis of cancer is 90 percent (figure 2).

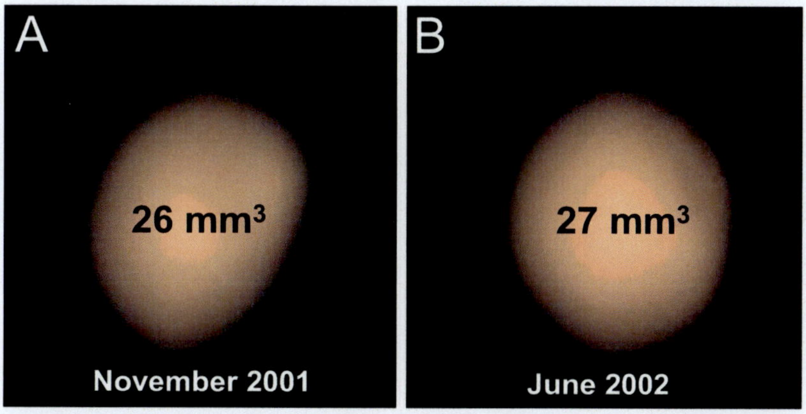


Figure 1. Images of a benign nodule obtained with the 3D volumetric CT software program in a 57-year-old patient. (A) Image obtained with the 3D volumetric software at baseline CT shows a nodule volume of 26 mm3. (B) Seven months later, the measured volume showed non significant increment, consistent with a doubling time of 117 years.

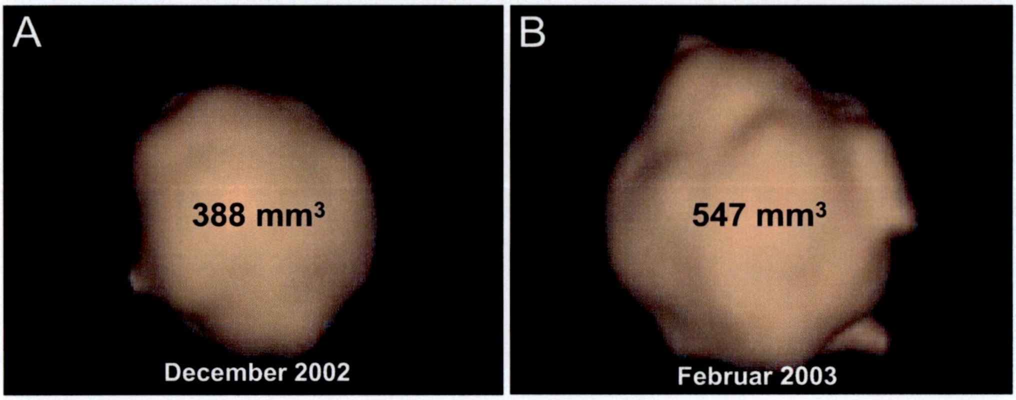


Figure 2. Images of a malignant nodule obtained with the 3D volumetric CT software program in a 63-year-old patient. (A) Image obtained with the 3D volumetric software at baseline CT showing a nodule volume of 388 mm3. (B) Two months later, the measured volume has significantly increased by 159mm3 consistent with a doubling time of 167 days.

Another proposed strategy is to use 18F-fluorodeoxyglucose positron emission tomography ($^{18}$F-FDG PET) for further evaluation of suspicious nodules of high-risk persons. For now, the largest meta-analysis for the performance of $^{18}$F-FDG PET in characterizing indeterminate pulmonary nodules larger than 1 cm and pulmonary mass lesions has yielded a sensitivity of 96 percent and specificity of 78 percent [21]. The high sensitivity figure is attributed to the fact that the vast majority of lung cancers are $^{18}$F-FDG avid. This tracer competes with glucose for uptake into cells, where it accumulates after being phosphorylated by hexokinase [22]. The amount of $^{18}$F-FDG accumulation over a fixed period is thus an indicator of the rate of cellular glucose metabolism and appears to correlate well with the malignant potential of most cancerous lesions. Noteworthy, however, is that the focal form of bronchioloalveolar carcinoma and typical carcinoid are two common sources of false negative PET findings [23, 24], owing to their unremarkable $^{18}$F-FDG uptake (figure 3). In contrast, the relatively lower specificity of $^{18}$F-FDG PET in characterizing indeterminate lung nodule and pulmonary mass lesions is due to the invariable $^{18}$F-FDG accumulation in active inflammatory or infectious lesions [25, 26]. Several reports have previously highlighted pathological $^{18}$F-FDG uptake in pulmonary granulomas (figure 4), histoplasmosis, tuberculosis, sarcoidosis, and Aspergillus infection [27, 28]. Furthermore, any injurious lesion that results in activation of granulocytes or macrophages within the lung parenchyma, like needle biopsy, recent radiotherapy and lung infarction, may equally induce pathologic $^{18}$F-FDG accumulation and consequently false positive PET interpretation [28, 29].

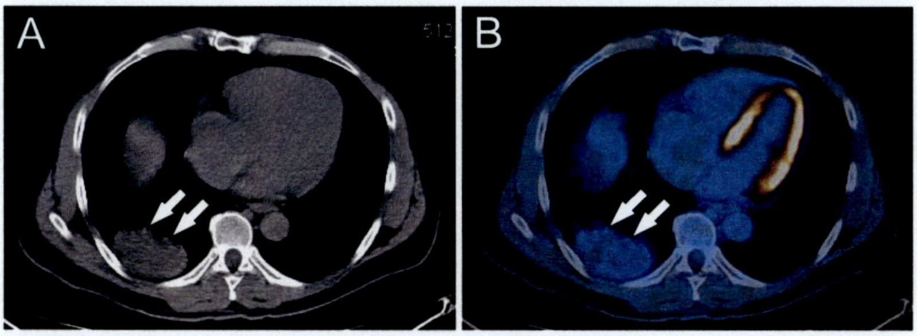


Figure 3. Focal form of bronchioloalveolar carcinoma in a 66-year-old patient. (A) CT image displays the primary tumor in the posterior segment of the right lower lobe (arrows). (B) PET/CT shows no significant $^{18}$F-FDG uptake by the tumor (arrows).

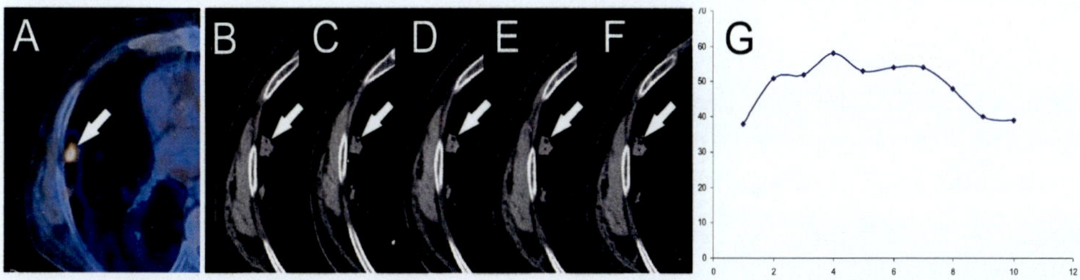


Figure 4. (A) False positive $^{18}$F-FDG PET/CT of a 15mm non necrotizing gigantocellular inflammatory granuloma (arrow) in a 76-year-old patient. (B-F) Dynamic CT scans and (G) time-density curve of nodule hemodynamics show a benign enhancement pattern (<25 HU wash-in with almost complete washout).

The recent introduction of PET/CT hybrid systems has dramatically improved lesions' characterization since the concomitantly acquired CT data has provided direct morphological correlation for each $^{18}$F-FDG signal [30-32]. Furthermore, the worthful role of dynamic contrast enhanced CT in characterizing indeterminate pulmonary nodules and pulmonary mass lesions is very promising [33, 34]. In this approach, dynamic acquisition centered over the questionable lesion is performed. It usually consists of a single native acquisition followed by multiple dynamic frames up to 15 minutes after I.V injection of iodinated contrast medium [33, 34]. Quantitative image analysis is established by creating a time density curve to study the kinetics of the contrast medium in the pulmonary lesion under investigation (figure 4). Currently, there is unanimous agreement that quantifying the wash-in and washout of a given pulmonary nodule is associated with a remarkable improvement in the overall specificity of CT analysis [34, 35]. In a study involved 107 patients with a solitary pulmonary nodule, when diagnostic criteria for malignancy of both wash-in of 25 Hounsfield Unit (HU) or greater and washout of 5-31 HU were applied, sensitivity, specificity, and accuracy for malignancy were, 94 percent, 90 percent, and 92 percent, respectively [34]. Accordingly, we may conclude that for indeterminate pulmonary lesions smaller than 8 mm, CT volumetric follow-up seems to be the examination of choice, which when reveals a significant volume increase, a reasonable second-step must be fine needle biopsy or surgical resection. For indeterminate lesions larger than 8 mm, the integration of dynamic contrast enhanced CT with $^{18}$F-FDG PET may optimize the overall specificity of lesion characterization. It has to be recognized, however, that surgical biopsy must always be considered whenever there is a high clinical or radiological suspicion of lung cancer or metastatic pulmonary lesion(s).

## Non Small-Cell Lung Cancer

According to the international TNM staging system (table), patients who present with early NSCLC (i.e., stage I-II) and selected patients with stage IIIA can be considered for curative surgical resection, whereas chemoradiotherapy and palliative care are reserved for those who present with stage IIIB and IV, respectively [36]. Since mediastinal lymph node involvement and extrathoracic metastases are found in 26 percent and 49 percent of patients with lung cancer at the time of diagnosis [37], accurate staging is crucial for selecting the most suitable therapeutic approach and for determining prognosis. With the successful introduction of PET/CT, a significant improvement in the diagnostic accuracy of lung cancer has been achieved, principally because of the more accurate topographic resolution provided by the concomitantly acquired CT [38-41]. Precise identification of mediastinal and distant metastases by $^{18}$F-FDG PET/CT has the potential to limit the number of tests and invasive procedures required for the metastatic workup of patients with lung cancer.

### Tumor (T) Status

The T status resumes the extent of the primary tumor by size and invasiveness to neighboring structures like the pleura, bronchovascular tree, and mediastinum (Table). While T1-T3 tumors are generally considered as resectable primary lesions, T4 status, in contrast, preclude surgical resection with curative intent [16, 42]. A notable exception for inoperability in T4 disease is the existence of metastatic nodule(s) in the same lobe as the main lesion [43]. Therefore, accurate T stage in NSCLC is an integral step for determining tumors' resectability and preoperative planning especially before en bloc resection of chest wall infiltrating tumors. Both CT and MRI are of equal diagnostic value for distinguishing T3-T4 tumors from T1-T2 tumors with sensitivity and specificity of 63 percent and 84 percent for the former and 56 percent and 80 percent for the later [44]. They have, however, some well recognized limitations: For instance, distinguishing neoplastic contiguity with the pleura, mediastinum or chest wall from definite invasion is quite challenging (figure 5) [45, 46]. Furthermore, variability in image interpretation may take place even among expert observers [47]. Accordingly, both CT and MRI may not be conclusive in some settings.

**Table 1 Currently applied staging algorithm of lung cancer according to the international TNM staging system[36]**

| Stage | Tumor | Node | Metastasis | General Description |
|---|---|---|---|---|
| Local | | | | |
| IA | T1 | N0 | M0 | T1 tumor:≤3 cm, surrounded by lung or pleura; no tumor more proximal than lobe bronchus |
| IB | T2 | N0 | M0 | T2 tumor: >3 cm, involving main bronchus ≥2cm distal to carina, invading pleura; atelectasis or pneumonitis extending to hilum but not entire lung |
| IIA | T1 | N1 | M0 | N1: involvement of ipsilateral peribronchial or hilar nodes and intra- pulmonary nodes by direct extension |
| Locally advanced | | | | |
| IIB | T2 | N1 | M0 | |
| | T3 | N0 | M0 | T3 tumor: invasion of chest wall, diaphragm, mediastinal pleura, pericardium, main bronchus <2cm distal to carina; atelectasis or pneumonitis of entire lung |
| IIIA | T1 | N2 | M0 | |
| | T2 | N2 | M0 | |
| | T3 | N1 | M0 | |
| | T3 | N2 | M0 | N2: involvement of ipsilateral mediastinal or subcarinal nodes |
| IIIB | Any T | N3 | M0 | N3: involvement of contralateral (lung) nodes or any supraclavicular node |
| Advanced | | | | |
| IIIB | T4 | Any N | M0 | T4 tumor; invasion of mediastinum, heart, great vessels, trachea, esophagus, vertebral body, carina; separate tumor nodules; malignant pleural effusion |
| IV | Any T | Any N | M1 | Distant metastasis |

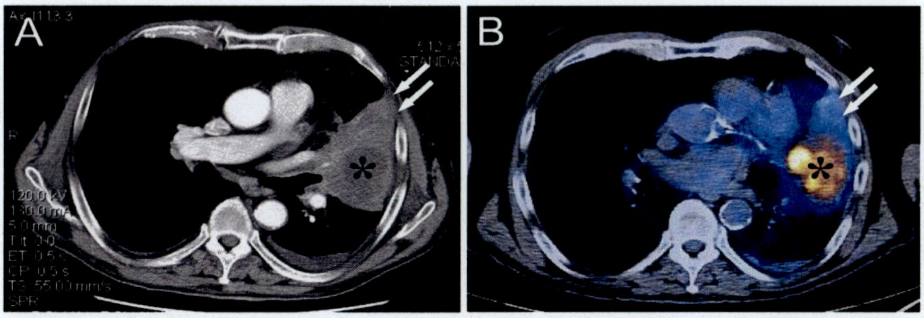


Figure 5. Adenocarcinoma of the left upper lobe in a 67-year-old patient. (A) Contrast enhanced CT shows that the mass (*) has a wide contact with the pleural surface with a questionable chest wall invasion (arrows). (B) 18F-FDG PET/CT reveals the true tumor extension, no chest wall invasion has been found and the contacting soft tissue density was confidently interpreted as post-stenotic atelectasis (arrows).

Studies that favor $^{18}$F-FDG PET/CT for the assessment of T stage in lung cancer are emerging. In a prospective study of 50 patients, integrated PET/CT was correct for T staging in 88 percent of patients, corresponding values for PET alone and CT alone were 40 percent and 58 percent, respectively [38]. Additional investigations by other research groups have reached similar conclusions [39, 40]. The added benefits of PET/CT in this setting are obvious since precise delineation of tumor boundaries for any potential chest wall infiltration or mediastinal invasion can be easily achieved by virtue of anatometabolic image fusion (figure 5). Despite the better performance of PET/CT over that of cross sectional imaging modalities, further comparative studies for T staging of special tumor entities like superior sulcus tumor or those that are at close proximity to the diaphragm are needed before standardizing PET/CT for T stage of lung cancer.

## Nodal (N) Status

Nodal status besides being a strong prognostic factor for resectable NSCLC, has also a remarkable impact on patient management and disease outcome. While surgical intervention with curative intent is the standard therapeutic approach for patients with resectable primary tumors and N1 nodal status, those who harbor N2 disease are potential candidates for neoadjuvant therapy protocols before applying any curative surgical intervention (Table). In contrast, N3 nodal status is considered unresectable [48]. Accordingly, accurate nodal staging has become of critical importance for patients with NSCLC. Computed tomography of the chest has been considered for a long time as the workhorse for noninvasive evaluation of the mediastinum in patients with NSCLC. However, the CT criteria for tumor involvement, that rely on the size or shape of the lymph nodes, have been shown to be far from ideal with a sensitivity and specificity in the range of 61 - 64 percent and 62 - 79 percent, respectively [49, 50]. These figures are related to the fact that normal sized lymph nodes (less than 1 cm in short-axis diameter) may harbor metastasis on histological examination, and nodal enlargement may be due to reactive hyperplasia or other benign condition like silicoanthracosis [51]. Several groups have investigated the role of $^{18}$F-FDG PET and PET/CT in evaluating the mediastinum of patients with NSCLC. With a range of sensitivity between 82 and 91 percent and specificity between 82 and 86 percent [51, 52], $^{18}$F-FDG PET has been shown to perform better than CT for mediastinal nodal staging (figure 6). These encouraging results have been optimized after the successful introduction of PET/CT. In fact, the diagnostic accuracy of $^{18}$F-FDG PET/CT in mediastinal nodal staging was significantly better than that of PET alone and CT alone [38-40]. This is not surprising since the morphologic data obtained from the CT part of PET/CT represents a cornerstone for the identification of the true origin of each $^{18}$F-FDG signal. It has to be recognized, however, that both false positive and false negative PET findings are not uncommon despite the remarkable improvement with PET/CT. Multiple studies have demonstrated positive predictive values for PET of 74 to 93 percent in mediastinal evaluation [51, 53], whereas, others revealed negative predictive values of 88 to 95 percent [52, 54]. These figures are explained by the lack of specificity of $^{18}$F-FDG, which accumulates in inflammatory and reactive lymph nodes, and by the limited spatial resolution of the currently available PET scanners that could miss lesions smaller than 8 mm [55]. Accordingly, for PET-positive mediastinal lymph nodes, both mediastinoscopy and endoscopic ultrasound guided biopsies must be considered as two complementary diagnostic approaches for an accurate staging of the mediastinum. However, in patients with clinical stage I tumors and negative mediastinal lymph nodes shown by PET/CT, mediastinoscopy can be omitted or better replaced by sentinel lymph node mapping and intraoperative frozen sections owing to the low (5.6 percent) likelihood of mediastinal involvement in this patient group [52, 56, 57]. It has to be recognized, however, that omitting mediastinoscopy in patients with central lung tumors and negative PET results in the mediastinum is still a debating subject since the tumor's activity may easily mask lower levels of abnormal activity in adjacent mediastinal lymph nodes, and consequently, may lead to false negative PET results [51].

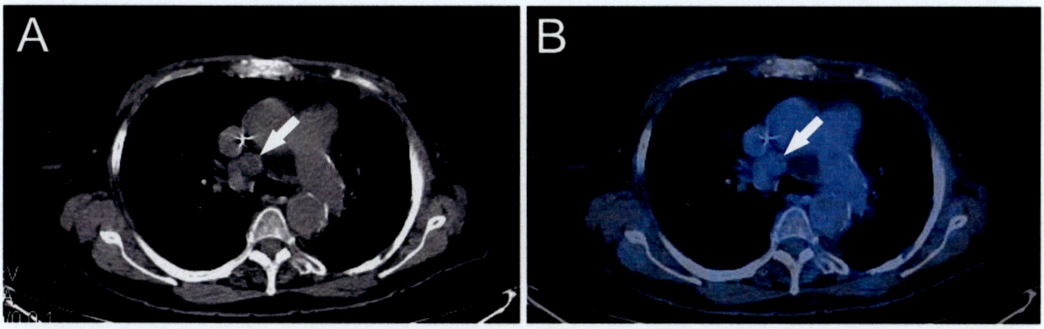


Figure 6. (A) CT image shows mediastinal lymphadenopathy (arrow) in a 76-year-old patient with right upper lobe adenocarcinoma. (B) PET/CT does not depict focally increased $^{18}$F-FDG accumulation, the false-positive CT finding was corrected on the basis of PET/CT result (arrow).

## Detection of Distant Metastasis (M Status)

The evaluation of distant metastases is also of paramount importance for determining the resectability of the tumor under investigation. In NSCLC, the brain, bone, liver and adrenal glands are common sites for distant metastases, and such extension is considered incompatible with curative surgical resection (i.e., M1 disease). Metastases to a different lung lobe, other than that where the primary tumor locates, are considered distant metastases as well [58, 59]. The frequency of occult metastasis at the time of presentation has been shown to be as high as 30 percent in patients with adenocarcinoma or large cell carcinoma [60], whereas, squamous cell carcinoma has a relatively lower frequency (15 percent) of occult metastasis at presentation [61]. Before the era of PET and PET/CT, a battery of noninvasive imaging modalities like CT, MRI, bone scan, and ultrasonography was required for the metastatic workup of NSCLC. Besides the considerable costs of these diagnostic tests combined, a dedicated diagnostic session is mandatory for each of them which may not always suit severely ill patients or those who are referred from remote areas. With regard to the thus far published data, $^{18}$F-FDG PET/CT has been proven superior to either PET alone or CT alone for the detection of distant metastases from NSCLC [38-40]. In fact, the integration of $^{18}$F-FDG PET/CT into the screening for extrathoracic metastases has resulted in a change of therapeutic management in about 20 percent of patients [62]. This can be reasoned by the distinguished ability of $^{18}$F-FDG PET to unmask occult metastatic sites and to avert futile surgery in patients with unresectable disease (figures 7and 8). However, because of the physiologic high uptake of $^{18}$F-FDG in the brain, MRI has been shown to be much more sensitive than $^{18}$F-FDG PET for detecting brain metastases and should be considered in patients with neurologic signs/symptoms or in asymptomatic patients with stage III disease [63, 64]. Furthermore, some conflicting results have been published regarding the performance of PET in detecting osseous metastases compared with bone scan, with some authors reporting better sensitivity and others reporting lower sensitivity than with bone scan [65-67]. However, it is generally agreed that PET has a better global accuracy (90 to 96 percent) than that of bone scan (66 to 78 percent) [65, 66]. Future applications of complementary PET tracers like $^{18}$F-fluoride may optimize the screening process for bone metastases in lung cancer patients [68].

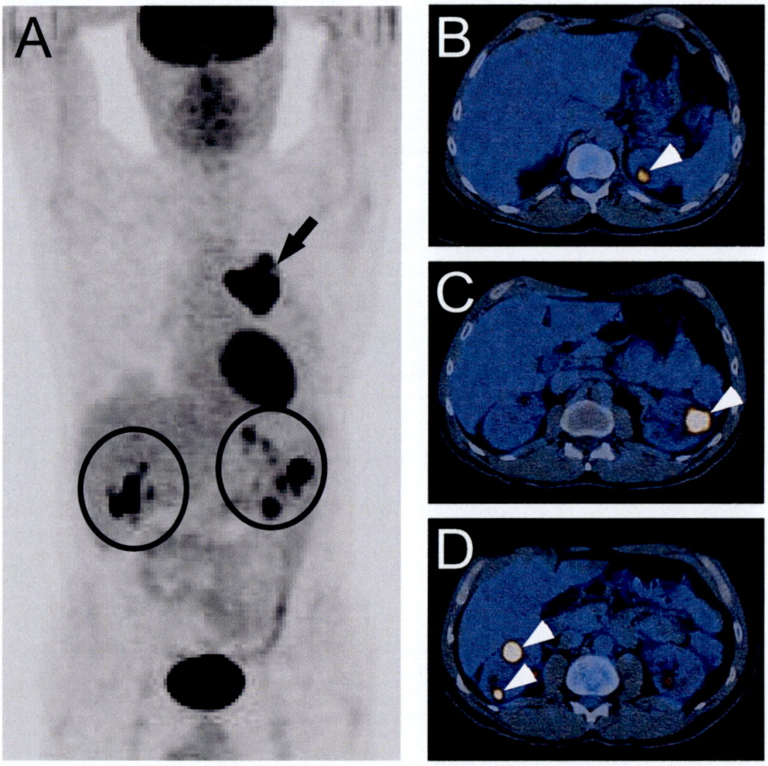


Figure 7. (A) $^{18}$F-FDG PET and (B-D) correlative PET/CT show a large 4x6 cm squamous cell carcinoma (arrow) of the left hilum, in a 53-year-old patient, that metastasizes to the renal parenchyma bilaterally (arrow heads). Renal metastases have been proven by needle biopsy.

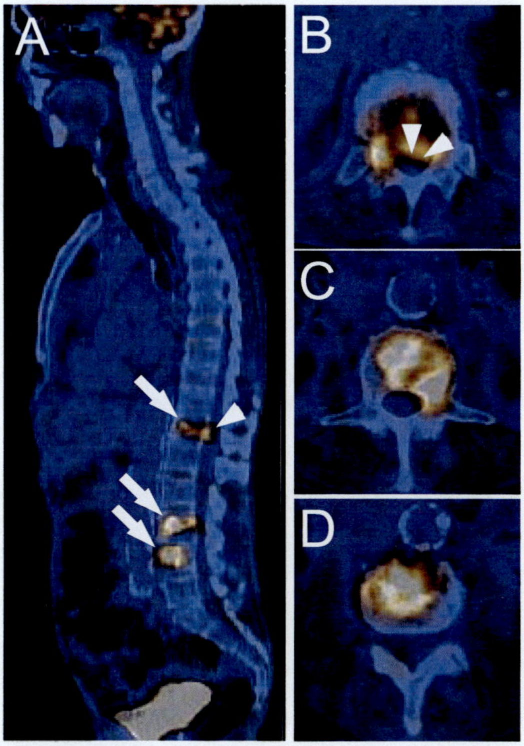


Figure 8. Bone metastases in a 63-year-old patient with large cell carcinoma. (A-D) $^{18}$F-FDG-avid soft-tissue mass in the lower dorsal and middle lumbar vertebrae (arrows) with an obvious encroachment on the spinal cord (arrow heads).

Being occasionally the only extrathoracic site of metastasis, the assessment of the adrenal glands for any potential metastatic involvement has gained special importance in patients with NSCLC. Given that up to 10 percent of patients with bronchogenic cancer have an adrenal mass on CT and that 2 to 8 percent of the general population has benign nonfunctioning cortical adenomas [69, 70], characterizing adrenal lesions in patients with lung cancer may be challenging since some adrenal lesions like adenomas and benign pheochromocytoma are $^{18}$F-FDG avid (figure 9) [71]. Both nonenhanced CT and MRI are complementary to PET in differentiating metastases from benign adrenal adenomas that accumulate $^{18}$F-FDG. This is primarily based on the augmented intracytoplasmic lipid contents of most adrenal adenomas that provoke a characteristic diagnostic signal upon nonenhanced CT or MRI examination [72, 73]. For instance, on nonenhanced CT, an attenuation value of less than 10 HU is considered sufficient for characterizing an adrenal mass as an adenoma with 79 percent sensitivity and 96 percent specificity [74, 75]. This diagnostic criterion, however, is not always valid since up to 30 percent of adenomas do not contain sufficient lipid to have low attenuation and many remains indeterminate and indistinguishable from nonadenomas on nonenhanced CT [76]. Chemical shift MRI has been shown to be more sensitive than CT for the diagnosis of adrenal adenoma with sensitivity and specificity range from 81 to 100 percent and 94 to 100 percent, respectively [75, 77], however, it may also misclassify some malignant lesions as benign [78]. This may imply that histopathologic verification of adrenal positive lesions on $^{18}$F-FDG PET must be considered to avoid omitting surgical intervention in an otherwise operable patient. However, histopathologic verification by fine needle biopsy is an invasive manoeuvre that should be avoided whenever possible. Fortunately, many authors have addressed the complementary role of delayed contrast-enhanced CT in characterizing indeterminate adrenal lesions [76, 79, 80]. In this approach, a series of images are acquired before and up to 10-15 minutes after I.V injection of iodinated contrast media then a time density curve is created to study the kinetics of the injected contrast media in the adrenal tissue under investigation. Several studies have reported that adrenal adenomas have a much earlier and more rapid contrast material washout than metastases [76, 79, 80]. Using a threshold value between 50 and 60 percent for absolute enhancement loss at 10-15 minutes after I.V injection of iodinated contrast media, a sensitivity of 98 to 100 percent and a specificity of 92 to 100 percent have been reported in differentiating adrenal adenomas from nonadenomatous lesions (figure 9) [76, 79].

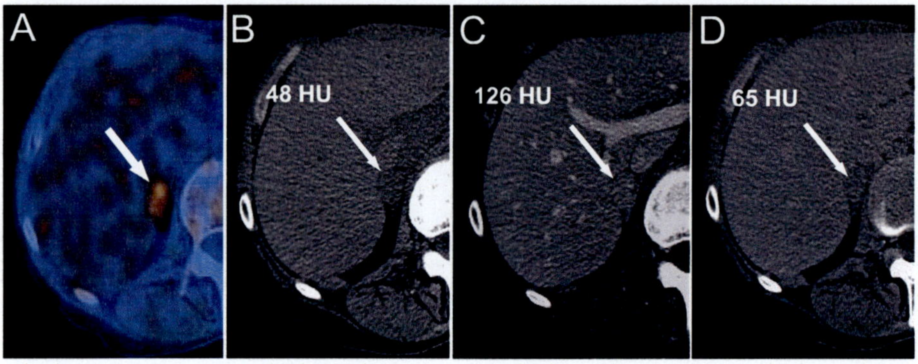


Figure 9. Images in a 56-year-old patient with adenocarcinoma of the right lung and biopsy-proved right adrenal adenoma. (A) $^{18}$F-FDG PET/CT shows pathological uptake in the right adrenal gland consistent with possible metastasis from lung cancer (arrow). (B) Precontrast, (C) portal venous phase enhanced, and (D) 10-minute delayed enhanced transverse CT images of right adrenal nodule (small arrows) show attenuation values of 48, 126, and 65 HU, respectively, the resultant absolute enhancement loss is 78%. These values are consistent with a benign adrenal lesion as proved by histological analysis.

## Therapy Monitoring

While patients with stage I-II NSCLC are suitable candidates for curative surgical resection, those who present with stage IIIA are considered for more aggressive therapeutic alternative like neoadjuvant chemotherapy and/or radiotherapy aiming at reducing their advanced locoregional tumor burden in order to reach an operable stage [36]. Complete pathological response to neoadjuvant treatment is an important prognostic indicator of favorable outcome and prolonged disease free survival. Given the potential toxicity of these regimens along with their considerable costs, a reliable response predictor in an early phase of neoadjuvant treatment that might allow using alternative regimen for non-responders or those who develop fulminating disease course would be of great clinical benefit.

$^{18}$F-FDG PET has been previously shown to be able to monitor therapy response of numerous malignant tumors like head and neck cancer, breast cancer, esophageal cancer and lymphoma [81], these results have encouraged many researchers to investigate its potential role in patients who undergo neoadjuvant treatment for locally advanced NSCLC. The vital role of $^{18}$F-FDG PET in therapy monitoring is obvious, since responding tumors have been shown to display a significant reduction in their initial $^{18}$F-FDG uptake even after the first cycle of induction chemotherapy [81]. This distinguished diagnostic criterion of PET is believed to be able to predict the subsequent histopathological tumor response and consequently disease outcome.

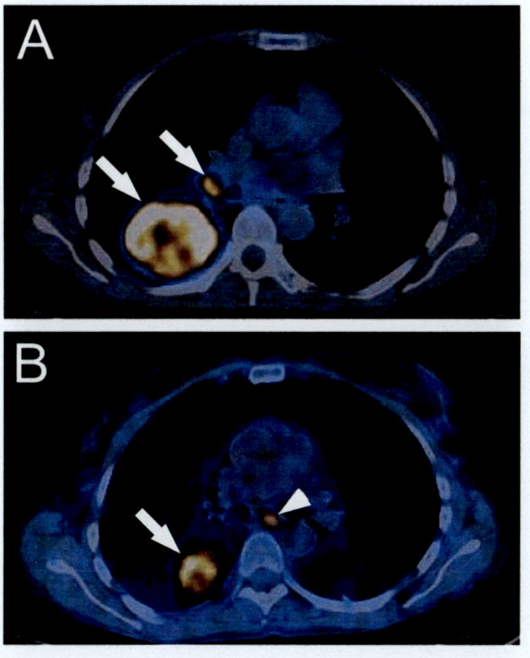


Figure 10. Large cell carcinoma in a 66-year-old patient. (A) A baseline $^{18}$F-FDG PET/CT image reveals hypermetabolic tumor mass in the right lower lobe associated with ipsi-lateral mediastinal lymph node metastasis (arrows). (B) Post-chemotherapy PET/CT displays significant reduction in both the $^{18}$F-FDG uptake as well as the size of the tumoral mass (arrow) along with a complete disappearence of the metastatic lymph node. Please note that the newly appearing focal hot spot (arrow head) was correctly identified by PET/CT to be the expression of a reflux oesophagitis and not of a cancer spread to the subcarinal nodal station.

Since CT has been considered for a long time as the backbone of assessing the treatment response of NSCLC, numerous studies have compared the performance of CT with that of $^{18}$F-FDG PET in this regard. As expected, the accuracy of $^{18}$F-FDG PET has surpassed that of CT for predicting the complete pathologic response after neoadjuvant therapy with a sensitivity, specificity, and accuracy of 100 percent, 95 percent, and 96 percent for $^{18}$F-FDG PET and 63 percent, 54 percent, and 57 percent for CT provided that a cutoff of $\geq$60 percent is used for the decrease in initial tumoral $^{18}$F-FDG uptake as measured by PET as well as for the reduction in tumor size as estimated by CT (figure 10) [82]. This can be reasoned by the fact that resistant viable cell clones may exist in a shrinking tumor mass, whereas on the other hand, residual masses can be completely necrotic or fibrotic, thus morphological criteria do not always provide reliable diagnostic information for therapy monitoring of locally advanced NSCLC.

In contrast to the primary tumor response, mediastinal restaging after induction chemotherapy or chemoradiotherapy for NSCLC remains a challenging task despite the tremendous improvement provided by $^{18}$F-FDG PET. Previously published reports have revealed sensitivity, specificity and accuracy of $^{18}$F-FDG PET for the detection of residual mediastinal nodal disease in the range of 58-64 percent, 93-96 percent, and 85-91 percent, respectively [83, 84]. Recently, these figures could be globally improved by using PET/CT which yielded sensitivity, specificity and accuracy of 77 percent, 92 percent, and 83 percent, respectively [85]. The rather low sensitivity is due to either residual microscopic cell nests within the lymph nodes that are beyond the spatial resolution capacity (~6mm) of the currently available PET scanners or a process of chemotherapy induced metabolic stunning for the $^{18}$F-FDG–avid tumor cells in these false negative lymph nodes. Furthermore, some false positive results have been reported owing to early reactive inflammatory changes after induction therapy. Accordingly, it has been recommended that at least 4 weeks must be elapsed after completion of chemotherapy (2 to 3 months after radiation or chemoradiation) to establish accurate $^{18}$F-FDG PET results [81]. However, it has to be recognized that despite these inherent limitations in $^{18}$F-FDG PET/CT imaging, the results obtained so far are better than those derived from mediastinal restaging using remediastinoscopy. In fact, postinduction remediastinoscopy has been previously shown to be inaccurate in up to 40 percent of patients owing to mediastinal fibrosis and adhesions from initial extensive mediastinoscopy [85]. Future comparative studies between $^{18}$F-FDG PET/CT and endoscopic ultrasound needle aspiration may come up with optimal results through integrating these 2 diagnostic procedures in postinduction mediastinal staging of NSCLC.

## Detection of Recurrence

After attempted curative treatment, patients with NSCLC have a risk of relapse and death exceeds 40% at five years [86]. Surgical re-treatment with curative intent offers the best chance for long term survival, with a 3-year survival rate of 38% [87], whereas, chemoradiotherapy is reserved for those with extensive tumor manifestations. Detection of recurrent disease using cross sectional imaging modalities like CT and MRI may be thwarted by the often extensive anatomic abnormalities induced by previous surgical treatment like parenchymal scarring, pleural thickening, pleural effusion, and mediastinal fibrosis. Furthermore, radiotherapy may induce slowly evolving parenchymal abnormalities in the lungs that may mimic local treatment failure owing to their nodular or masslike appearance [88]. The development of $^{18}$F-FDG PET has taken the evaluation of locoregional structural abnormalities beyond morphologic analysis to functional and metabolic analysis of disease. Studies that favor $^{18}$F-FDG PET and PET/CT for the diagnostic workup of patients with suspected relapse of NSCLC after curative treatment with surgery, chemotherapy, or radiotherapy are emerging. Recently, two clinical trials have yielded quite convincing results in this regard with sensitivities of 93 to 98 percent, specificities of 82 to 89 percent, and accuracies of 86 to 92 percent [87, 89]. Another property of $^{18}$F-FDG PET is the ability to simultaneously detect unsuspected tumor foci in order to avoid futile re-surgery in patients with extensive locoregional tumor burden or those with distant metastases. Integrating $^{18}$F-FDG PET in the diagnostic workup of patients with suspected recurrence of lung cancer has been shown to impact patient management in more than 50 percent of cases [89, 90].

## Small-Cell Lung Cancer

Small cell lung cancer (SCLC) is the most aggressive form of lung cancer. At presentation, 30 to 40 percent of patients with SCLC present with limited disease (LD), whereas, 60 to 70 percent present with extensive disease (ED) [91]. According to the Veterans Administration Lung Cancer Study Group, LD is defined as disease confined to one hemithorax, mediastinum, and regional lymph nodes, which can be encompassed within a single tolerable radiation port. Disease extension outside the thorax or the existence of malignant pleural effusion is categorized as ED [92]. Currently, most patients with LD SCLC are treated with a combination of chemotherapy and chest irradiation. This dual-modality therapy has been shown to increase complete response rate and to decrease local treatment failure [93, 94]. In selected patients with very limited-stage disease (T1–T2, N0), surgical resection may be feasible [95, 96]. In extensive stage SCLC, chemotherapy remains the standard therapeutic approach [97]. For patients who achieved complete response, prophylactic cranial irradiation is believed to improve the overall disease-free survival through reducing the risk of brain metastasis [98].

### Initial Staging

Accurate tumor staging is a prerequisite for choosing the appropriate therapeutic approach in SCLC. The primary role of diagnostic imaging is to separate patients with LD from those with ED. On the basis of the widespread dissemination of SCLC, a battery of imaging tests is performed, such as CT of the chest and abdomen, CT or MRI of the brain, and bone scan [99]. Despite the high sensitivity of morphological cross-sectional imaging modalities to structural changes, identification of tumor tissue can be challenging in some settings (e.g., in normal-sized lymph nodes). Furthermore, morphologic imaging modalities are mostly used to evaluate a given anatomical region rather than the entire body. Metastases outside the imaging field are thus missed. The potential of $^{18}$F-FDG PET in initial staging of SCLC has been investigated by many authors [100-105]. In fact, $^{18}$F-FDG PET has been proven superior to conventional staging procedures with an accuracy of 100, 99, and 96 percent for the detection of the primary lesions, regional lymph node metastases, and extracranial distant metastases, respectively [105]. Corresponding values for conventional staging procedures are 100, 83, and 81 percent [105]. Of note, is the remarkable impact of $^{18}$F-FDG PET on patient management that reached 29 percent in some series [103]. The better performance of $^{18}$F-FDG PET can be explained by the known high avidity of SCLC to $^{18}$F-FDG owing to its high proliferation potential and short doubling time. This allows PET to detect occult tumor nests in normal sized lymph nodes, in bone/bone marrow and in visceral organs (figure 11). Furthermore, PET has the potential to exclude malignancy in many indeterminate lesions that may be detected by morphologic cross-sectional imaging modalities. This effect can certainly alleviate the need for a further diagnostic workup to prove or disprove such indeterminate radiologic findings. However, it has to be recognized that because of the high physiologic accumulation of $^{18}$F-FDG in the brain, PET scans is not sensitive enough for the detection of brain metastases [103, 105]. This suggests that, in patients who are found to have LD with PET, if brain metastases need to be excluded, a gadolinium-enhanced MRI scan of the brain remains necessary. Despite the limited number of published studies on the utility of $^{18}$F-FDG PET/CT in SCLC, it is obvious that combining functional and anatomical data would maximize the specificity and consequently the overall diagnostic accuracy by virtue of referring each individual $^{18}$F-FDG signal to its true origin. Recently, this hypothesis has been confirmed in a prospective study composed of 34 patients in which $^{18}$F-FDG PET/CT yielded a specificity of 100 percent in comparison with 83 percent for $^{18}$F-FDG PET alone [106].

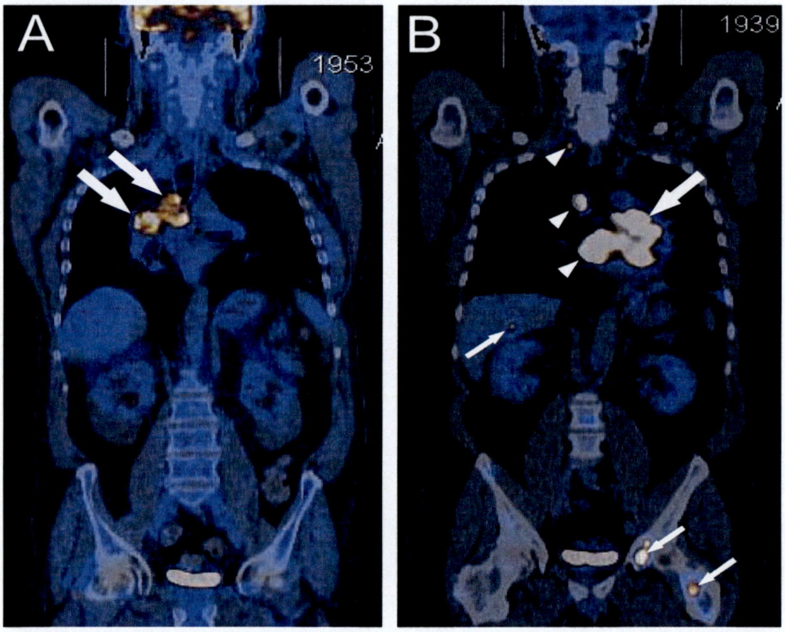


Figure 11. (A) Limited disease SCLC in a 53-year-old patient, PET/CT shows pathological $^{18}$F-FDG uptake in a right hilar mass, as well as in mediastinal lymph node metastases (arrows). (B) Extensive disease SCLC in a 67 -year- old patient, PET/CT shows pathological $^{18}$F-FDG uptake in a left hilar mass (arrow), with mediastinal and right supraclavicular lymph node metastases (arrow heads), and hepatic and osseous metastases (small arrows).

## Therapy Monitoring

Being one of the most chemosensitive malignancies, tumor shrinkage under chemotherapy can easily be established in patients with SCLC using CT or MRI. Confirming complete remission of SCLC may allow prophylactic cranial irradiation to be performed, this has been shown to offer complete responders a significant improvement in both overall and disease free survival through reducing the potential occurrence of brain metastases [98]. After treatment completion, however, the nature of any residual mass or lymph nodes can not be confidently determined by CT or MRI since post-therapy consolidation or fibrosis may structurally resemble viable tumor residue. In contrast, the metabolic characters of lesion detection by $^{18}$F-FDG PET can be used to predict the true nature of any residual mass in SCLC [103]. Consequently, early salvage therapy can be given to patients with persisting tumors, whereas, the administration of unnecessary toxic therapy to patients with a nonviable mass can be confidently withheld. In a recent study, $^{18}$F-FDG PET could identify 5/5 (100 percent) patients with complete remission, 11/12 (91 percent) patients with residual disease and 3/3 (100 percent) patients with fulminating disease course under chemotherapy and was able to change therapeutic management in 15 percent of the studied population [103]. Similar encouraging results were reported in another prospective study composed of 20 patients [107].

## Detection of Recurrence

Despite a remarkable initial response rate to chemotherapy (45 to 75 percent in patients with LD and 20 to 30 percent in patients with ED), SCLC has a progression-free survival time of 12 months for patients with LD and approximately 4 months for those with ED [108]. Recurrent SCLC after initial therapy has an extremely poor prognosis. Patients who have a relapse more than 4 months after the initial treatment have a 20 to 30 percent response to additional chemotherapy, whereas those with relapse less than 4 months after therapy have only 10 to 15 percent response rate. In patients with a relapse occurring later than 8 months after initial therapy, long term survival may be possible after second-line therapy [109]. Therefore, a close follow-up schedule for patients with SCLC during the first 3 years after therapy has been recommended [109]. Recurrent SCLC can be revealed by clinical symptoms, physical examination, laboratory tests, chest radiography, and computed tomography. The role of $^{18}$F-FDG PET and PET/CT is certainly promising but, unfortunately, has not been well studied in recurrent SCLC. However, since $^{18}$F-FDG PET is known by its very high sensitivity for the detection of primary SCLC, its integration in the follow-up schedule of this patient group may allow early identification of tumor recurrence in order to apply the appropriate therapeutic intervention before further disease progression. Whether the integration of PET results will ameliorate the overall outcome of recurrent SCLC, needs to be established.

## RADIATION THERAPY PLANNING

An essential parameter for careful planning of radiotherapy is to know whether the primary tumor and the nodal metastases will be included within a suitable radiation port in such a manner that critical organ doses are not exceeded. For that purpose, cross sectional imaging modalities like CT and MRI have widely been applied. However, CT and MRI are not always able to delineate the limits between malignant tumor and adjacent normal tissue and the same hold true for determining regional lymph node involvement. Radiation treatment planning based only on CT or MRI findings is likely to miss regions of macroscopic tumor in some patients and may lead to the irradiation of unnecessarily large volumes in others [110-112]. Incomplete irradiation may cause poor local control and high rate of relapse [113], whereas, irradiating adjacent normal tissue (i.e., collapsed lung) may result in a considerable morbidity besides the non ignorable risk of developing a second radiation induced primary tumor that may adversely affect long-term outcome. The innovation of 3-dimentional radiotherapy and intensity-modulated radiation therapy (IMRT) has enabled the delivery of radiation doses with high degree of accuracy. The implementation of these 2 modalities, however, requires an adequate selection and delineation of target volumes on the basis of a reliable imaging procedure [114]. One imaging modality with the potential to distinguish accurately between benign and malignant lesions and to precisely define the extent of disease is whole-body PET with $^{18}$F-FDG. In a recent study of 101 patients, the incorporation of $^{18}$F-FDG PET results into radiotherapy planning and the use of radiotherapy simulation using PET/CT image fusion has been shown to modify the size of the gross tumor volume in up to 49 percent of cases [112]. These results can be reasoned by the unique ability of $^{18}$F-FDG PET/CT to discriminate between tumor tissue and atelectasis or necrotic areas and by its high sensitivity and negative predictive value for the detection or exclusion of disease spread to mediastinal lymph nodes regardless the size of these nodes [114]. Another study went further to conclude that contrast enhanced PET/CT was superior to low dose unenhanced PET/CT in the assessment of lesion delineation especially in case of mediastinal and chest wall invasion [115]. Furthermore, many groups have reported a significant reduction in both inter- as well as intra-observer variability when $^{18}$F-FDG PET data was available for tumor volume delineation [116, 117]. Despite these encouraging results, the impact on treatment outcome and the cost-effectiveness of PET/CT remain to be established.

## RISK STRATIFICATION/OUTCOME PREDICTION

The overall outcome of NSCLC is strongly related to the international TNM staging system. However, some patients with relatively earlier TNM stage infrequently develop post operative disease relapse and die ahead of their illness [118]. Understanding the biological behavior of lung cancer may help to identify high-risk patient groups who could benefit from alternative or aggressive therapeutic pathways aiming at an optimal disease free survival. Since $^{18}$F-FDG PET has the potential to gauge the global metabolic state of each individual tumor, it is obvious that it could play a pivotal role in predicting the outcome of patients with lung cancer as it has been previously shown for other tumors types like breast, head and neck, and pancreatic cancers in addition to lymphoma and sarcoma [119-123]. Using different cutoff points ranged from 5 to 10, the standardized uptake value (SUV), which is a semiquantitative measure of $^{18}$F-FDG uptake, has been proven an independent prognostic factor in NSCLC whatever had been the applied therapeutic approach [124-127]. In fact, patients who harbored tumors that are characterized by a relatively low SUV, such as focal form of bronchioloalveolar carcinoma and well differentiated adenocarcinoma, had a significantly better disease free survival rate than those who had tumors that display higher values. In a study involved 498 patients with lung cancer, gradual increase in SUV was associated with a remarkable decrease in patients' survival that reached 37 percent at 24 months for those with tumors that displayed SUV between 17 and 48 [128]. Recently, other investigators have confirmed the same observations for SCLC as well as for any residual tumor tissue of pulmonary origin after concluding chemo- or radio-therapy [129-131].

## FUTURE PERSPECTIVES

The development trials of alternative radiotracers and diagnostic tools for lung cancer are of great clinical importance. For instance, the proliferation potential of lung cancer can be assessed in vivo by using tracers that target the process of DNA synthesis like 3'-$^{18}$F-fluoro-3'-deoxy-L-thymidine ($^{18}$F-FLT). Although the sensitivity of $^{18}$F-FDG has far surpassed that of $^{18}$F-FLT in initial staging of lung cancer [132], the tumoral uptake of $^{18}$F-FLT has been shown to correlate with Ki-67 labeling index, a distinguished criterion that may permit $^{18}$F-FLT PET to monitor treatment of lung cancer with cytostatic drugs [133]. Likewise, non invasive monitoring of tumor apoptosis after induction therapy has been shown to be feasible using $^{99m}$Tc-Annexin V scintigraphy [134]. Marked tumoral uptake of Annexin V after treatment was a reliable predictor of complete response rate [135]. Furthermore, Annexin V scintigraphy could separate responders from non responders in an early phase with an accuracy of 94 percent [136]. Another radiopharmaceutical of potential prognostic benefit is $^{18}$F-fluoromisonidazole ($^{18}$F-FMISO). This tracer has been shown to be a true hypoxia marker both in vitro and in vivo [137, 138]. Identifying the regional distribution of tumor hypoxia is mandatory for careful radiotherapy planning. Preliminary results have revealed that a steady tumoral accumulation of $^{18}$F-FMISO over the time is a predictor of unsuccessful radiotherapy and high recurrence rate that exceeds 90 percent [139]. Identifying this high risk group before radiotherapy planning may allow them to benefit from intensified treatment protocols to obtain long term disease remission.

## REFERENCES

[1] Jemal A, Siegel R, Ward E, et al. Cancer statistics, 2006. *CA Cancer J. Clin.* 2006;56:106-130.

[2] Patel JD, Bach PB, Kris MG. Lung cancer in US women: a contemporary epidemic. *JAMA*. 2004;291:1763-1768.

[3] Patel JD. Lung cancer in women. *J. Clin. Oncol.* 2005;23:3212-3218.

[4] Risch HA, Howe GR, Jain M, Burch JD, Holowaty EJ, Miller AB. Are female smokers at higher risk for lung cancer than male smokers? A case-control analysis by histologic type. *Am. J. Epidemiol.* 1993;138:281-293.

[5] Zang EA, Wynder EL. Differences in lung cancer risk between men and women: examination of the evidence. *J. Natl. Cancer Inst.* 1996;88:183-192.

[6] Wei Q, Cheng L, Amos CI, et al. Repair of tobacco carcinogen-induced DNA adducts and lung cancer risk: a molecular epidemiologic study. *J. Natl. Cancer Inst.* 2000;92:1764-1772.

[7] Belani CP, Marts S, Schiller J, Socinski MA. Women and lung cancer: Epidemiology, tumor biology, and emerging trends in clinical research. *Lung Cancer*. 2006;55:15-23.

[8] Stabile LP, Davis AL, Gubish CT, et al. Human non-small cell lung tumors and cells derived from normal lung express both estrogen receptor alpha and beta and show biological responses to estrogen. *Cancer Res*. 2002;62:2141-2150.

[9] Taioli E, Wynder EL. Re: Endocrine factors and adenocarcinoma of the lung in women. *J Natl Cancer Inst*. 1994;86:869-870.

[10] Pauk N, Kubik A, Zatloukal P, Krepela E. Lung cancer in women. *Lung Cancer*. 2005;48:1-9.

[11] Muscat JE, Wynder EL. Lung cancer pathology in smokers, ex-smokers and never smokers. *Cancer Lett*. 1995;88:1-5.

[12] Cerfolio RJ, Bryant AS, Scott E, et al. Women with pathologic stage I, II, and III non-small cell lung cancer have better survival than men. *Chest*. 2006;130:1796-1802.

[13] Mulshine JL, Sullivan DC. Clinical practice. Lung cancer screening. *N. Engl. J. Med.* 2005;352:2714-2720.

[14] Erasmus JJ, McAdams HP, Connolly JE. Solitary pulmonary nodules: Part II. Evaluation of the indeterminate nodule. *Radiographics*. 2000;20:59-66.

[15] Mack MJ, Hazelrigg SR, Landreneau RJ, Acuff TE. Thoracoscopy for the diagnosis of the indeterminate solitary pulmonary nodule. *Ann. Thorac Surg*. 1993;56:825-830; discussion 830-832.

[16] Bunyaviroch T, Coleman RE. PET evaluation of lung cancer. *J. Nucl. Med.* 2006;47:451-469.

[17] Wormanns D, Kohl G, Klotz E, et al. Volumetric measurements of pulmonary nodules at multi-row detector CT: in vivo reproducibility. *Eur. Radiol.* 2004;14:86-92.

[18] Wormanns D, Diederich S. Characterization of small pulmonary nodules by CT. *Eur. Radiol.* 2004;14:1380-1391.

[19] MacMahon H, Austin JH, Gamsu G, et al; Fleischner Society. Guidelines for management of small pulmonary nodules detected on CT scans: a statement from the Fleischner Society. *Radiology.* 2005;237:395-400.

[20] Henschke CI, Yankelevitz DF, Naidich DP, et al. CT screening for lung cancer: suspiciousness of nodules according to size on baseline scans. *Radiology.* 2004;231:164-168.

[21] Gould MK, Maclean CC, Kuschner WG, Rydzak CE, Owens DK. Accuracy of positron emission tomography for diagnosis of pulmonary nodules and mass lesions: a meta-analysis. *JAMA.* 2001;285:914-924.

[22] Weissleder R. Molecular imaging in cancer. *Science.* 2006;312:1168-1171.

[23] Heyneman LE, Patz EF. PET imaging in patients with bronchioloalveolar cell carcinoma. *Lung Cancer.* 2002;38:261-266.

[24] Belhocine T, Foidart J, Rigo P, et al. Fluorodeoxyglucose positron emission tomography and somatostatin receptor scintigraphy for diagnosing and staging carcinoid tumours: correlations with the pathological indexes p53 and Ki-67. *Nucl. Med. Commun.* 2002;23:727-734.

[25] Kaim AH, Weber B, Kurrer MO, Gottschalk J, Von Schulthess GK, Buck A. Autoradiographic quantification of 18F-FDG uptake in experimental soft-tissue abscesses in rats. *Radiology.* 2002;223:446-451.

[26] Yamada S, Kubota K, Kubota R, Ido T, Tamahashi N. High accumulation of fluorine-18-fluorodeoxyglucose in turpentine-induced inflammatory tissue. *J. Nucl. Med.* 1995;36:1301-1306.

[27] Asad S, Aquino SL, Piyavisetpat N, Fischman AJ. False-positive FDG positron emission tomography uptake in nonmalignant chest abnormalities. *AJR. Am. J. Roentgenol.* 2004;182:983-989.

[28] Chang JM, Lee HJ, Goo JM, et al. False positive and false negative FDG-PET scans in various thoracic diseases. *Korean J. Radiol.* 2006;7:57-69.

[29] Kamel EM, McKee TA, Calcagni ML, et al. Occult lung infarction may induce false interpretation of 18F-FDG PET in primary staging of pulmonary malignancies. *Eur. J. Nucl. Med. Mol. Imaging.* 2005;32:641-646.

[30] Kamel EM, Goerres GW, Burger C, von Schulthess GK, Steinert HC. Recurrent laryngeal nerve palsy in patients with lung cancer: detection with PET-CT image fusion -- report of six cases. *Radiology.* 2002;224:153-156.

[31] Kostakoglu L, Hardoff R, Mirtcheva R, Goldsmith SJ. PET-CT fusion imaging in differentiating physiologic from pathologic FDG uptake. *Radiographics.* 2004;24:1411-1431.

[32] Rosenbaum SJ, Lind T, Antoch G, Bockisch A. False-positive FDG PET uptake--the role of PET/CT. *Eur. Radiol.* 2006;16:1054-1065.

[33] Yi CA, Lee KS, Kim EA, et al. Solitary pulmonary nodules: dynamic enhanced multi-detector row CT study and comparison with vascular endothelial growth factor and microvessel density. *Radiology*. 2004;233:191-199.

[34] Jeong YJ, Lee KS, Jeong SY, et al. Solitary pulmonary nodule: characterization with combined wash-in and washout features at dynamic multi-detector row CT. *Radiology*. 2005;237:675-683.

[35] Yi CA, Lee KS, Kim BT, et al. Tissue characterization of solitary pulmonary nodule: comparative study between helical dynamic CT and integrated PET/CT. *J. Nucl. Med*. 2006;47:443-450.

[36] Spira A, Ettinger DS. Multidisciplinary management of lung cancer. *N. Engl. J. Med*. 2004;350:379-392.

[37] Jemal A, Thomas A, Murray T, Thun M. Cancer statistics, 2002. *CA Cancer J. Clin*. 2002;52:23-47.

[38] Lardinois D, Weder W, Hany TF, et al. Staging of non-small-cell lung cancer with integrated positron-emission tomography and computed tomography. *N. Engl. J. Med*. 2003;348:2500-2507.

[39] Antoch G, Stattaus J, Nemat AT, et al. Non-small cell lung cancer: dual-modality PET/CT in preoperative staging. *Radiology*. 2003;229:526-533.

[40] Shim SS, Lee KS, Kim BT, et al. Non-small cell lung cancer: prospective comparison of integrated FDG PET/CT and CT alone for preoperative staging. *Radiology*. 2005;236:1011-1119.

[41] von Schulthess GK, Steinert HC, Hany TF. Integrated PET/CT: current applications and future directions. *Radiology*. 2006;238:405-422.

[42] Herman SJ, Winton TL, Weisbrod GL, Towers MJ, Mentzer SJ. Mediastinal invasion by bronchogenic carcinoma: CT signs. *Radiology*. 1994;190:841-846.

[43] Osaki T, Sugio K, Hanagiri T, et al. Survival and prognostic factors of surgically resected T4 non-small cell lung cancer. *Ann. Thorac Surg*. 2003;75:1745-1751.

[44] Webb WR, Gatsonis C, Zerhouni EA, et al. CT and MR imaging in staging non-small cell bronchogenic carcinoma: report of the Radiologic Diagnostic Oncology Group. *Radiology*. 1991;178:705-713.

[45] Glazer HS, Duncan-Meyer J, Aronberg DJ, Moran JF, Levitt RG, Sagel SS. Pleural and chest wall invasion in bronchogenic carcinoma: CT evaluation. *Radiology*. 1985;157:191-194.

[46] Kuriyama K, Tateishi R, Kumatani T, et al. Pleural invasion by peripheral bronchogenic carcinoma: assessment with three-dimensional helical CT. *Radiology*. 1994;191:365-369.

[47] Webb WR, Sarin M, Zerhouni EA, Heelan RT, Glazer GM, Gatsonis C. Interobserver variability in CT and MR staging of lung cancer. *J. Comput. Assist. Tomogr*. 1993;17:841-846.

[48] Kelly RF, Tran T, Holmstrom A, Murar J, Segurola RJ Jr. Accuracy and cost-effectiveness of [18F]-2-fluoro-deoxy-D-glucose-positron emission tomography scan in potentially resectable non-small cell lung cancer. *Chest.* 2004;125:1413-1423.

[49] McLoud TC, Bourgouin PM, Greenberg RW, et al. Bronchogenic carcinoma: analysis of staging in the mediastinum with CT by correlative lymph node mapping and sampling. *Radiology.* 1992;182:319-323.

[50] Gould MK, Kuschner WG, Rydzak CE, et al. Test performance of positron emission tomography and computed tomography for mediastinal staging in patients with non-small-cell lung cancer: a meta-analysis. *Ann. Intern. Med.* 2003;139:879-892.

[51] Pieterman RM, van Putten JW, Meuzelaar JJ, et al. Preoperative staging of non-small-cell lung cancer with positron-emission tomography. *N. Engl. J. Med.* 2000;343:254-261.

[52] Kernstine KH, Mclaughlin KA, Menda Y, et al. Can FDG-PET reduce the need for mediastinoscopy in potentially resectable nonsmall cell lung cancer? *Ann. Thorac Surg.* 2002;73:394-401; discussion 401-402.

[53] Vansteenkiste JF, Stroobants SG, De Leyn PR, et al. Lymph node staging in non-small-cell lung cancer with FDG-PET scan: a prospective study on 690 lymph node stations from 68 patients. *J. Clin. Oncol.* 1998;16:2142-2149.

[54] Gonzalez-Stawinski GV, Lemaire A, Merchant F, et al. A comparative analysis of positron emission tomography and mediastinoscopy in staging non-small cell lung cancer. *J. Thorac. Cardiovasc. Surg.* 2003;126:1900-1905.

[55] Takamochi K, Yoshida J, Murakami K, et al. Pitfalls in lymph node staging with positron emission tomography in non-small cell lung cancer patients. *Lung Cancer.* 2005;47:235-242.

[56] Liptay MJ, Grondin SC, Fry WA, et al. Intraoperative sentinel lymph node mapping in non-small-cell lung cancer improves detection of micrometastases. *J. Clin. Oncol.* 2002;20:1984-1988.

[57] Meyers BF, Haddad F, Siegel BA, et al. Cost-effectiveness of routine mediastinoscopy in computed tomography- and positron emission tomography-screened patients with stage I lung cancer. *J. Thorac. Cardiovasc. Surg.* 2006;131:822-829.

[58] Mountain CF. The international system for staging lung cancer. *Semin. Surg. Oncol.* 2000;18:106-115.

[59] Carretta A, Ciriaco P, Canneto B, Nicoletti R, Del Maschio A, Zannini P. Therapeutic strategy in patients with non-small cell lung cancer associated to satellite pulmonary nodules. *Eur. J. Cardiothorac. Surg.* 2002;21:1100-1104.

[60] Sider L, Horejs D. Frequency of extrathoracic metastases from bronchogenic carcinoma in patients with normal-sized hilar and mediastinal lymph nodes on CT. *AJR. Am. J. Roentgenol.* 1988;151:893-895.

[61] Stitik FP. Staging of lung cancer. *Radiol. Clin. North Am.* 1990;28:619-630.

[62] Goerres GW, von Schulthess GK, Steinert HC. Why most PET of lung and head-and-neck cancer will be PET/CT. *J. Nucl. Med.* 2004;45 Suppl 1:66S-71S.

[63] Rohren EM, Provenzale JM, Barboriak DP, Coleman RE. Screening for cerebral metastases with FDG PET in patients undergoing whole-body staging of non-central nervous system malignancy. *Radiology.* 2003;226:181-187.

[64] Ludwig V, Komori T, Kolb D, Martin WH, Sandler MP, Delbeke D. Cerebral lesions incidentally detected on 2-deoxy-2-[18F]fluoro-D-glucose positron emission tomography images of patients evaluated for body malignancies. *Mol. Imaging Biol.* 2002;4:359-362.

[65] Bury T, Barreto A, Daenen F, et al. Fluorine-18 deoxyglucose positron emission tomography for the detection of bone metastases in patients with non-small cell lung cancer. *Eur. J. Nucl. Med.* 1998;25:1244-1247.

[66] Gayed I, Vu T, Johnson M et al. Comparison of bone and 2-deoxy-2-[18F]fluoro-D-glucose positron emission tomography in the evaluation of bony metastases in lung cancer. *Mol. Imaging Biol.* 2003;5:26-31.

[67] Fujimoto R, Higashi T, Nakamoto Y, et al. Diagnostic accuracy of bone metastases detection in cancer patients: comparison between bone scintigraphy and whole-body FDG-PET. *Ann. Nucl. Med.* 2006;20:399-408.

[68] Hetzel M, Arslandemir C, Konig HH et al. F-18 NaF PET for detection of bone metastases in lung cancer: accuracy, cost-effectiveness, and impact on patient management. *J. Bone Miner Res.* 2003;18:2206-2214.

[69] Macari M, Rofsky NM, Naidich DP, Megibow AJ. Non-small cell lung carcinoma: usefulness of unenhanced helical CT of the adrenal glands in an unmonitored environment. *Radiology.* 1998;209:807-812.

[70] Mitnick JS, Bosniak MA, Megibow AJ, Naidich DP. Non-functioning adrenal adenomas discovered incidentally on computed tomography. *Radiology.* 1983;148:495-499.

[71] Yun M, Kim W, Alnafisi N, Lacorte L, Jang S, Alavi A. 18F-FDG PET in characterizing adrenal lesions detected on CT or MRI. *J. Nucl. Med.* 2001;42:1795-1799.

[72] Bae KT, Fuangtharnthip P, Prasad SR, Joe BN, Heiken JP. Adrenal masses: CT characterization with histogram analysis method. *Radiology.* 2003;228:735-742.

[73] Glazer GM, Woolsey EJ, Borrello J, et al. Adrenal tissue characterization using MR imaging. *Radiology.* 1986;158:73-79.

[74] Korobkin M, Giordano TJ, Brodeur FJ, et al. Adrenal adenomas: relationship between histologic lipid and CT and MR findings. *Radiology.* 1996;200:743-747.

[75] Mayo-Smith WW, Boland GW, Noto RB, Lee MJ. State-of-the-art adrenal imaging. *Radiographics.* 2001;214:995-1012.

[76] Szolar DH, Korobkin M, Reittner P, et al. Adrenocortical carcinomas and adrenal pheochromocytomas: mass and enhancement loss evaluation at delayed contrast-enhanced CT. *Radiology.* 2005;234:479-485.

[77] Israel GM, Korobkin M, Wang C, Hecht EN, Krinsky GA. Comparison of unenhanced CT and chemical shift MRI in evaluating lipid-rich adrenal adenomas. *AJR. Am. J. Roentgenol.* 2004;183:215-219.

[78] Outwater EK, Siegelman ES, Huang AB, Birnbaum BA. Adrenal masses: correlation between CT attenuation value and chemical shift ratio at MR imaging with in-phase and opposed-phase sequences. *Radiology.* 1996;200:749-752.

[79] Caoili EM, Korobkin M, Francis IR, et al. Adrenal masses: characterization with combined unenhanced and delayed enhanced CT. *Radiology.* 2002;222:629-633.

[80] Korobkin M, Brodeur FJ, Francis IR, Quint LE, Dunnick NR, Londy F. CT time-attenuation washout curves of adrenal adenomas and nonadenomas. *AJR. Am. J. Roentgenol.* 1998;170:747-752.

[81] Juweid ME, Cheson BD. Positron-emission tomography and assessment of cancer therapy. *N. Engl. J. Med.* 2006;354:496-507.

[82] Cerfolio RJ, Bryant AS, Winokur TS, Ohja B, Bartolucci AA. Repeat FDG-PET after neoadjuvant therapy is a predictor of pathologic response in patients with non-small cell lung cancer. *Ann. Thorac Surg.* 2004;78:1903-1909.

[83] Ryu JS, Choi NC, Fischman AJ, Lynch TJ, Mathisen DJ. FDG-PET in staging and restaging non-small cell lung cancer after neoadjuvant chemoradiotherapy: correlation with histopathology. *Lung Cancer.* 2002;35:179-187.

[84] Hellwig D, Graeter TP, Ukena D, Georg T, Kirsch CM, Schafers HJ. Value of F-18-fluorodeoxyglucose positron emission tomography after induction therapy of locally advanced bronchogenic carcinoma. *J. Thorac Cardiovasc. Surg.* 2004;128:892-899.

[85] De Leyn P, Stroobants S, De Wever W, et al. Prospective comparative study of integrated positron emission tomography-computed tomography scan compared with remediastinoscopy in the assessment of residual mediastinal lymph node disease after induction chemotherapy for mediastinoscopy-proven stage IIIA-N2 Non-small-cell lung cancer: a Leuven Lung Cancer Group Study. *J. Clin. Oncol.* 2006;24:3333-2339.

[86] Sugimura H, Yang P. Long-term Survivorship in Lung Cancer: A Review. *Chest.* 2006; 129:1088-1097.

[87] Hellwig D, Groschel A, Graeter TP, et al. Diagnostic performance and prognostic impact of FDG-PET in suspected recurrence of surgically treated non-small cell lung cancer. *Eur. J. Nucl. Med. Mol. Imaging.* 2006;33:13-21.

[88] Bruzzi JF, Munden RF. PET/CT imaging of lung cancer. *J. Thorac Imaging.* 2006;21:123-136.

[89] Hicks RJ, Kalff V, MacManus MP, et al. The utility of (18)F-FDG PET for suspected recurrent non-small cell lung cancer after potentially curative therapy:

impact on management and prognostic stratification. *J. Nucl. Med.* 2001;42:1605-1613.

[90] Roberts KB, Manus MP, Hicks RJ, et al. PET imaging for suspected residual tumour or thoracic recurrence of non-small cell lung cancer after pneumonectomy. *Lung Cancer.* 2005;47:49-57.

[91] Tas F, Aydiner A, Topuz E, Camlica H, Saip P, Eralp Y. Factors influencing the distribution of metastases and survival in extensive disease small cell lung cancer. *Acta Oncol.* 1999;38:1011–1015

[92] Abrams J, Doyle LA, Aisner J. Staging, prognostic factors, and special considerations in small cell lung cancer. *Semin. Oncol.* 1988;15:261-277.

[93] Warde P, Payne D. Does thoracic irradiation improve survival and local control in limited-stage small-cell carcinoma of the lung? a meta-analysis. *J. Clin. Oncol.* 1992;10:890-895.

[94] Pignon JP, Arriagada R, Ihde DC, et al. A meta-analysis of thoracic radiotherapy for small-cell lung cancer. *N. Engl. J. Med.* 1992;327:1618-1624.

[95] Shepherd FA, Ginsberg RJ, Feld R, Evans WK, Johansen E. Surgical treatment for limited small-cell lung cancer: The University of Toronto Lung Oncology Group experience. *J. Thorac Cardiovasc. Surg.* 1991;101:385-393.

[96] Simon GR, Wagner H. Small cell lung cancer. *Chest.* 2003;123:259S-271S.

[97] Johnson DH. Management of small cell lung cancer: current state of the art. *Chest.* 1999;116:525S-530S.

[98] Auperin A, Arriagada R, Pignon JP, et al. Prophylactic cranial irradiation for patients with small-cell lung cancer in complete remission: Prophylactic Cranial Irradiation Overview Collaborative Group. *N. Engl. J. Med.* 1999;341:476-484.

[99] Argiris A, Murren JR. Staging and clinical prognostic factors for small-cell lung cancer. *Cancer J.* 2001;7:437-447.

[100] Schumacher T, Brink I, Mix M, et al. FDG-PET imaging for the staging and follow-up of small cell lung cancer. *Eur. J. Nucl. Med.* 2001;28:483-488.

[101] Chin R Jr, McCain TW, Miller AA, et al. Whole body FDG-PET for the evaluation and staging of small cell lung cancer: a preliminary study. *Lung Cancer.* 2002;37:1-6.

[102] Shen YY, Shiau YC, Wang JJ, Ho ST, Kao CH. Whole-body $^{18}$F-2-deoxyglucose positron emission tomography in primary staging small cell lung cancer. *Anticancer Res.* 2002;22:1257-1264.

[103] Kamel EM, Zwahlen D, Wyss MT, Stumpe KD, von Schulthess GK, Steinert HC. Whole-body (18)F-FDG PET improves the management of patients with small cell lung cancer. *J. Nucl. Med.* 2003;44:1911-1917.

[104] Bradley JD, Dehdashti F, Mintun MA, Govindan R, Trinkaus K, Siegel BA. Positron emission tomography in limited-stage small-cell lung cancer: a prospective study. *J. Clin. Oncol.* 2004;22:3248-3254.

[105] Brink I, Schumacher T, Mix M, et al. Impact of [18F]FDG-PET on the primary staging of small-cell lung cancer. *Eur. J. Nucl. Med. Mol. Imaging*. 2004;31:1614-1620.

[106] Fischer BM, Mortensen J, Langer SW, et al. A prospective study of PET/CT in initial staging of small-cell lung cancer: comparison with CT, bone scintigraphy and bone marrow analysis. *Ann. Oncol.* 2006 Oct 23; [Epub ahead of print]

[107] Fischer BM, Mortensen J, Langer SW, et al. PET/CT imaging in response evaluation of patients with small cell lung cancer. *Lung Cancer*. 2006;54:41-49.

[108] Simon GR, Wagner H; American College of Chest Physicians. Small cell lung cancer. *Chest.* 2003;123(1 Suppl):259S-271S.

[109] Adjei AA, Marks RS, Bonner JA. Current guidelines for the management of small cell lung cancer. *Mayo Clin. Proc*. 1999;74:809-816.

[110] Dizendorf EV, Baumert BG, von Schulthess GK, Lutolf UM, Steinert HC. Impact of whole-body 18F-FDG PET on staging and managing patients for radiation therapy. *J. Nucl. Med.* 2003;44:24-29.

[111] Ciernik IF, Dizendorf E, Baumert BG, et al. Radiation treatment planning with an integrated positron emission and computer tomography (PET/CT): a feasibility study. *Int. J. Radiat. Oncol. Biol. Phys.* 2003;57:853-863.

[112] Deniaud-Alexandre E, Touboul E, Lerouge D, et al. Impact of computed tomography and 18F-deoxyglucose coincidence detection emission tomography image fusion for optimization of conformal radiotherapy in non-small-cell lung cancer. *Int. J. Radiat. Oncol. Biol. Phys.* 2005;63:1432-1441.

[113] Tada T, Minakuchi K, Koda M, et al. Limited-stage small cell lung cancer: local failure after chemotherapy and radiation therapy. *Radiology.* 1998;208:511-515.

[114] Gregoire V, Haustermans K, Geets X, Roels S, Lonneux M. PET-Based Treatment Planning in Radiotherapy: A New Standard? *J. Nucl. Med.* 2007;48(1 Suppl):68S-77S.

[115] Pfannenberg AC, Aschoff P, Brechtel K, et al. Low dose non-enhanced CT versus standard dose contrast-enhanced CT in combined PET/CT protocols for staging and therapy planning in NSCLC. *Eur. J. Nucl. Med. Mol. Imaging*. 2007;34:36-44.

[116] Ashamalla H, Rafla S, Parikh K, et al. The contribution of integrated PET/CT to the evolving definition of treatment volumes in radiation treatment planning in lung cancer. *Int. J. Radiat. Oncol. Biol. Phys.* 2005;63:1016-1023.

[117] Fox JL, Rengan R, O'Meara W, et al. Does registration of PET and planning CT images decrease interobserver and intraobserver variation in delineating tumor volumes for non-small-cell lung cancer? *Int. J. Radiat. Oncol. Biol. Phys.* 2005;62:70-75.

[118] Okada M, Nishio W, Sakamoto T, Harada H, Uchino K, Tsubota N. Long-term survival and prognostic factors of five-year survivors with complete resection of non-small cell lung carcinoma. *J. Thorac. Cardiovasc. Surg.* 2003;126:558-562.

[119] Cachin F, Prince HM, Hogg A, Ware RE, Hicks RJ. Powerful prognostic stratification by [18F]fluorodeoxyglucose positron emission tomography in patients with metastatic breast cancer treated with high-dose chemotherapy. *J. Clin. Oncol.* 2006;24:3026-3031.

[120] Allal AS, Dulguerov P, Allaoua M, et al. Standardized uptake value of 2-[(18)F] fluoro-2-deoxy-D-glucose in predicting outcome in head and neck carcinomas treated by radiotherapy with or without chemotherapy. *J. Clin. Oncol.* 2002;20:1398-1404.

[121] Lyshchik A, Higashi T, Nakamoto Y, et al. Dual-phase 18F-fluoro-2-deoxy-D-glucose positron emission tomography as a prognostic parameter in patients with pancreatic cancer. *Eur. J. Nucl. Med. Mol. Imaging.* 2005;32:389-397.

[122] Spaepen K, Stroobants S, Dupont P, et al. Prognostic value of pretransplantation positron emission tomography using fluorine 18-fluorodeoxyglucose in patients with aggressive lymphoma treated with high-dose chemotherapy and stem cell transplantation. *Blood.* 2003;102:53-59.

[123] Hawkins DS, Schuetze SM, Butrynski JE, et al. [18F]Fluorodeoxyglucose positron emission tomography predicts outcome for Ewing sarcoma family of tumors. *J. Clin. Oncol.* 2005; 23:8828-8834.

[124] Vansteenkiste JF, Stroobants SG, Dupont PJ, et al. Prognostic Importance of the Standardized Uptake Value on $^{18}$F-Fluoro-2-Deoxy-Glucose–Positron Emission Tomography Scan in Non–Small-Cell Lung Cancer: An Analysis of 125 Cases. *J. Clin. Oncol.* 1999; :3201-3206.

[125] Higashi K, Ueda Y, Arisaka Y, et al. 18F-FDG uptake as a biologic prognostic factor for recurrence in patients with surgically resected non-small cell lung cancer. *J. Nucl. Med.* 2002;43:39-45.

[126] Downey RJ, Akhurst T, Gonen M, et al, Preoperative F-18 fluorodeoxyglucose-positron emission tomography maximal standardized uptake value predicts survival after lung cancer resection. *J. Clin. Oncol.* 2004;22:3255-3260.

[127] Sasaki R, Komaki R, Macapinlac H, et al. [$^{18}$F]Fluorodeoxyglucose Uptake by Positron Emission Tomography Predicts Outcome of Non–Small-Cell Lung Cancer. *J. Clin. Oncol.* 2005;1136-1143.

[128] Davies A, Tan C, Paschalides C, et al. FDG-PET maximum standardised uptake value is associated with variation in survival: Analysis of 498 lung cancer patients. *Lung Cancer.* 2007;55:75-78.

[129] Pandit N, Gonen M, Krug L, Larson SM. Prognostic value of [18F]FDG-PET imaging in small cell lung cancer. *Eur. J. Nucl. Med. Mol. Imaging.* 2003;30:78-84.

[130] Hoekstra CJ, Stroobants SG, Smit EF, et al. Prognostic relevance of response evaluation using [18F]-2-fluoro-2-deoxy-D-glucose positron emission tomography in patients with locally advanced non-small-cell lung cancer. *J. Clin. Oncol.* 2005;23:8362-8370.

[131] Pottgen C, Levegrun S, Theegarten D, et al. Value of 18F-fluoro-2-deoxy-D-glucose-positron emission tomography/computed tomography in non-small-cell lung cancer for prediction of pathologic response and times to relapse after neoadjuvant chemoradiotherapy. *Clin. Cancer Res.* 2006;12:97-106.

[132] Cobben DC, Elsinga PH, Hoekstra HJ, et al. Is 18F-3'-fluoro-3'-deoxy-L-thymidine useful for the staging and restaging of non-small cell lung cancer? *J. Nucl. Med.* 2004;45:1677-1682.

[133] Yap CS, Czernin J, Fishbein MC, et al. Evaluation of thoracic tumors with 18F-fluorothymidine and 18F-fluorodeoxyglucose-positron emission tomography. *Chest.* 2006;129:393-401.

[134] Belhocine T, Steinmetz N, Green A, Rigo P. In vivo imaging of chemotherapy-induced apoptosis in human cancers. *Ann. N Y Acad. Sci.* 2003;1010:525-529.

[135] Kartachova M, Haas RL, Olmos RA, Hoebers FJ, van Zandwijk N, Verheij M. In vivo imaging of apoptosis by 99mTc-Annexin V scintigraphy: visual analysis in relation to treatment response. *Radiother. Oncol.* 2004;72:333-339.

[136] Rottey S, Slegers G, Van Belle S, Goethals I, Van de Wiele C. Sequential 99mTc-hydrazinonicotinamide-annexin V imaging for predicting response to chemotherapy. *J. Nucl. Med.* 2006;47:1813-1818.

[137] Sorger D, Patt M, Kumar P, et al. [18F]Fluoroazomycinarabinofuranoside (18FAZA) and [18F]Fluoromisonidazole (18FMISO): a comparative study of their selective uptake in hypoxic cells and PET imaging in experimental rat tumors. *Nucl. Med. Biol.* 2003;30:317-326.

[138] Foo SS, Abbott DF, Lawrentschuk N, Scott AM. Functional imaging of intratumoral hypoxia. *Mol. Imaging Biol.* 2004;6:291-305.

[139] Eschmann SM, Paulsen F, Reimold M, et al. Prognostic impact of hypoxia imaging with 18F-misonidazole PET in non-small cell lung cancer and head and neck cancer before radiotherapy. *J. Nucl. Med.* 2005;46:253-260.

In: Lung Cancer in Women
Editor: Varetta N. Torres, pp. 309-333
ISBN: 978-1-60021-659-6


*Chapter XIV*

# LUNG CANCER IN WOMEN: FINE NEEDLE ASPIRATION (FNA) CYTOLOGY DIAGNOSIS

***Dilip K. Das****

Associate Professor, Department of Pathology,
Faculty of Medicine, Kuwait University, Kuwait

## ABSTRACT

Lung cancer is not only the most common cancer in the world, a wide variety of secondaries affect this organ too. Although females are affected much less compared to males, the lung cancer prevalence has been reported to increase among females during the recent years in parallel to the increment in cigarette consumption. Various tissue diagnostic techniques used for lung cancer are conventional cytologic and histopathologic methods as well as fine needle aspiration (FNA) cytology. Of all the diagnostic tools, FNA cytology is simple, safe, accurate and cost effective, which can be practiced on an out patient basis. In a review of literature, the adequacy rate of material obtained by FNA in thoracic lesions, ranged from 68.9% to 95.5% with an average of 82.4% and the diagnostic yield ranged from 67.4% to 91.7% with an average of 81.7%. Examination of routinely stained smears (by Papanicolaou and May-Grünwald-Giemsa/ Diff-Quik methods) showed that nearly two thirds of the intrathoracic FNAs are malignant (36.3% to 88.5% with an average of 65.6%). Where as adenocarcinoma and epidermoid (squamous cell) carcinoma are common primary cancers, small-cell carcinoma (SCC) is relatively less frequent and large cell carcinoma is rare. In our material, the male to female ratio was 2.6:1 for malignancies of the lung. It was 7:1 for squamous cell carcinoma, 2.25:1 for adenocarcinoma, and 4:0 for small cell carcinoma.

In a review of 15 studies, the sensitivity of FNA for intrathoracic lesions ranged from 76.0% to 99.0% (average, 87.7%), the specificity from 68.0% to 100.0% (average, 96.8%), and diagnostic accuracy from 65.0% to 99.0% (average, 88.9%). The clinical

* Address for Corresspondence: Dr. Dilip K. Das, MBBS, MD, PhD, DSc, FRCPath. Department of Pathology, Faculty of Medicine, Kuwait University, P.O. Box: 24923; Safat 13110, Kuwait. Tel: 00965-4986019, 00965-5319476; Fax: 00965-5338905; E-mail: dilip76@hotmail.com, dilip@hsc.edu.kw

utility of FNA, especially in patients with mediastinal compression syndrome and those with poor surgical risk, can be realized from the fact that the rate of more invasive diagnostic methods such as diagnostic mediastinoscopy and futile thoracotomies are greatly reduced by FNA cytology, which provides a tissue diagnosis in minutes with high degree of success.

The major limitation of FNA includes complication like pneumothorax. Sampling and interpretation errors in the hands of inexperienced cytopathologists also contribute to limitations of this diagnostic tool. Diagnostic dilemma may be due to inflammatory pseudo-tumors and cytologic atypia in benign tumors. Diagnostic difficulty may also be encountered in small round cell tumors and poorly differentiated carcinomas/malignancies. In such situations, adoption of ancillary studies like cytochemistry, immuno cytochemistry, florescent insituhybridization (FISH), and electron microscopy can improve the diagnosis of lung cancer.

## Introduction

Lung cancer is not only the most commonly diagnosed cancer in the world (1.35 million new cases) but also the most common cause of cancer deaths [1]. The incidence of lung cancer in men, however, has slowly decreased since the late 1980s and has began to plateau in women at the end of last decade (1990s) [2]. Although more men than women die of lung cancer at present, there is a rising trend in female lung cancer mortality in the developed countries, which has been observed to parallel with the past and current prevalence of cigarette smoking among women in the United States and elsewhere [3]. In a developing county like India, data from major Population Based Cancer Registries show that lung cancer is the 1$^{st}$ or 2$^{nd}$ most common cancer in males and 6$^{th}$ to 10$^{th}$ most common cancer in females [4]. Epidemiologic evidence, supported by recent biochemical and genetic data, suggest that women are more susceptible to tobacco-induced carcinogenesis than men [5].

Obtaining a definite preoperative diagnosis plays a critical role in deciding upon the treatment approach for lung carcinoma, the prognosis of which depends upon its histology and the time of its first diagnosis [6]. The diagnostic methods used for lung cancer are sputum cytology, transbronchial biopsy and lavage, thoracocentesis and pleural biopsy, transthoracic fine needle aspiration (FNA), and open lung biopsy [7]. Of these, FNA biopsy of pulmonary lesions is not only cost effective, but highly sensitive and specific with high diagnostic yield and few complications[8]. It is a technically simple and relatively safe procedure, which allows early diagnosis of lung tumors and thereby, may improve the long term prognosis [9].

## Diagnostic Techniques for Lung Cancer

Since early 1980s, flexible bronchoscopy with forceps biopsy and transbronchial aspiration (TBNA); computed tomography (CT)-guided transthoracic fine-needle aspiration (FNA); and endoscopic ultrasonography (EUS)-guided FNA have revolutionized lung cancer diagnosis and staging by facilitating precise biopsy of lung lesions and virtually all lymph-node stations[10]. For FNA of intrathoracic lesions, a 10 to 20 ml disposable plastic syringe and a diposable fine needle (21 to 23 gauge) fitted with a syringe pistol (Franzen's syringe handle, Cameco) are required. The selection of the length of needle depends upon the depth of the mass lesion in thorax. Although FNA of thorax can be attempted without sophisticated imaging guidance [11, 12], in most studies it is performed under fluoroscopy [13-15], CT [16-18], and US guidance [19-21]. The route of needle aspiration can be percutaneous transthoracic [22-24], transtracheal/bronchial [25-27], and transesophageal [28-30]. Supraclavicular and suprasternal percutaneous approach have been adopted under US guidance for pancost tumors and apical lung lesions [31] and under CT guidance for mediastinal lesions [32], respectively. The routine stains used for cytodiagnosis are May-Grünwald-Giemsa (MGG) or Diff-Quik and Papanicolaou stain. Whereas Papanicolaou stain highlights the nuclear features such as chromatin pattern and nuclear outline, the cytoplasmic color and contents are better displayed by MGG or Diff- Quik.

CT-guided trans-thoracic fine needle aspiration (FNA) cytology is a rapid, reliable, and cost-effective method for the diagnosis of lung lesions and has served as a useful tool in evaluating both neoplastic and inflammatory lung nodules [24]. The two diagnostic approaches most useful in evaluating the CT-detected, small, non-calcified nodule are short-term observation of nodule and CT-guided FNA [33]. In case of small lung lesions, CT-guided FNA is an equally safe and effective procedure in inpatients and outpatients. Further, outpatient performance of CT-guided FNA can decrease costs [34]. The use of coaxial technique for CT-guided lung FNA biopsy reduces the number of pleural passes significantly [35] and the possibility of quick and effective performance of transthoracic biopsy shortens the diagnostics considerably [36]. According to Iwasaki et al [37], video-assisted thoracic fine needle aspiration (VAT-FNA) cytology, which can be applied to the peripheral lung lesions, is not only useful, cost-beneficial, safe and minimally invasive but also accurate. Endoscopic ultrasound (EUS)-guided fine-needle aspiration (FNA) cytology, on the other hand, is an accurate, safe, and minimally invasive technique for the analysis of mediastinal lymph nodes (LNs) and can additionally detect tumor invasion (T4), suspected by CT in patients with centrally located tumors [38, 39]. Cervical ultrasonography and FNA is a safe and cost effective procedure of evaluating the status of impalpable cervical lymph nodes in lung cancer patients, and also helps in staging of lung cancer [40].

## ADEQUACY AND DIAGNOSTIC YIELD OF MATEIAL

Adequacy of sample and diagnostic yield of aspirated material are important factors in the diagnosis of cancers and its further characterization by FNA. Adequacy rate of aspirated material in FNA of thoracic lesions ranges from 68.9% to 95.5% with an average of 82.4% [16, 17, 19, 23, 41-44]. Even if the aspirated material is adequate, in a small fraction of cases, it may be non- diagnostic/inconclusive. The overall diagnostic yield of FNA material in literature ranges from 67.4% to 91.7% with an average of 81.7% [11, 14, 18, 19, 23, 26, 45-50]. The lowest diagnostic yield of 67.7% was observed in a study based on FNA without US- or CT-guidance [11]. Significant improvement in adequacy and diagnostic accuracy can be achieved by presence of cytopathologist at the time of aspiration and by rapid staining technqiue to certify that the aspirate is adequate before releasing the patient [49, 51-53]. It has been observed that the diagnostic yield of malignancy cases is slightly higher (average 88.3%) than the benign lesions (average 79.9%) of the thorax [45, 46, 54]. In a study by Shimizu et al [55], the diagnostic yield was found to improve with increase in size of the lesion (48.5% for <10 mm lesions, 62.5% for 11-15 mm lesions, and 83.9% for 16-20 mm lesions). It is further observed that the adequacy rate of combined FNA and core biopsy is more than FNA or core biopsy alone [43, 48].

## Cytologic Characterization of Material

Reported frequency of malignancies in thoracic FNAs shows a wide variation. As revealed from 15 studies over a period of 25 years (table 1), the frequency of malignant lesions in intra-thoracic FNA ranged from 36.3% to 88.5% with an average of 65.6% [12-14, 17, 18, 24, 44, 45, 56-62]. Besides the primary lesions, the secondaries form a significant proportion of malignancies in the lung. The ratio of primary tumor to metastatic deposit is about 2.5 to 3.5:1 [13, 61].

**Table 1. Frequency of Distribution of Lesions in Transthoracic Fine Needle Aspiration**

| Author(s) Year | No. of cases | Frequency distribution in percentages | | | |
|---|---|---|---|---|---|
| | | Malignancy | Suspicious | Benign | Inadequate |
| Mazza et al (2005) [18] | 321 | 72.0 | 2.5 | 11.2 | 14.3 |
| Haq et al (2004) [12] | 59 | 59.3 | 8.5 | 16.9 | 15.2 |
| Tan et al (2002) [24] | 114 | 65.8 | 0.0 | 27.2 | 7.0 |
| Wallace et al (2002) [17] | 61 | 47.5 | 4.9 | 24.6 | 23.0 |
| Dahlstrom et al (2001) [56] | 288 | 64.6 | 2.1 | 23.2 | 10.1 |
| Knudson et al (1996) [57] | 128 | 64.8 | 1.6 | 26.6 | 7.0 |
| Das et al (1995) [44] | 190 | 36.3 | 1.1 | 31.6 | 31.1 |
| Zhai (1990) [45] | 50 | 68.0 | 0 | 32.0 | 0 |
| Rajwanshi et al (1989) [58] | 186 | 64.5 | 2.7 | 10.8 | 22.0 |
| Young et al (1987) [59] | 255 | 75.7 | 4.7 | 11.4 | 8.2 |
| Kaufman et al (1987) [14] | 342 | 83.0 | 0 | 6.5 | 10.5 |
| Linder et al (1986) [60] | 32 | 56.3 | 12.5 | 15.6 | 15.6 |
| Johnston (1984) [61] | 1015 | 63.5 | 0 | 31.1 | 5.4 |
| Pilotti et al (1982) [13] | 130 | 88.5 | 0 | 11.5 | 0 |
| Janieson et al (1981) [62] | 81 | 74.1 | 0 | 25.9 | 0 |
| Total | 217 | 65.6±13.00 | 2.7± 3.65 | 20.4±8.78 | 11.3±9.07 |

As per a standard text book in pathology [63], squamous cell carcinoma was probably the most common type of bronchogenic carcinoma (30% to 35%), followed by adenocarcinoma (20% to 30%), small cell carcinoma (20% to 25%), and large cell undifferentiated carcinoma (7% to 15%), between 1950s and 1980s. The frequencies of different types of lung cancers, however, appear to be changing. According to Pirozynski [64], adenocarcinoma has become the most frequent histologic type (approx 50%) while squamous cell carcinoma, previously the most common, accounts for approximately one third of lung cancer cases, and small cell cancer 15%. Analysis of 69 malignancy cases of lung diagnosed by us [65] showed that adenocarcinoma was the most common malignancy (37.7%), followed by squamous cell carcinoma (23.2%), sarcomas (7.2%), small cell carcinoma (5.8%), lymphomas (5.8%), mesothelioma (4.3%), and malignant germ cell tumors (4.3%) (table 2). Thirty five malignant lesions of the lung described by Haq et al [12], however, showed completely different frequencies and included 20 (57.14%) cases of squamous cell carcinoma, 1 (2.86%) adenocarcinoma, 8 (22.86%) large cell carcinoma, and 6 (17.14%) small cell carcinoma.

**Table 2. Malignancies of the Lung Diagnosed FNA Cytology at the Institute of Cytology and Preventive Oncology (ICMR), New Delhi during 1985-1990**

| FNA cytodiagnosis | No of cases | | |
|---|---|---|---|
| | Total | Male | Female |
| Squamous cell carcinoma | 16 | 14 | 2 |
| Adenocarcinoma | 26 | 18 | 8 |
| Small cell carcinoma | 4 | 4 | 0 |
| Large cell carcinoma | 1 | - | 1 |
| Miscellaneous carcinomas | 2 | 2 | - |
| Mesothelioma | 3 | 1 | 2 |
| Sarcomas | 5 | 3 | 2 |
| Lymphomas | 4 | 2 | 2 |
| Malignant germ cell tumor | 3 | 3 | - |
| Misccellaneous malignancies | 4 | 2 | 2 |
| Malignancy (not otherwise specified) | 1 | 1 | - |
| Total | 69 | 50 | 19 |

From the management point of view, it is important to classify the primary epithelial malignancies of the lung into small cell cancer (SCC) and non-small cell cancer (NSCC). In FNA cytologic material, the ratio of SCC to NSCC ranges from 1: 3.3 to 1: 4.8 (average 1: 4.4) [12, 50, 65, 66]. Arora et al [66] diagnosed 76 malignant lesions of lung by percutaneous FNA and bronchial washings, and categorized them cytomorphologically into 50 NSCC, 15 SCC, 1 NHL, 1 carcinoid, and 9 undifferentiated/ poorly differentiated carcinoma. The common primary non-small cell carcinomas of lung include squamous cell carcinoma (figure 1.A and B) and adenocarcinoma (figure 2 A and B). Less common NSCC of the lung diagnosed by FNA cytology include bronchioloalveolar carcinoma, which can have usual and unusual features [67, 68] and large cell anaplastic carcinoma. Rare variants are bronchial mucoepidermoid carcinoma [69], adenocarcinoma of fetal type [70], adenoid cystic carcinoma [71], and amphicrine carcinoma [72], which shows dual differentiation i.e.

glandular and endocrine. Small cell carcinoma (figure 3 A) forms part of neuroendocrine neoplasms, which includes typical carcinoid, atypical carcinoid and small cell anaplastic carcinoma [73]. It also forms part of small round cell tumors (SRCT) in the thoracic cavity, which includes neuroblastoma, ganglioneuroblastoma, Ewing's sarcoma, pulmonary blastoma and non-Hodgkin's lymphoma [74]. The FNA cytologic features of small cell anaplastic carcinomas [74-76] and NHL [77] in the thorax, and pulmonary blastoma [78] have been reported independently or as a part of small round cell tumors.

Sarcomas, either primary or metastatic form a small but significant component of intrathoracic malignancies. In general sarcomas are characterised by losely cohesive, rather flat, cellular aggregates and isolated cells [79]. The reported primary sarcomas diagnosed by transthoracic FNA include chondrosarcoma [80], liposarcoma [81] and Ewings sarcoma [74] (figure 3B and C) and alveolar rhabdomyosarcoma. Even rare mixed tumors like carcinosarcomas have been diagnosed by FNAC [82, 83]. The metastatic mesenchymal tumors diagnosed by FNA of thorax include malignant fibrous histiocytoma [84], dermatofibrosarcoma protuberans [85], and malignant schwannoma [86]. Kim et al [79] diagnosed 17 metastatic sarcomas in the lung by FNA which included malignant fibrous histiocytoma (5 cases), fibrosarcoma (3), leiomyosarcoma (3), endometrial stromal sarcoma (3), osteogenic sarcoma (1) and poorly differentiated sarcomas (2). The germ cell tumors of thorax, both primary and metastatic, have been diagnosed by FNA cytology [87, 88]. Another group of neoplasms diagnosed by FNA cytology of mediastinal mass includes thymomas, either benign or malignant [89, 90].

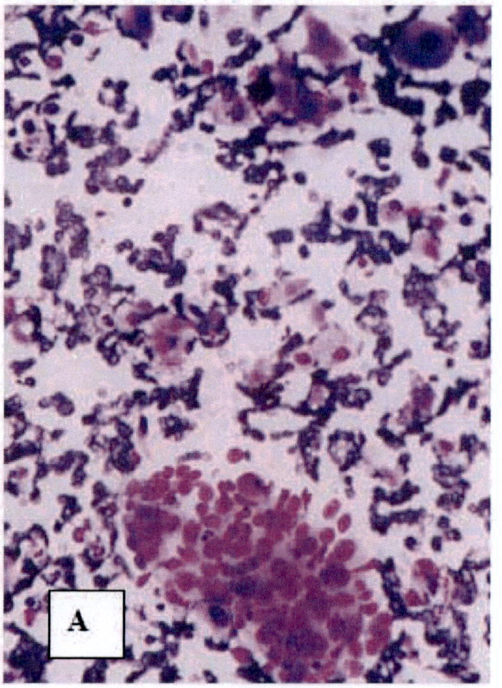


Figure 1A. Squamous cell carcinoma: FNA smear from the left lung (upper zone) mass of a 60-year-old woman. A cluster of malignant cells along with a few dispersed tumor cells showing evidence of keratinization and a few alveolar macrophages (May-Grünwald-Giemsa x 200).

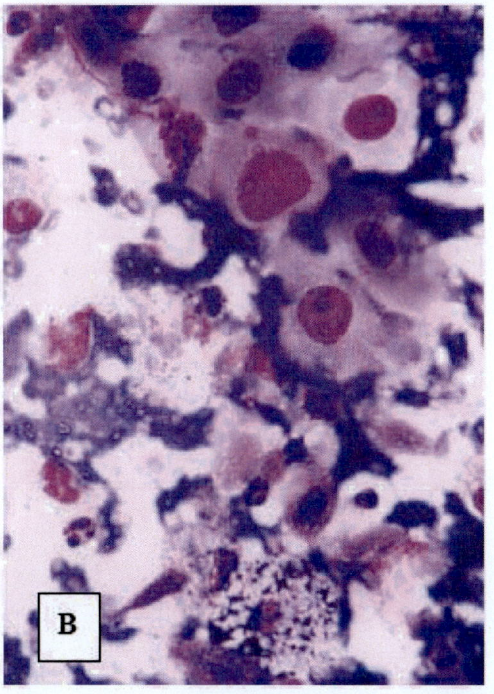


Figure 1B. Squamous cell carcinoma: Higher magnification of the case shown in Figure 1A. A group of tumor cells with evidence of keratinization and a carbon laden alveolar macrophage (May-Grünwald-Giemsa x 500).

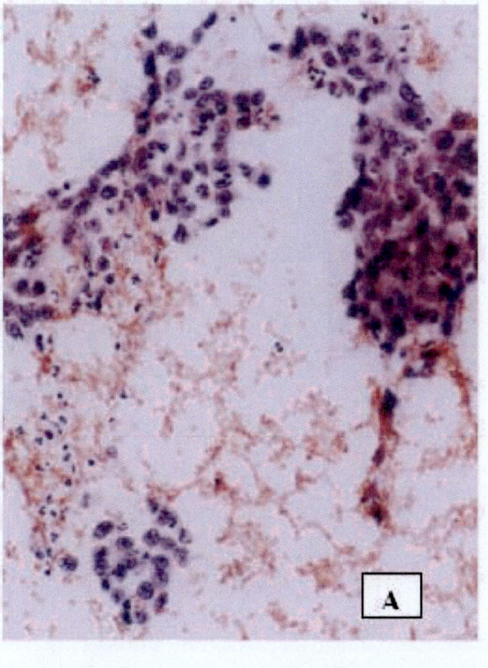


Figure 2A. Adenocarcinoma: FNA smear from the right lung mass of a 50-year-old woman. Groups of tumor cells with prominent nucleoli show microacinar formation (Papanicolaou x 200).

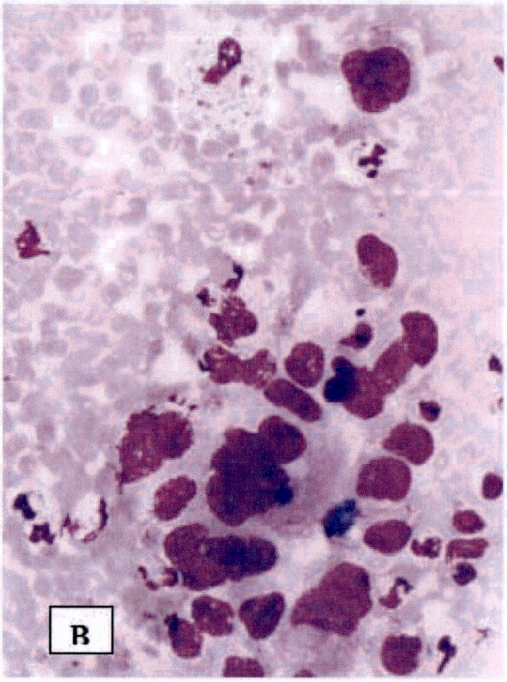


Figure 2B. Adenocarcinoma: Pleomorphic malignant cells show vague microacinar formation. An alveolar macrophage is seen in the background. Same case as shown in Figure 2A (May-Grünwald-Giemsa x 400).

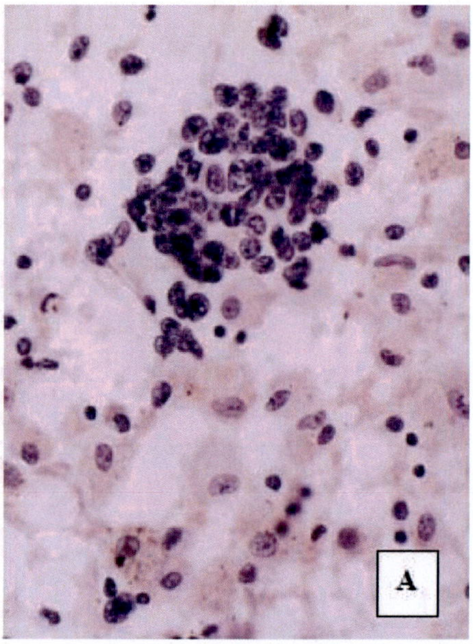


Figure 3A. Small cell carcinoma: FNA smear from the left lung mass in a 65-year-old woman. A group of tumor cells, which are small in size and have salt and pepper chromatin, show nuclear moulding. Numerous alveolar macrophages and a few lymphocytes are seen in the back ground (Papanicolaou x 400).

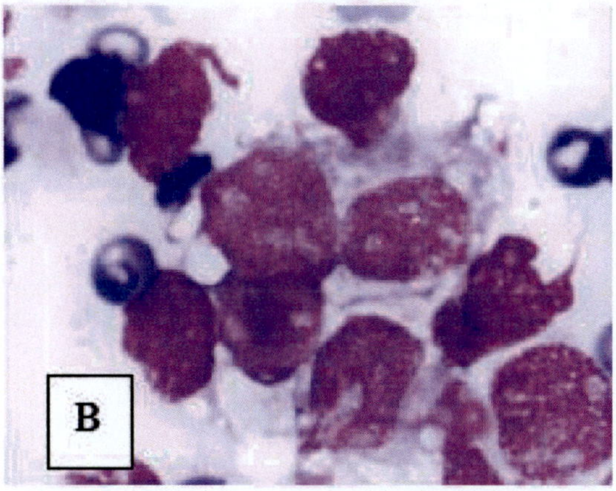


Figure 3B. Ewings sarcoma: FNA smear from the right lung mass in a 23-year-old woman. Small round tumor cells with abundant cytoplasmic vacuoles due to glycogen (May-Grünwald-Giemsa x 1000).

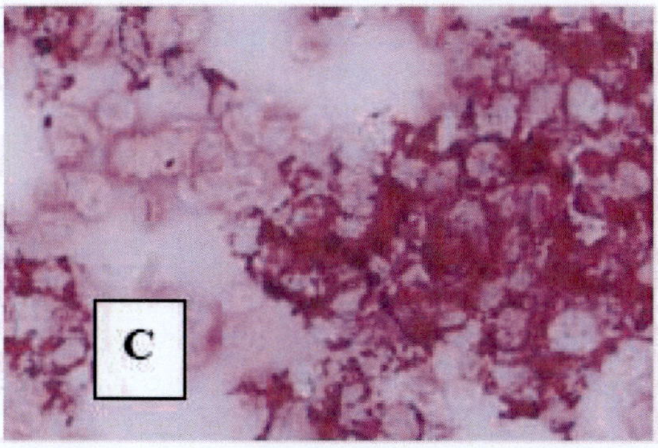


Figure 3C. Ewings sarcoma: PAS staining shows intense positive reaction, which was sensitive to diastase, indicating that the contents of the vacuoles was glycogen. Same case as shown in Figure 3B (x 400).

## Lung Cancer in Women: The Emerging Trends

The emerging data demonstrate sex specific differences in lung cancer susceptibility and prognosis. The patient population of lung cancer is changing from mostly male smokers to include women and non-smokers, which implies that development of lung cancer is modulated by complex interactions between genetic, hormonal, behavioral, and environmental factors [91]. The SEER Cancer Statistics Review (1975-2003) [92] revealed that the age adjusted incidence rate of lung cancer in males of USA reached a peak in the year 1984 (102.0 per 100,000) followed by a steady decline till 2003 (78.5 per 100,000). On the other hand, the females showed a rising trend from 24.5 per 100,000 in 1975 to 52.9 per 100,000 in 1998, followed by minimal decline till 2003 (51.3 per 100,000). Cerfolio et al [93] found that women with pathologic stages I, II, and III non-small cell cancer had better survival than men. In a study by Das [65], the male to female ratio was 2.63:1 among 69 malignanciy cases of lung diagnosed by FNA cytology. The male to female ratios in squamous cell carcinoma, adenocarcinoma, and small cell carcinoma were 7:1, 2.25:1 and 4:0, respectively. Okutan et al [7], observed that 44 (11.2%) of 393 primary lung cancer patients were female and the cell type distribution was as follows: adenocarcinoma 45.4%, squamous cell cancer 29.5%, small cell cancer 20.5%, and large cell cancer 4.6%. The authors found a low rate of smokers but a high rate of adenocarcinoma among their female patients. According to Baldini and Strauss [94], women who smoke appear to be at higher risk of developing small cell carcinoma than squamous cell cancer, whereas men who smoke have a similar risk for the two histologic types. Furthermore, women smokers are more likely to develop adenocarcinoma of the lung, possibly due to the effect of estrogens.

## DIAGNOSTIC EFFICACY OF FNA CYTOLOGY IN THORACIC LESIONS

In general, the efficacy of FNA in diagnosis of thoracic lesions has been very good. The sensitivity, specificity, and diagnostic accuracy of FNA cytology in 15 studies, over a period of 28 years (1978-2005) (table 3) based on various imaging guidance modalities, ranged from 76 to 99% (87.7± 6.76%), 68 to 100% (96.8± 8.21%), and 65 to 99% (88.9± 8.66%), respectively [8, 13, 16-18, 21, 24, 27, 38, 39, 95-99]. It is observed that the diagnostic efficacy of thoracic FNA is affected by factors such as diagnostic modalities employed, lesion size, and histologic type of tumor.

**Table 3. Sensitivity, Specificity and Diagnostic Accuracy of FNA Cytology in Intra Thoracic Lesions**

| Author (s) and year | Site | No of cases | Sensitivity (%) | Specificity (%) | Diagnostic accuracy (%) |
|---|---|---|---|---|---|
| Mazza et al (2005) [18] | Lung | 321 | 99 | 95 | 99 |
| Annema et al (2005) [38] | Med | 242 | 91 | 100 | 93 |
| Rintoul et al (2005) [27] | Med | 20 | 85 | 100 | 89 |
| Caddy et al (2005) [95] | Med | 52 | 93 | 100 | 95 |
| Tan et al (2002) [24] | Lung | 114 | 93.4 | 95.8 | 94 |
| Wallace et al (2002) [17] | Lung | 57 | 82 | 100 | 88 |
| Larsen et al (2002) [39] | Med | 79 | 92 | 100 | 94 |
| Wiersema et al (2001) [21] | Med | 82 | 96 | 100 | 98 |
| Dewan et al (1995) [96] | Lung | 33 | 81 | 100 | 86 |
| Saa-Gandi and Mearns (1991) [8] | Lung | 74 | 81 | 100 | 83.3 |
| Pacella et al (1991) [16] | Thorax | 75 | 76 | 68 | 81 |
| Caya et al (1984) [97] | Thorax | 82 | 79 | 100 | 83 |
| Montali et al (1983) [98] | Lung | 302 | 88.4 | 99.9 | 89.4 |
| Pilloti et al (1982) [13] | Thorax | 56 | 91 | 95 | 65* |
| Sagel et al (1978) [99] | Thorax | 1211 | 87 | 99 | 96 |
| Total | | 187 | 87.7±6.76 | 96.8±8.21 | 88.9±8.66 |
| Med= mediastinum, * for subtyping | | | | | |

### Diagnostic Techniques and Their Efficacy

The sensitivitity, specificity, and diagnostic accuracy of CT-guided FNA of pulmonary lesions in 4 studies were 84.5± 10.02, 90.8± 15.35, and 87.8± 8.00, respectively [8, 16-18]. The sensitivity, specificity, and accuracy of EUS-FNA in 4 other studies were even better, i.e., 93.0± 2.16%, 100%, and 95.0± 2.16%, respectively [21, 38, 39, 95]. In a study by Baba et al [100], the sensitivity of preoperative cytodiagnosis was 43.7% for trans-bronchial biopsy, 52.9% for trans-bronchial forceps biopsy-stamp cytology, 66.6% for trans-bronchial fine needle aspiration, and 85.0% for percutaneous fine needle aspiration. It is observed that various diagnostic modalities are complimentary and supplementary to each other in improving the diagnostic efficacy. In a study by Iyoda et al [101], the sensitivity of the diagnostic procedures for primary lung cancers were as follows: 64.8% for brushings, 56.1% for trans-bronchial forceps biopsy (TBFB), 72.0% for trans-bronchial forceps biopsy-stamp cytology (TBFB-SC), and 86.4% for trans-bronchial fine needle aspiration (TBFNA). The four transbronchial biopsy procedures (brushings, TBFB, TBFB-SC, and TBFNA) had a combined overall sensitivity of 92.7%. According to Kim et al [48], the sensitivity for transthoracic FNA, core biopsy, and both were 94.6%, 88.3%, and 97.2%, respectively. Yamagami et al [43] offered a precise diagnosis in 79.7% by FNA, 91.3% by core biopsy, and 94.2% cases by combined use of both techniques.

### Lesion Size and Diagnostic Efficacy

Yamagami et al [43] observed diagnostic accuracy of 100% for lesions of size 31-100 mm, whereas the lesions below 30 mm had diagnostic accuracy $\leq$ 93.8%. In another study, the diagnostic efficacy was better for 0.8 -1.0 cm lesions (sensitivity, 88%; accuracy, 92%) than those for 0.5-0.7 cm lesions (sensitivity, 50%; Accuracy, 70%) [17].

### Histologic Type of Tumor and Diagnostic Efficacy

Among 106 bronchogenic carcinoma (BC) and 6 neuroendocrine tumors of the lung, the cytodiagnostic accuracy rates were 75.5%, 72%, 100%, 53%, and 50% for bronchogenic adenocarcinoma, squamous-cell carcinoma, small-cell carcinoma, large-cell carcinoma, and mixed carcinomas [102]. For NSCC, Caddy et al [95] observed the sensitivity, specificity, and diagnostic accuracy of 92%, 100%, and 94%, respectively. The efficacy of transthoracic FNA for small cell carcinoma vs. other lung malignancies was as follows: sensitivity 67% vs. 81%, equal specificity 100%, and accuracy 96% vs. 88% [6].

## Impact of FNA of Thorax on Surgical Management

Patients with intrathoracic mass lesions often present with pleural effusion or mediastinal obstruction syndrome in a state of respiratory distress requiring immediate therapeutic management. In such a situation the FNA cytology has the potential to play the important role of providing a quick tissue diagnosis [77]. Because of FNA, patients who are with poor surgical risk are spared a thoracotomy in many instances and patients who are clinically inoperable can receive chemotherapy and radiation therapy without major surgery done solely for diagnostic purposes [103]. Romano et al [34] observed that CT-guided FNAB of small lung lesions (<15 mm) is an equally safe and effective procedure in inpatients and outpatients. Further, outpatient performance of FNAB can decrease costs. Routine diagnosis provided by transthoracic FNA helps to plan the management of cases, either medically or surgically. According to Delgado et al [6] if a diagnosis of small cell carcinoma of lung is made, the surgical treatment approach is no longer considered and chemotherapy becomes the treatment of choice. On the other hand, exact mediastinal evaluation of patients with non-small-cell lung cancer (NSCLS) is mandatory to improve selection of resectable and curable patients for surgery [30].

Endoscopic ultrasound guided fine needle aspiration biopsy (EUS-FNA) qualifies as the next diagnostic step in patients with suspected lung cancer and a non-diagnostic bronchoscopy, if the intrapulmonary mass is located adjacent or near the esophagus. EUS-FNA also permits the surgeon to assess the extent of malignancy [104]. EUS-FNA was superior to mediastinoscopy (MS) in examination of lymph nodes (particularly paratracheal and subcarinal) of patients considered for resection of lung cancer [30]. It is suggested that EUS-FNA (with diagnostic accuracy as high as 97%), may replace CT-guided biopsies and reduce the number of exploratory thoracotomies [29]. As a result of EUS-FNA, a thoracotomy was avoided in 49% patients and in 68%, a mediastinoscopy was avoided [39]. According to Annema et al [38] EUS-FNA prevented 70% of scheduled surgical procedures because of the demonstration LN metastasis in non-small-cell lung cancer (52%), tumor invasion (T4) (4%), tumor invasion and lymph node metastasis (5%), SCLC (8%), or benign diagnoses (1%). Larsen et al [105] observed that the addition of routine-EUS-FNA to standard workup in routine clinical practice improved selection of surgically curable patients with NSCLC (9% futile thoracotomies by EUS-FNA versus 25% by standard workup, $p<0.03$).

## Complications Folowing Guided FNA of Thorax

The major limitation of FNA biopsy of thorax includes the high rate of complications, especially pneumothorax with frequency ranging from 1.6% to 46.0%, and an average of 17.0% [11, 18, 31, 36, 41, 46, 50, 75, 96, 99, 106-110]. Although, the frequency of pneumothorax is much less (<10%) in some studies and ranges from 1.6% to 6.3%, with an average of 3.8 % [11, 31, 50, 106-108], others have reported a relatively higher frequency (>10%) of pneumothorax (table 4), ranging from 12.8% to 46%, with an average of 24.9%. Chest tube drainage was necessary in 3.9% to 26% (average of 9.5%) of these patients [9, 18, 36, 41, 46, 75, 96, 99, 109, 110]. It is observed that the average depth of inserting the needle was significantly higher in a drained pneumothorax (8.9± 2.17 cm) than in a non-drained pneumothorax (7.7± 1.3 cm, $p= 0.024$) [36]. Pneumothorax was detected in only 10% when a "protective" technique (iatrogenic-controlled pneumothorax or creation of saline solution injected salinoma) was used but 60% when traversing the lung parenchyma in transthoracic FNA of mediastinal lymph nodes of >1.5 cm in diameter [47]. Other less common or rare complications related to the technique of FNAB includes hemoptysis [9, 11, 75, 108], hemothorax [9, 108], post-procedural fever [21, 36], and needle tract implantation or spread of tumor along the needle tract [108, 111-115]. In a study by Wong et al [46], bleeding occurred in 6 (8%) and there was one death in a patient with abnormal hematologic parameters. FNA performed on resected lung lobes involved by lung carcinoma showed malignant cells prior to aspiration in 10% and following FNA in 60% (p=0.002), indicating that FNAC has the potential to spread cells to the pleural space [114]. However, according to Kim et al [115], the incidence of chest wall implantation metastasis after FNAB is extremely rare (8 of 4365 percutaneous FNAB of indeterminate pulmonary nodules). There are also some studies, which record very minimal or no complications of thoracic FNAs [13, 19, 22, 104, 109, 116, 117].

**Table 4. Studies Showing Higher Frequency of Pneumothorax (>10%) and Patients Requiring Chest Tube Drainage in FNAB of Thorax**

| Author(s) and year | No.of cases | Frequency of pneumothorax (%) | Frequency of chest tube drainage (%) |
|---|---|---|---|
| Mazza et al (2005) [18] | 321 | 13.1 | 6.6 |
| Wong et al (2002) [46] | 67 | 20.9 | 6.0 |
| Wojtas et al (2001) [36] | 406 | 12.8 | 3.9 |
| Dennie et al (2001) [109] | 506 | 22.9 | 6.5 |
| Dewan et al (1995) [96] | 33 | 46.0 | 26.0 |
| Steenskov et al (1982) [110] | 500 | 25.0 | 4.4 |
| Todd et al (1981) [41] | 2114 | 39.9 | 10.4 |
| Stamfel (1979) [9] | 120 | 17.5 | 9.2 |
| Sagel et al (1978) [99] | 1211 | 24.0 | 14.0 |
| Sinner (1976) [111] | 2726 | 27.2 | 7.7 |
| Total | 800 | 24.9±10.73 | 9.5±6.53 |

## Diagnostic Dilemma

Besides complications of the FNA techniques, the other limitations of FNA thorax relates to sampling and interpretation errors. In a study by Caya et al [97], 11 of the 13 negative diagnoses were due to sampling errors. Excavated squamous cell carcinoma and scar adenocarcinoma, accompanying tuberculosis can also lead to false negative diagnosis by FNA [118]. Various benign conditions that may be confused with or mimic malignancy in FNA cytology are inflammatory pseudo tumor [119], aspergillus infection [120], sclerosing hemangioma with cytologic atypia (with well-differentiated adenocarcinoma, especially bronchioloalveolar carcinoma) [121]. Lack of familiarity with uncommon lesions such as thymoma, pulmonary hamartoma, pulmonary pseudolymphoma, typical carcinoid and spindle cell carcinoid mimicking oat cell carcinoma may also result in erroneous interpretation [122]. Similarly, malignancy cases may be misdiagnosed as benign lesions. Adenocarcinoma and bronchioloalveolar carcinoma cases can be diagnosed as atypia or negative in FNA smears or BAL [120]. The discrepancy between cytology and histology may also be mainly due to poorly differentiated carcinoma [108]. According to Yilmaz et al [123], cell typing by transthoracic FNA (TFNA) may lead to incorrect results in the presence of poor differentiation, mixed tumors and peripheral epidermoid carcinoma. Further, the likelihood of a correct diagnosis using the TFNA specimens was 6.2-fold higher for well-differentiated tumors than for poorly differentiated tumors ($p< 0.005$) [123]. Small round cell tumors may also prove a difficult diagnostic problem in FNA cytology, especially when poorly differentiated. Bavikatty and Michael [124] observed that the presence of nuclear molding was the single most useful feature in differentiating small-cell carcinoma from other small round cell tumors on thinprep (TP). According to Arora et al [66] nuclear molding, cell size and scant, basophilic cytoplasm were highly sensitive and specific by univariate analysis for distinguishing SCC from NSCC. Small-cell-like large-cell neuroendocrine carcinoma can be mistaken for small-cell carcinoma. The most important differentiating features between these two entities are nuclear size and perceptibility of nucleoli of tumor cells [125]. Fine needle aspiration cytology of pulmonary blastoma may be suggestive of neuroblastoma [126]. Thus, when the SRCT is poorly differentiated, it may be impossible to characterize it based on morphological features alone. In such difficult situations, ancillary studies may be of help to arrive at a correct diagnosis.

## Contribution of Ancillary Techniques

Improvement in cytodiagnosis can be achieved by adoption of ancillary studies. Lung, being a common site for metastatic carcinoma, differentiation of primary from metastatic carcinomas becomes difficult at times based on cytomorphology alone. FNA smears (stained previously with the Pap technique) of 12/14 adenocarcinoma, and 6/8 small cell carcinomas were positive for thyroid transcription factor-1 (TTF-1) but 11/12 squamous cell carcinoma, and all metastatic tumors were negative [127]. Mucinous and mixed bronchioloalveolar carcinomas (BAC) have an immunohistochemical phenotype (FNA material stained with Ck7 and 20, and TTF-1) that is different from that of conventional pulmonary adenocarcinoma. Knowledge of these staining patterns is crucial for distinguishing mucinous and mixed BACs from metastatic adenocarcinoma involving the lungs [128]. Use of immunocytochemistry (ICC) and electron microscope (E/M) may help in classifying the poorly differentiated tumors, determine neuroendocrine differentiation and establish primary site in suspected metastatic malignancies [129]. ICC or ICC with EM are helpful in confirming neoplasms like metastatic prostatic carcinoma [130], metastasis for intracranial meningioma [131], metastatic adamantinoma [132], and metastatic malignant schwannoma [86]. These ancillary studies are also useful in the diagnosis of primary tumors like chondroblastoma [133], amphicrine carcinoma [72], and pulmonary carcinosarcoma [82]. In a study of ancillary techniques by O'Reilly et al [129], ICC provided significant additional information in 40% cases and confirmed the light microscopic impression in 36% cases. E/M on the other hand provided significant additional information in 67% cases.

Nakamura et al [134] found that the ability of florescent insitu hybridization (FISH) to detect cancer cells was superior to conventional cytology for the diagnosis of lung cancer (specificity 100% for both but sensitivity 71.8% for conventional cytology versus 87.1% for FISH). Ludovini et al [135] found that p53 positivity (p=0.005) and Rb negativity (p=0.016) were associated with chemotherapy response. In a microarray analysis by Lim et al [136], RNA amplification was successful and gene expression profile from NSCLC could determine malignancy. A small volume tissue from NSCLC obtained by FNA had gene expression profile, different from normal and similar to tumor profiles. E-cadherin (a cell surface molecule that mediates cell-cell adhesion in normal epithelium) expression of FNAB specimens can be helpful in predicting tumor cell differentiation (decreased expression of 33% in low-grade adenocarcinoma vs. 100% in high-grade adenocarcinoma, p< 0.005), invasiveness, and defining a subpopulation of patients with primary lung adenocarcinoma with possible poor outcome [137].

## Conclusion

Thus, imaging-guided FNA of thoracic lesions is a safe and accurate diagnostic tool, with high degree of sensitivity and specificity for lung cancer at any intrathoracic station.

## References


[1] Parkin DM, Bray F, Ferlay J, Pisani P. Global cancer statistics, 2002. *CA Cancer J. Clin.* 2005; 55: 74- 108.

[2] Williams MD, Sandler AB. The epidemiology of lung cancer. *Cancer Treat Res.* 2001; 105: 31- 52.

[3] Pauk N, Kubik A, Zatloukal P, Krepela E. Lung cancer in women. *Lung Cancer.* 2005; 48: 1- 9.

[4] [No authors listed]. Consolidated Report of the Population Based Cancer Registries: Incidence and Distribution of Cancer (1990-1996). New Delhi. National Cancer Registry Programme, Indian Council of Medical Research. 2001.

[5] Stabile LP, Siegfried JM. Sex and gender differences in lung cancer. *J. Gend. Specif. Med.* 2003; 6: 37- 48.

[6] Delgado PI, Jorda M, Ganjei-Azar P. Small cell carcinoma versus other lung malignancies: diagnosis by fine needle aspiration cytology. *Cancer.* 2000; 90: 279-285.

[7] Okutan O, Kartaloglu Z, Ilvan A, Kunter E, Cerrahoglu K, Capraz F. *Bull Cancer.* 2004; 91: 201- 210.

[8] SaaGandi FW, Mearns AJ. Fine needle aspiration biopsy of pulmonary lesions: A 2-year experience in a district general hospital with a literature review. *J. R. Coll. Surg. Edinb.* 1991; 36: 309-311.

[9] Stampfel G. X-ray controlled percutaneous needle aspiration biopsy of the lungs. *Rongenblatter.* 1979; 32: 481-485.

[10] Savage C, Morrison RJ, Zwischenberger JB. Bronchoscopic diagnosis and staging of lung cancer. *Chest Surg. Clin. N. Am.* 2001; 11: 701- 721.

[11] Suri JC, Goel A, Bhatia A. Safety and efficacy of unguided transthoracic fine needle aspiration biopsy (FNAB) in outdoor patients. *Indian J. Chest. Dis. Allied. Sci.* 1991; 33: 129-132.

[12] Haq MH, Talukder SI, Haque MA, Sarker CB, Saleh AF, Debnath CR. Role of fine needle aspiration cytology in the diagnosis of pulmonary lesions. *Mymensingh. Med. J.* 2004; 13: 16-19.

[13] Pilotti S, Rilke F, Goribauchi G, Damascelli B. Fine needle aspiration biopsy cytology of primary and metastatic pulmonary tumors. *Acta Cytol.* 1982; 26: 661-666.

[14] Kaufman M, Schwartz I, Weissberg D. Fine needle aspiration biopsy in diagnosis of pulmonary masses. *Am. Surg.* 1987; 53: 339-341.

[15] Swinburn CR, Veale D, Peel ET, Wadehra V, Elliot ST, Sumerling MD, Cornis PA, Gibson GT. A prospective randomized comparison of fine needle aspiration biopsy and fiberoptic bronchoscopy in the investigation of peripheral pulmonary opacities. *Respir. Med.* 1989; 83: 493-495.

[16] Pacella CM, Papini E, Valle D, Buffa E, Bizzarri G, Rossi Z, Nardi F. Fine needle aspiration biopsy (FNAB) guided with tomodensitometry of pulmonary and mediastinal masses: Personal experience. *Radiol. Med. Torino.* 1991; 82: 89-94.

[17] Wallace MJ, Krishnamurthy S, Broemeling LD, Gupta S, Ahrar K, Morello FA Jr, Hicks ME. CT-guided percutaneous fine-needle aspiration biopsy of small (< or =1-cm) pulmonary lesions. *Radiology.* 2002; 225: 823- 828.

[18] Mazza E, Madau C, Ricciardi A, Falchini M, Matucci M, Ciarpallini T. On-site evaluation of percutaneous CT-guided fine needle aspiration of pulmonary lesions. *Radiol. Med.* (Torino) 2005; 110: 141- 148.

[19] Pedersen OM, Aasen TB, Gulsvik A. Fine needle aspiration biopsy of mediastinal and peripheral pulmonary masses guided by real time sonography. *Chest.* 1986; 89: 504-508.

[20] Chen CC, Hsu WH, Huang CM, Hsu JY, Chiang CD. Ultrasound guided fine needle aspiration biopsy of small pulmonary nodules abutting to the chest wall. Chang Hua I Hsueh Chih. *Chinese Med. J.* 1996; 57: 106-111.

[21] Wiersema MJ, Vazquez-Sequeiros E, Wiersema LM. Evaluation of mediastinal lymphadenopathy with endoscopic US-guided fine-needle aspiration biopsy. *Radiology.* 2001; 219: 252- 257.

[22] Liu GS, Wu YL, Zeng CG, Yang MT, Cai YH, Rong TH, Huang ZF, Liang XM. Percutaneous super fine needle aspiration biopsy of intrathoracic lesions. *J. Surg. Oncol.* 1989; 40: 135-138.

[23] Colquhoun SD, Rosenthal DL, Morten DL. Role of percutaneous fine needle aspiration biopsy in suspected intrathoracic malignancy. *Ann. Thorac. Surg.* 1991; 51: 390-393.

[24] Tan KB, Thamboo TP, Wang SC, Nilsson B, Rajwanshi A, Salto-Tellez M. Audit of transthoracic fine needle aspiration of the lung: cytological subclassification of bronchogenic carcinomas and diagnosis of tuberculosis. *Singapore Med. J.* 2002; 3: 570- 575.

[25] de Vivo F, Pond GD, Rhenman B, Icenogle TB, Vasu MA, Copeland JG. Transtracheal aspiration and fine neele aspiration biopsy for the diagnosis of pulmonary infection in heart transplant patients. *J. Thorac. Cardiovasc. Surg.* 1988; 96: 696-699.

[26] Bhat N, Bhagat P, Pearlman ES, Kane G, Figueroa W, Kannan V, Kline TS. Transbronchial needle aspiration biopsy in the diagnosis of pulmonary neoplasms. *Diagn. Cytopathol.* 1990; 6: 14-17.

[27] Rintoul RC, Skwarski KM, Murchison JT, Wallace WA, Walker WS, Penman ID. Endobronchial and endoscopic ultrasound-guided real-time fine-needle aspiration for mediastinal staging. *Eur. Respir. J.* 2005; 25: 416- 421.

[28] Weirsema MJ, Kochman ML, Cramer HM, Wiersema LM. Preopertive staging of non-small cell lung cancer by transesophageal US guided fine needle aspiration biopsy of mediastinal lymph nodes. *Radiology.* 1994; 190: 239-242.

[29] Annema JT, Veselic M, Rabe KF. EUS-guided FNA of centrally located lung tumours following a non-diagnostic bronchoscopy. *Lung Cancer.* 2005; 48: 357-361.

[30] Larsen SS, Vilmann P, Krasnik M, Dirksen A, Clementsen P, Skov BG, Jacobsen GK. Endoscopic ultrasound guided biopsy versus mediastinoscopy for analysis of paratracheal and subcarinal lymph nodes in lung cancer staging. *Lung Cancer.* 2005; 48: 85- 92.

[31] Hsu WH, Chiang CD, Wang RC, Chiang CS, Hsu JY. Apical malignancies diagnosed by ultrasound guided fine needle aspiration biopsy. *J. Formos. Med. Assoc.* 1993; 92: 983-987.

[32] Belfiore G, Camera L, Moggio G, Vetraeni A, Fraioli G, Salvatore M. Middle mediastinum lesions. Preliminary experience with CT-guided fine needle aspiration biopsy with suprasternal approach. *Radiology.* 1997; 202: 870-873.

[33] Libby DM, Smith JP, Altorki NK, Pasmantier MW, Yankelevitz D, Henschke CI. Managing of small pulmononary nodule discovered by CT. *Chest.* 2004; 125: 1522-1529.

[34] Romano M, Griffo S, Gentile M, Mainenti PP, Tamburrini O, Iaccarino V, Salvatore M. CT guided percutaneous fine needle biopsy of small lung lesions in out patients. Safety and efficacy of the procedure compared to inpatients. *Radiol. Med.* (Torino) 2004; 108: 275- 282.

[35] Mullan CP, Kelly BE, Ellis PK, Hughes S, Anderson N, Mc Cluggage WG. CT-guided fine-needle aspiration of lung nodules: effect on outcome of using coaxial technique and immediate cytological evaluation. *Ulster. Med. J.* 2004; 73: 32- 36.

[36] Wojtas G, Jahnz-Rozyk K, Plusa T, Hussein N. Frequency of complications after transthoracic fine needle biopsy of lung tumors. *Pol. Merkuriusz. Lek.* 2001; 11: 314-319.

[37] Iwasaki A, Kamihara Y, Yoneda S, Kawahara K, Shirakusa T. Video-assisted thoracic needle aspiraton cytology for malignancy of the peripheral lung. *Thorac. Cardiovasc. Surg.* 2003; 51: 89- 92.

[38] Anema JT, Versteegh MI, Veselic M, Voigt P, Rabe KF. Endoscopic ultrasound-guided fine-needle aspiration in the diagnosis and staging of lung cancer and its impact on surgical staging. *J. Clin. Oncol.* 2005; 23: 8283- 8285.

[39] Larsen SS, Krasnik M, Vilmann P, Jacobsen GK, Pedersen JJ, Faurschou P, Folke K. Endoscopic ultrasound-guided biopsy of suspected malignancy in the mediastinum has a major impact on the clinical decision process. *Thorax.* 2002; 57: 98- 103.

[40] Sihoe AD, Lee TW, Ahuja AT, Yim AP. Should cervical ultrasonography be a routine staging investigation for lung cancer patients with impalpable cervical lymph nodes? *Eur. J. Cardiothorac. Surg.* 2004; 25: 486- 491.

[41] Todd TR, Weesbroad G, Tao LC, Sanders DE, Delaru NC, Chamberlain DW, Ilves R, Pearson FG, Cass W, Cooper JD. Aspiration biopsy of the thoracic lesions. *Ann. Thorac. Surg.* 1981; 32: 134-161.

[42] Johnson RD, Gobien RP, Valicenti JF Jr. Current status of radiologically directed pulmonary thin needle aspiration biopsy: An analysis of 200 consecutive biopsies and review of the literature. *Ann. Clin. Lab. Sci.* 1983; 13: 225-239.

[43] Yamagami T, Iida S, Kato T, Tanaka O, Nishimura T. Combining fine-nedle aspiration and core biopsy under CT fluoroscopy guidance: better way to treat patients with lung nodules? *Am. J. Roentgenol.* 2003; 180: 811- 815.

[44] Das DK, Pant CS, Pant JN, Sodhani P. Transthoracic (percutaneous) fine needle aspiration cytology diagnosis of pulmonary tuberculosis. *Tuberc. Lung Dis.* 1995; 76: 84-89.

[45] Zhai RY. Fine needle aspiation biopsy of intrathoracic mass guided by real time sonography: analysis of 50 cases. *Chung Hua Chung Liu Tsa Chih.* 1990; 12: 114-116.

[46] Wong PW, Stefanec T, Brown K, White DA. Role of fine-needle aspirates of focal lung lesions in patients with hematologic malignancies. *Chest.* 2002; 121: 527- 532.

[47] Zwischenberger JB, Savage C, Alpard SK, Anderson CM, Marroquin S, Goodacre BW. Mediastinal tranthoracic needle and core lymph node biopsy: should it replace mediastinoscopy? *Chest.* 2002; 121: 1165- 1170.

[48] Kim HK, Shin BK, Cho SJ, Moon JS, Kim MK, Kim CY, Park SH, Kim KT, In KH, Oh YH, Kang EY, Park SH, Kim I. Transthoracic fine needle aspiration and core

biopsy of pulmonary lesions. A study of 296 patients. *Acta Cytol.* 2002; 46: 1061-1068.

[49] Emery SC, Savedes TJ, Behling CA. Utility of immediate evaluation of endoscopic ultrasound-guided transesophageal fine needle aspiration of mediastinal lymph nodes. *Acta Cytol.* 2004; 48: 630- 634.

[50] Kowalewsky J, Sir J, Dancewicz M, Swiniarska J, Peplinski J. Fine-needle aspiration biopsy under CT-guidance—usefulness in diagnosis of malignant lung tumors. *Pneumonol. Alergol. Pol.* 2004; 72: 177- 180.

[51] Austin JH, Cohen MB. Value of having a cytopathologist present during percutaneous fine needle aspiration biopsy of lung: report of 55 cancer patients and meta-analysis of the literature. *Am. J. Roentgenol.* 1993; 160: 175-177.

[52] Santambrogio L, Nosotti M, Bellaviti N, Pavani G, Radice F, Caputo V. CT- guided fine needle aspiration cytology of solitary pulmonary nodules: A prospective, randomized study of immediate cytologic evaluation. *Chest.* 1997; 112: 423-425.

[53] Kucuk CU, Yilmaz A, Yilmaz A, Akkaya E. Computed tomography-guided transthoracic fine-needle aspiration in diagnosis of lung cancer: A comparision of single-pass needle and multiple-pass coaxial needle systems and the value of immediate cytologic assessment. *Respirology.* 2004; 9: 392- 396.

[54] Wung KP, Kelly SI, Britt JE. Percutaneous needle aspiration biopsy of chest lesions: New instrument and new technique. *Chest.* 1988; 93: 993-997.

[55] Shimizu K, Ikeda N, Tsuboi M, Hirano T, Kato H. Percutaneous CT-guided fine needle aspiration for lung cancer smaller than 2 cm and revealed by ground-glass opacity at CT. *Lung Cancer.* 2006; 51: 173-179.

[56] Dahlstrom JE, Langdale-Smith GM, James DT. Fine needle aspiration cytology of pulmonary lesions: a reliable diagnostic test. *Pathology.* 2001; 33: 13-16.

[57] Knudsen DU, Nielsen SM, Hariri J, Christensen J, Kristensen S. Ultrasonographically guided fine needle aspiration biopsy of intra thoracic tumors. *Acta Radiol.* 1996; 37: 327-331.

[58] Rajwanshi A, Jayaram N, Behra D, Gupta SK, Malik SK. Fine needle aspiration cytology of intrathoracic lesions – a reappraisal. *Indian J. Pathol. Microbiol.* 1989; 32: 306-309.

[59] Young GP, Young I, Cowan DF. Blei RL. The reliability of fine needle aspiration biopsy in the diagnosis of deep lesions of the lung and mediastinum: experience with 250 cases using a modified technique. *Diagn. Cytopathol.* 1987; 3: 1-7.

[60] Linder J, Olsen GA, Johnsten WW. Fine needle aspiration biopsy of the mediastinum. *Am. J. Med.* 1986; 81: 1005-1008.

[61] Johnston WW. Percutaneous fine needle aspiration biopsy of the lung: A study of 1015 patients. *Acta Cytol.* 1984; 28: 218-224.

[62] Jamieson WR, Suen KC, Hicken P, Martin AL, Burr LH, Munro AI. Reliability of percutaneous needle aspiration biopsy for diagnosis of bronchogenic carcinoma. *Cancer Detect. Prev.* 1981; 4: 331-336.

[63] Kuhn III C, Askin FB. Lung and Mediastinum. In JM Kissane, editor. Andersons Pathology. St Louis: *The CV Mosby Co.* 1990; pp 920- 1046.

[64] Pirozynski M. 100 years of lung cancer. *Respir. Med.* 2006; 100: 2073- 2084.

[65] Das DK. Fine needle aspiration (FNA) cytology of thorax: value and limitations. In: Fine needle Fine needle aspiration cytology (FNAC): Its value and limitations with special reference to a developing country (India). *Thesis for the degree of Doctor of Science (DSc) in Pathology (Medicine)* from Utkal University, Bhubaneswar, India. 2001, PP: 139-166.

[66] Arora VK, Singh N, Chaturvedi S, Bhatia A. Significance of cytologic criteria in distinguishing small cell from non-small cell carcinoma of the lung. *Acta Cytol.* 2003; 47: 216- 220.

[67] Silverman JF, Finely JL, Park HK, Strausbauch P, Unverforth M, Carney M. Fine needle aspiration cytology of bronchioloalveolar cell carcinoma of the lung. *Acta Cytol.* 1985; 29: 887-894.

[68] Tao LC, Weisbrod GL, Pearson FG, Sanders DE, Danat EE, Filipetto L. Cytologic diagnosis of bronchioloalveolar carcinoma by fine needle aspiration biopsy. *Cancer.* 1986; 57: 1565-1570.

[69] Tao LC, Robertson DI. Cytologic diagnosis of bronchial mucoepidermoid carcinoma by fine needle aspiration biopsy. *Acta Cytol.* 1978; 22: 221-224.

[70] Lee KG, Cho NH. Fine needle aspiration cytology of pulmonary adenocarcinoma of fetal type: report of a case with immunohistochemical and ultrastructural studies. *Diagn. Cytopathol.* 1991; 7: 408-414.

[71] Smith RC, Amy RW. Adenoidcystic carcinoma metastatic to the lung. Report of a case diagnosed by fine needle aspiration biopsy cytology. *Acta Cytol.* 1985; 29: 533-534.

[72] Reddy V, Gattuso P, Reyes CV, Chinoy M. Amphicrine carcinoma of the lung: Diagnosis by fine needle aspiration cytology. *Cytopathology.* 1990; 1: 45-48.

[73] Szyfelbein NM, Ros JS. Carcinoids, atypical carcinoid and small cell carcinoma of the lung: differential diagnosis of fine needle aspiration biopsy specimens. *Diagn. Cytopathol.* 1988; 4: 1-8.

[74] Das DK, Bhambhani S, Chachra KL, Murthy NS, Tripathi RP. Small round cell tumors of abdomen and thorax: Role of fine needle aspiration cytologic features in diagnosis and differential diagnosis. *Acta Cytol.* 1997; 41: 1035-1047.

[75] Sinner WN, Sandstedt B. Small cell carcinoma of the lung. Cytological, roentgenologic and clinical findings in a consecutive series diagnosed by fine needle aspiration biopsy. *Radiology.* 1976; 121: 269-274.

[76] Silverman JF, Raab SS, Park HK. Fine needle aspiration cytology of primary large cell lymphoma of the mediastinum: Cytomorphologic findings with potential pitfalls in diagnosis. *Diagn. Cytopathol.* 1993; 9: 209-214.

[77] Das DK, Gupta SK, Dutta U, Sharma SC, Datta BN. Malignant lymphoma of convoluted lymphocytes: Diagnosis by fine needle aspiration cytology and cytochemistry. *Diagn. Cytopathol.* 1986; 2: 307-311.

[78] Cosgrove MM, Chandrasoma PT, Martin SE. Diagnosis of pulmonary blastoma by fine needle aspiration biopsy: Cytologic and immunocytochemical findings. *Diagn. Cytopathol.* 1991; 7: 83-87.

[79] Kim K, Naylor B, Han IH. Fine needle aspiration cytology of sarcomas metastatic to the lung. *Acta Cytol.* 1986; 30: 688-694.

[80] Stanfield BL, Powers CW, Desch CE, Brooks JW, Frable WJ. Fine needle aspiration cytology of an unusual primary lung tumor, chondrosarcoma: Case report. *Diagn. Cytopathol.* 1991; 7: 423-426.

[81] Attal H, Jensen J, Reyes CV. Myxoid liposarcoma of the anterior mediastinum: Diagnosis by fine needle aspiration biopsy. *Acta Cytol.* 1995; 39: 511-513.

[82] Finley JL, Silverman JK, Dabbs DJ. Fine needle aspiration cytology of pulmonary carcinosarcoma with immunocytochemical and ultrastructure observations. *Diagn. Cytopathol.* 1988; 4: 239-243.

[83] Tao CW, Chen CH, Chiu MH, Shyu HL, Li WY, Perng RP. Pulmonary carcinosarcoma: diagnostic approach by fine needle aspiration biopsy. *Chung Hua I Hsuch Tsa Chih Taipei.* 1993; 51: 235-237.

[84] Nguyen GK, Jeannot A. Cytopathologic aspects of pulmonary metastasis of malignant fibrous histiocytoma, myxoid variant: Fine needle aspiration biopsy of a case. *Acta Cytol.* 1982; 26:349-353.

[85] Perry MD, Furlong JW, Johnston WW. Fine needle aspiration cytology of metastatic dermatofibrosarcoma protuberans: A case report. *Acta Cytol.* 1986; 30: 507-512.

[86] Saleh HA, Beydoun R, Masood S. Cytology of malignant schwannoma metastatic to lung: Report of a case with diagnosis by fine needle aspiration biopsy. *Acta Cytol.* 1993; 37: 409-412.

[87] Motoyama T, Yamamoto O, Twamoto H, Watanabe H. Fine needle aspiration cytology of primary mediastinal germ cell tumors. *Acta Cytol.* 1995; 39: 725-732.

[88] Das DK, Rath B, Gondal R. Mediastinal teratoma: Preoperative diagnosis by fine needle aspiration cytology. *Diagn Oncol.* 1992; 2: 113-116.

[89] Dahlgren S, Sanstedt B, Sundstrom C. Fine needle aspiration cytology of thymic tumors. *Acta Cytol.* 1983; 27: 1-6.

[90] Finley JL, Silverman JF, Stausbauch PH, Dabbs DJ, West RL, Weaver MD, Norris HT. Malignant thymic neoplasms: Diagnosis by fine needle aspiration biopsy with histologic, immunocytochemical and ultrastructural confirmation. *Diagn. Cytopathol.* 1986; 2: 118-125.

[91] Belani CP, Marts S, Schiller J, Socinski MA. Women and lung cancer: Epidemiology, tumor biology, and emerging trends in clinical research. *Lung Cancer.* 2007; 55: 15-23.

[92] [No authors listed]. Lung and bronchus cancer (invasive): Age adjusted SEER incidence rates by year, race, and sex. SEER Cancer Statistic Review (1975-2003), SEER 9 areas census. National Cancer Institute (htpp://srab.cancer.gov/ jointpoint/).2006, P25-1130.

[93] Cerfolio RJ, Bryant AS, Scott E, Sharma M, Robert F, Spencer SA, Garner RI. Women with pathologic stage I, II, and III non-small cell lung cancer have better survival than men. *Chest.* 2006; 130: 1796- 1802.

[94] Baldini EH, Strauss GM. Women and lung cancer: waiting to exhale. *Chest.* 1997; 112: 229S-234S.

[95] Caddy G, Conron M, Wright G, Desmond P, Hart D, Chen RY. The accuracy of EUS-FNA in assessing mediastinal lymphadenopathy and staging patients with NSCLC. *Eur. Respir. J.* 2005; 25: 410- 415.

[96] Dewan NA, Reeb SD, Gupta NC, Gobar LS, Scott WJ. PET-FDG imaging and transthoracic needle lung aspiration biopsy in evaluation of pulmonary lesions: A comparative risk-benefit analysis. *Chest.* 1995; 108: 441-446.

[97] Caya JG, Clowry LG, Wollenberg NJ, Tieu TM. Transthoracic fine needle aspiration cytology: Analysis of 82 patients with detailed verification criteria and evaluation of false negative cases. *Am. J. Clin. Pathol.* 1984; 82: 100-103.

[98] Montali G, Croce F, Ravetto C, Ghiringhelli G, Solbiati L. Percutaneous pulmonary needle biopsy using thin-needle aspiration. Experience with 302 patients. *Radiol. Med. Torino.* 1983; 69: 559-565.

[99] Sagel SS. Ferguson TB, Forrest JV, Roper CL, Weldon CS, Clark RE. Percutaneous transthoracic aspiration needle biopsy. *Am. Thorac. Surg.* 1978; 26: 399-405.

[100] Baba M, Iyoda A, Yasufuku K, Hoshino H, Sekine Y, Shibuya K, Iizasa T, Saith Y, Hiroshima K, Fujisawa T. Preoperative cytodiagnosis of very small-sized peripheral-type primary lung cancer. *Lung Cancer.* 2002; 37: 277- 280.

[101] Iyoda A, Baba M, Shibuya K, Moriya Y, Yasufuku K, Sekine Y, Izasa T, Hiroshima K, Nakatani Y, Fujisawa T. Transbronchial fine needle aspiration cytological examination: a useful tool for diagnosing primary lung cancer. *Thorac. Cardiovasc. Surg.* 2006; 54: 117-119.

[102] Nguyen GK, Gray JA, Wong EY, Crocket JA, McNamee C. Cytodiagnosis of bronchogenic carcinoma and neuroendocrine tumor of the lung by transthoracic fine needle aspiration. *Diagn. Cytopathol.* 2000; 23: 431- 434.

[103] Bonfiglio TA. Fine needle aspiration biopsy of the lung. *Pathol. Annu.* 1981; 16 (Pt.1): 159-180.

[104] Pantzar P, Meurala H, Koivuniemi A, Laustela E. Peroperative fine needle aspiation biopsy of lung tumors. *Scand.. J. Thorac. Cardiovasc. Surg.* 1983; 17: 51-53.

[105] Larsen SS, Vilmann P, Krasnik M, Dirksen A, Clemensten P, Maltbaek N, Lassen U, Skov BG, Jacobsen GK. Endoscopic ultrasound guided biopsy performed routinely in lung cancer staging spares futile thoracotomies: preliminary results from a randomized clinical trial. *Lung cancer.* 2005; 49: 377- 385.

[106] Targhetta R, Bourgeois JM, Marty-Double C, Coste E, Proust A, Balmes P, Pourcelot L. Peripheral pulmonary lesions: Ultrasonic features and ultrasonically guided fine needle aspiration biopsy. *J. Ultrasound. Med.* 1993; 12: 369-374.

[107] Khan J, Akhtar M, Von Sinner WM, Bouchama A, Buzarbashi M. CT guided fine needle aspiration biopsy in the diagnosis of mediastinal tuberculosis. *Chest.* 1994; 106: 1329-1332.

[108] Hsu WH, Chiang CD, Hsu JY, Kwan PC, Chen CL, Chen CY. Ultrasound guided fine needle aspiation biopsy of lung cancers. *J. Clin. Ultrasound.* 1996; 24: 225-233.

[109] Dennie CJ, Matinzer FR, Marriner JR, Maziak DE. Tranthoracic needle biopsy of the lung: results of early discharge in 506 patients. *Radiology.* 2001; 219: 247- 251.

[110] Steenskov V, Frederiksen P, Thommesen P. Clinical value of perctuaneous intrathoracic fine needle aspiration biopsy: An analysis of 500 cases. *Scand.. J. Thorac. Cardiovasc. Surg.* 1982; 16: 289-291.

[111] Sinner WN. Complications of percutaneous transthoracic needle aspiration biopsy. *Acta Radiol. Diagn. Stockh.* 1976; 17: 813-828.

[112] Moloo Z, Finley RJ, Lefcae MS, Turner Smith L, Craig ID. Possible spread of bronchogenic carcinoma to the chest wall after a transthoracic fine needle aspiration biopsy. A case report. *Acta Cytol.* 1985; 29: 167-169.

[113] Seyfer AE, Walsh DS, Graeber GM, Nuno IN, Eliassen AH. Chest wall implantation of lung cancer after thin needle aspiration biopsy. *Ann. Thorac. Surg.* 1989; 48: 284-286.

[114] Sawabata N, Ohta M, Maeda H. Fine-needle aspiration cytologic technique for lung cancer has a high potential of malignant cell spread through the tract. *Chest.* 2000; 118: 936- 939,

[115] Kim JH, Kim YT, Lim HK, Kim YH, Sung SW. Management of chest wall implantation of non-small cell lung cancer after fine needle aspiration biopsy. *Eur. J. Cardiothorac. Surg.* 2003; 23: 828- 832.

[116] Castelain G, Salignac P, Hamasson JP. Fine needle aspiration biopsy in pneumology: 351 punctures. *Sem. Hop.* 1979; 55: 36-38.

[117] Sloth M, Andersson MJ, Bartholdy NJ, Thommesen P. Fine needle aspiration biopsy of the thoracic cage including the pleura-clinical value. *Roentgenblatter.* 1986; 39: 5-6.

[118] Michiels E, Demedts M. Pitfalls of transthoracic needle aspiration biopsy. *Acta Clin. Belg.* 1991; 46: 359-363.

[119] Hosler GA, Steinberg DM, Sheth S, Hamper UM, Erozan YS, Ali SZ. Inflammatory pseudo tumor: a diagnostic dilemma in cytopathology. *Diagn. Cytopathol.* 2004; 31: 267- 270.

[120] Crapanzano JP, Zakowski MF. Diagnostic dilemmas in pulmonary cytology. *Cancer.* 2001; 93: 364- 375.

[121] Ng WK, Fu KH, Wang E, Tang V. Sclerosing hemangioma of lung: A close cytologic mimicker of pulmonary adenocarcinoma. *Diagn. Cytopathol.* 2001; 25: 316- 320.

[122] Suen KC, Quenville NF. Fine needle aspiration cytology of uncommon thoracic lesions. *Am. J. Clin. Pathol.* 1981; 75: 803-809.

[123] Yilmaz A, Uskul TB, Bayramgurler B, Baran R. Cell type accuracy of transthoracic fine needle aspiration material in primary lung cancer. *Respirology.* 2001; 6: 91-94.

[124] Bavikatty NR, Michael CW. Cytologic features of small-cell carcinoma on Thin Prep. *Diagn. Cytopathol.* 2003; 29: 8- 12.

[125] Yang YJ, Steele CT, Ou XL, Snyder KP, Kohman LJ. Diagnosis of high-grade pulmonary neuroendocrine carcinoma by fine-needle aspiration biopsy: nonsmall-cell or small-cell type? *Diagn. Cytopathol.* 2001; 25: 292- 300.

[126] Ishikawa N, Sato H, Tsunezuka Y, Hiranuma C, Ueno Y, Kurumaya H. Pulmonary blastoma in a child: report of a case. *Surg. Today.* 2001; 31: 705- 707.

[127] Liu J, Farhood A. Immunostaining for thyroid transcription factor-1 on fine needle aspiration specimens of lung tumors: a comparision of direct smears and cell block preparations. *Cancer.* 2004; 102: 109-114.

[128] Simsir A, Wei XJ, Yee H, Moreira A, Cangiarella J. Differential expression of cytokeratins 7 and 20, and thyroid transcription factor-1 in bronchioloalveolar carcinoma: an immunohistochemical study in fine-needle aspiration biopsy specimens. *Am. J. Clin. Pathol.* 2004; 121: 350- 357.

[129] O'Reilly PE, Breveckner J, Silverman JF. Value of ancillary studies in fine needle aspiration cytology of the lung. *Acta Cytol.* 1994; 38: 144-150.

[130] Chen LT, Tseng HH, Hwang WS. Occult prostate adenocarcinoma with pulmonary metastasis: Diagnosis by fine needle aspiration biopsy of the lung and immuno cytochemistry. *Taiwan I Hsueh Hui Tsa Chih.* 1989; 88: 940-942.

[131] Jha RC, Weisbrod GL, Dardick I, Herman SJ, Chamberlain D. Intracranial meningioma with pulmonary metastasis: Diagnosis of by percutaneous fine needle aspiration biopsy and electron microscopy. *Can. Assos. Radiol. J.* 1991; 42: 287-290.

[132] Perez Ordonez B, Berard YC. Metastatic adamantinoma diagnosed by fine needle aspiration biopsy of the lung. *Diagn. Cytopathol.* 1994; 10: 347-351.

[133] Ascoli V, Faccialo F, Muda AO, Martelli M, Nardi F. Chondroblastoma of the rib presenting as an intrathoracic mass: Report of a case with fine needle aspiration biopsy, immunocytochemistry and electron microscopy. *Acta Cytol.* 1992; 36: 423-429.

[134] Nakamura H, Aute I, Kawasaki N, Taguchi M, Ohira T, Kato H. Quantitative detection of lung cancer cells by fluorescence insitu hybridization: comparision with conventional cytology. *Chest.* 2005; 128: 906- 911.

[135] Ludovini V, Gregorc V, Pistola L, Mihaylova Z, Floriani I, Darwish S, Stracci F, Tofanetti FR, Ferraldeschi M, Di Carlo L, Ragusa M, Daddi G, Tonato M. Vascular endothelial growth factor, p53, Rb, Bcl-2 expression and response to chemotherapy in advance non-small cell lung cancer. *Lung Cancer.* 2004; 46: 77- 85.

[136] Lim EH, Aggarwal A, Agasthian T, Wong PS, Tan C, Sim E, Tan L, Goh PS, Wang SC, Khoo KL, Mukherjee A, Khoo SM, Chua G, Nilsson B, Lee KH, Tan P. Feasibility of using low-volume tissue samples for gene expression profiling of advanced non-small cell lung cancers. *Clin. Cancer Res.* 2003; 9: 5980- 5987.

[137] Kalogeraki A, Bouros D, Zoras O, Karabekios S, Chalkiadakis G, Stathopoulos E, Siafakas N, Delides GS. E-cadherin expression on fine-needle aspiration biopsies in primary lung adenocarcinomas is related to tumor differentiation and invasion. *Anticancer Res.* 2003; 23: 3367- 3371.

In: Lung Cancer in Women
Editor: Varetta N. Torres, pp. 335-357

ISBN: 978-1-60021-659-6


*Chapter XV*

# EMPLOYMENT PARTICIPATION AND WORK EXPERIENCE OF FEMALE BREAST CANCER AND LYMPHOMA SURVIVORS FROM THE NORDIC STUDY OF CANCER AND WORK (NOCWO)

***Holmfridur K. Gunnarsdottir[1], Gudbjorg Linda Rafnsdottir[1,2], Jon Gunnar Bernburg[2] and Marja-Liisa Lindbohm***

[1] Research Center for Occupational Health and Working Life, Iceland.
[2] Faculty of Social Sciences, University of Iceland.
[3] Center of Expertise for Health and Work,
Finnish Institute of Occupational Health.

## ABSTRACT

### Purpose

The aim of our study was to analyze the effect of cancer diagnosis on employment status, social interactions at work, commitment to the organization, and motives for work among women who have been diagnosed with breast cancer or Hodgkin's or Non-Hodgkin's lymphoma.

### Methods

Survivors, aged 25-57 at the time of diagnosis, were selected from female breast and lymphoma cancer survivors in four Nordic countries listed at registers of hospitals or in cancer registers. The reference group was a random sample, with the same age distribution as the cancer survivors, taken from the national population registers. A questionnaire was sent to 2247 cancer survivors and 4710 referents. Ordinary least squares multiple regression was used for continuous dependent variables. Binary logistic regression was used for dichotomous dependent variables.

### Results

In all 1580 cancer survivors (70.3%), 1490 diagnosed with breast cancer, 90 diagnosed with Hodgkin's or Non-Hodgkin's lymphoma, and 2516 (53.4%) of the referents answered the questionnaire. The employment participation of breast cancer survivors in our study was not less than that of the referents whereas the lymphoma survivors were less likely to be working. Breast cancer survivors were on average less committed to the organization, perceived less social support at work and scored lower on work motives, but experienced less discrimination than the referents. The lymphoma survivors were less content with the working climate in their unit/department than the referents and like the breast cancer survivors, perceived less social support at work.

### Conclusions

Our study provides information on differences between cancer survivors and a non-cancer reference group regarding factors that are important for return to and well-being at work. It also shows that the cancer type plays a role, therefore all cancer survivors can not be grouped together.

## Introduction

The prognosis of many cancer patients has changed for the better (Engeland et al., 1998) and some cancers are rapidly becoming chronic conditions that are diagnosed in working-age individuals (Bradley et al., 2005). In the USA the 5-year survival rate for all cancer in the years 1974-1998 was 62% (American Cancer Society, 2003). Thus many survive their initial diagnosis and treatment and an increasing number of cancer patients can be expected to be able to return to work after their treatment or continue to work during their treatment (Bouknight, Bradley, and Luo, 2006; Bradley, Bednarek, and Neumark, 2002; Satariano, and DeLorenze, 1996; Short, Vasey, and Tunceli, 2005; Taskila-Åbrandt et al., 2004). Of interest now are the long-term consequences of being treated for cancer (Kornblith, 1998) and research on the work impact of cancer is therefore necessary (Steiner, Cavender, Main, and Bradley, 2004). A population-based study of Finnish cancer survivors, which included all working aged cancer survivors in certain years, showed that they were slightly less often employed than their referents, mainly because of their higher retirement rate, however, a strong variation in the employment rate between persons with different cancer types was seen (Taskila-Åbrandt, Pukkala, Martikainen, Karjalainen, and Hietanen, 2005).

Two reviews have provided an overview of studies on factors that influence the return to work of cancer survivors and work outcomes after cancer diagnosis (Spelten, Sprangers, and Verbeek, 2002; Steiner et al., 2004). According to the studies reviewed, factors negatively associated with return to work are non-supportive work environment and work posing physical demands. Discretion over work-hours or amount of work and positive attitude of co-workers are, on the other hand, positively associated with return to work.

## Labour Market Participation

Labour market participation is important for the individuals and for the society as a whole. The employment rates among women in the Nordic countries are high compared to other Western countries, 71.9% in Denmark, 66.5% in Finland, 80.5% in Iceland, and 71.7% in Norway (Eurostat, 2005). Women are thus a substantial part of the Nordic work-force.

Return to work is dependent on many factors like the nature of the social system and many other social and cultural factors (Spelten et al., 2003). It has been claimed that cancer survivors might be forced to continue working to maintain health insurance coverage (Bradley, and Bednarek,, 2002; Bradley et al., 2002), and in some cases they have been rejected for medical insurance (Chirikos, Russell-Jakobs, and Jacobsen, 2002). Having alternative resources might play an important role for whether or not people return to the labour market (Abrahamsen, Loge, Hannisdal, Holte, and Kvalöy, 1998).

Even though Denmark, Finland, Iceland, and Norway do not have quite the same type of welfare systems with respect to the structure and amounts of benefits and use of income-testing in the social security system (Ólafsson, 1999; Ólafsson, 2005), all the Nordic countries have an extensive welfare system with public health insurance and reasonable safety-nets for the least fortunate.

For most people, work is more than a paycheck (Clark, and Landis, 1989; Peteet, 2000). Work is perceived as a measure of self-worth, competence, independence, maturity, and responsibility; it provides social contacts, interactions, and group affiliation but on the other hand cancer serves as a stimulus for the employee to re-evaluate career and life priorities and to make changes (Clark, and Landis, 1989; Main, Nowels, Cavender, Etschmaier, and Steiner, 2005; Peteet, 2000).

Because of the strong gender segregation in the labour market, women and men do not usually work side by side. According to Charles and Grusky (2004) the sex segregation is especially prominent in the Nordic countries, with egalitarian ideological climates, family-friendly state policies and other institutional practices such as low levels of fertility and high rates of female labour force participation.

Gender differences in the vulnerability to life events have been detected, suggesting that women may be more affected by negative events within the family than men (Kivimäki, Vahtera, and Pentti, 1998). Jobs and families are complex variables with good and bad effects on physical and mental health. Both are arenas for social support, which is beneficial to health, both are sometimes hazardous environments. The job and the home – the double shift – paid work plus housework can each produce high levels of psychological stress, especially for women (Lorber, and Moore, 2002).

Because women and men often do different kinds of work, they are vulnerable to different kinds of job-related injuries and illnesses and should be analyzed separately for labour market outcomes (Doyal, 1995; Lorber, and Moore, 2002; Steiner et al., 2004).

## Support and Discrimination at Work

A study among Finnish cancer patients showed that people with different diagnoses and in different occupations received an unequal amount of support from co-workers and supervisors, and the people whose cancer was treated with chemotherapy received more support than people who had other treatments. Women received more support than the men, but they also needed more support. Both among men and women, there was a clear need for more support especially from occupational health services (Taskila et al., 2006). Supportive work environment seems to have a pivotal role in the cancer survivors' successful return to work (Bouknight et al., 2006; Spelten et al., 2002).

Older studies show that cancer survivors expressed a fear of facing co-workers, subordinates and employers after returning to work and were afraid of discrimination in the form of rejection because of the cancer diagnosis (Clark, and Landis, 1989; Hoffman, 1991). A more recent study found little evidence that women diagnosed with breast cancer experience discrimination at work (Maunsell et al, 2004).

Even if it is assumed that the attitude of society and thereby employers has changed with more knowledge, many factors may hinder a successful re-entry to the workforce like fear of job loss, changes in tasks, problems with employer and co-workers, personal changes in attitudes to work, diminished physical capacity, and discrimination when it exists (Bouknight et al., 2006; Maunsell, Brisson, Dubois, Lauzier, and Fraser, 1999).

## Employment of Female Cancer Survivors

According to Kauppinen (1998) the scale of problems related to work stress is on the increase across the European Union (EU). One reason is that the character of work has changed. These changing working conditions, with heated competition and atypical or precarious work forms are leading to a harder working life. Today, the labour market demands flexibility, social competence and adaptability. Kauppinen points out that these changes affect both women and men, but that women are particularly vulnerable.

According to this, the labour market is becoming more disadvantageous for women who are unwell by some reason. However, recent studies of breast cancer survivors indicate that cancer diagnosis does not have a great impact on women's labour participation, even if they may have poorer self-assessed physical or mental work capacity (Bouknight et al., 2006; Bradley, and Bednarek, 2002). Only a slightly less employment participation was observed among Finnish breast cancer survivors (Taskila-Åbrandt et al., 2005). Bradley et al. (2002) studied labour participation of American women after breast cancer and found that the probability of breast cancer survivors working was 10% less than for women without breast cancer but they surprisingly found that those women who returned to the labour market worked three more hours per week than women who had not had cancer. The reason for this was not clear but one of the suggestions of the authors was that for women, who continue to work, the morbidity associated with cancer and its treatment did not interfere with work.

In studying work absence after breast cancer diagnosis Drolet et al. (2005) found that women who had been diagnosed with breast cancer in Canada often took some time off work after the diagnosis but three years later those women were not absent from work more often or for longer periods of time than other working women.

Even if breast cancer survivors return to work they are more likely than their cancer-free, age- and work status-matched peers to be functionally impaired, to have reduced work effort and to experience downturns in market earnings (Chirikos et al, 2002) and especially for the younger survivors breast cancer diagnosis is likely to have a negative impact on work life or career and financial situation (Ganz et al., 2002). Not only the patient's functional status has impact on returning to work after breast cancer but also other factors as the physical demands of the job (Bouknight et al., 2006; Satariano, and DeLorenze, 1996).

According to our knowledge there are few studies on the employment pattern of female survivors of Hodgkin's and non-Hodgkin's disease and the results are rather conflicting. All the subsequent studies included both women and men. One study found no decrease in the number of employed among responding survivors of lymphatic tumours (van der Wouden et al., 1992), another study showed that of the patients in remission and able to go back to work, only 54% had done so (Razavi et al., 1993). A study among Hodgkin's survivors showed that most survivors enjoy good health, however, some physical, role and cognitive functional impairments may persist that limit their activities (Joly et al., 1996). Survivors of Non-Hodgkin's lymphoma in Finland were less likely to be employed than their referents but the difference between survivors of Hodgkin's disease and their referents was not significant (Taskila-Åbrandt et al., 2005). A Norwegian study showed that most long-term survivors of Hodgkin's disease had returned to their job or studies after 18 months from start of treatment, except a number of permanently disabled patients (Abrahamsen et al., 1998).

Despite its importance, there are few studies on the impact of cancer and its treatment on return to work with high numbers of survivors and a population based reference group (Spelten et al., 2002; Steiner et al., 2004). Having this in mind it was considered valuable to collaborate between Nordic countries in order to profit from the experience and knowledge available and to strengthen the study with a sufficient sample size. The Nordic Study on Cancer and Work Life (NOCWO) was initiated in the following Nordic countries: Denmark, Finland, Iceland, and Norway. The study was coordinated by an expert group with representatives from each country. The general aim of NOCWO was to clarify the problems people with cancer face in working life and to examine the effect of cancer in returning to work.

The types of cancers that were chosen for NOCWO were: breast cancer in women, Hodgkin's and Non-Hodgkin's disease (lymphomas) in women and men, prostate and testicular cancer in men. These cancer types were chosen as they usually have high survival rate and therefore the patients are likely to return to the labour market after or even during their treatment. As it turned out only Finland and Iceland collected data on lymphoma survivors, the breast cancer survivors on the other hand are from all the four countries.

The specific aim of our study was to analyze the effect of cancer diagnosis on employment status, social interactions at work, commitment to the organization, and motives for work among women who have been diagnosed with breast cancer or Hodgkin's or Non-Hodgkin's lymphoma.

# MATERIAL AND METHODS

## Criteria for Selecting the Survivors

The eligibility criteria of NOCWO were:

1. A good prognosis and no previous cancer. 2. The age range of the selected patients should be 25-57 years at the time of the diagnosis. This age range was selected in order to get to persons of working age. Older age groups were not included because of higher co-morbidity of other chronic diseases. 3. Cancer cases should be selected from patients, who had been diagnosed 1 – 6 years ago. 4. The treatment of cancer (chemotherapy and radiotherapy) should have been finished at the time of the survey and the disease should not have recurred.

As it turned out not all the countries could fulfill this criteria. For example in Iceland all cancer cases diagnosed with the respective cancers 25-57 of age at diagnoses in the years 1998-2002 were included as it was not possible to distinguish between those who had good prognosis and those who had not and those who were still receiving treatment and those who were not. In addition, as it took time in some of the countries to get needed permissions from the respective Scientific Ethics Committees and Data Protection Commissions, the time span between sending out the questionnaires and the diagnosis can vary from 2– 9 years. In Denmark the study period was 1997-2001, follow-up until 2005. In Finland the study period was 1997-2001, follow-up until 2003. In Iceland the study period was 1998-2002, follow-up until 2005. In Norway the study period was 1998-2002, follow-up until 2004.

## Recruitment of the Cancer Survivors and Referents

The cancer survivors were recruited from the patient registers of oncological units (Finland, Norway) or from national cancer registers (Denmark, Iceland). The sample size of survivors was decided to be about 1000 in each country (except Iceland). Separate reference groups, with the same sex and age distribution as the cancer survivors, about 1500 persons in each country, were selected from the national population registers. In Iceland, where the eligible group of survivors was only 423, it was decided to have the reference group about 4 times bigger. Referents with cancer were excluded based on the questionnaires or register data.

## Questionnaires

Questionnaire data were collected from cancer survivors and their referents in all four countries. Previously validated series of questions were utilized in planning the questionnaire for the study participants.

The questionnaire covered the following topics:

- Personal background data: sex, marital status, year of birth, number of children in the home, annual income of the family, education, employment participation, and occupation.
- General health: physical and psychological well-being, absence from work due to cancer or treatment.
- Telling about the illness at the workplace: to whom (colleagues, managers, occupational health care personnel) and possible reasons for telling or keeping the illness a secret.
- Changes in work activity, work ability.
- Organizational culture, discrimination, commitment to the organization.
- Social interactions, opportunities for participation and employment security.
- Wellbeing at work, motives for work.

In the present study we used the subsequent questions.

Questions on changes in work activity that were used in a Finnish study on the prevalence of work-related asthma symptoms (Saarinen et al., 2001). Have you changed employer or occupation during the last 6/7 years? (Alternatives: yes/no). If yes: Was the cancer the cause for the change? (Alternatives: no – yes, partly – yes, mainly). To what extent was the change of the employer or occupation influenced by: 1. Physical demands of the former employment. 2. Your own voluntary choice. 3. Negative attitude of your superior. 4. Negative attitude of the working community. 5. Reorganization at your workplace/organization (e.g. fusion or bankruptcy); 6. Other reason, what? (Alternatives: not at all – to some extent – much).

The measurement of discrimination was partly based on the Social Impact Scale, which was used in the study of Fife and Wright (2000). The specific questions were developed on the basis of a qualitative interview study carried out in Finland among 25 cancer survivors (unpublished data).

How do the following statements correspond to your situation? 1. My colleagues doubt my ability to carry out my tasks. 2. My supervisor doubts my ability to carry out my tasks. 3. My colleagues avoid me. 4. My superior avoids me. 5. My colleagues do not inform me of work-related issues. 6. My supervisor does not inform me of work-related issues. 7. My colleagues belittle my problems. 8. My supervisor belittles my problems. 9. I feel isolated from my colleagues. (Alternatives: not at all – a little – to some extent – rather well – well).

Following questions were all based on the General Nordic questionnaire for psychological and social factors at work, QPSNordic, (Lindström et al., 2000) and were all five faceted. The individual values of the items measuring the same factor were summed up for the analyses.

Commitment to the organization: *The following statements deal with organizational commitment. Please indicate the extent to which you personally agree or disagree with each of these statements.* To my friends I praise this organization a great place to work. My values are very similar to the organization's values. This organization really inspires me to give my very best job performance. (Alternatives: disagree totally – disagree to some extent – indifferent – agree to some extent – agree totally).

Social interactions: If needed, can you get support and help with your work from your co-workers? If needed, can you get support and help with your work from your immediate superior? If needed, are your co-workers willing to listen to your work-related problems? If needed, is your immediate superior willing to listen to your work-related problems? Are your work achievements appreciated by your immediate superior? (Alternatives: very seldom or never – rather seldom – sometimes – rather often – very often or always).

Organizational culture (*What is the climate like in your work unit?*). Alternatives: 1. Competitive. 2. Encouraging and supportive. 3. Distrustful and suspicious. 4. Relaxed and comfortable. 5. Rigid and rule-based. (Alternatives: very little or not at all – rather little – somewhat – rather much – very much).

Work motives: *How important are the following considerations in relation to your ideal job?* 1. To develop my own personality. 2. To have good pay and material benefits. 3. To have a peaceful and orderly job. 4. To get a sense of accomplishing something worthwhile. 5. That the work is secure and provides regular income. 6. To have a safe and healthy physical work environment. 7. To be able to put my imagination and creativity to good use at work. (Alternatives: unimportant – not so important – rather important – very important – absolutely necessary).

The following variables from the questionnaires were also used in the regression analysis: marital status (dichotomized into paired and non-paired); age at survey; education (compulsory school, 1 – 9 years = low education; secondary/vocational school/college 10 – 16 years = medium education; higher university degree > 16 years = high education); employment status (employed/not employed, the unemployed includes unemployed persons, homemakers, students, military conscripts, and those on disability pension, retired or unknown). The occupational status was based on the international standard classification of occupation (International Labour Office, 1990) but in this chapter divided into three occupational classes as was done in a Norwegian study based on much the same questionnaire (Gudbergsson, Fosså, Borgeraas, and Dahl, 2006). Accordingly the sample was grouped as follows. High occupational status [higher-grade professionals, directors, and higher legislators, seniors officials, managers, self-employed higher-grade professionals, and liberal professionals, (e.g. physicians, teachers, and lawyers); technicians, associate, professionals, (e.g. opticians, and superiors at bank and post offices]. Medium occupational status [clerks (e.g. bank clerks and secretaries), service and care workers, shop and market sales worker (e.g. cooks, waiters, hairdressers, police officers, and salespersons). Low occupational status: workers [other self-employed, skilled agricultural and fishery workers, craft and related trade workers (e.g. bricklayers, painters, and machinery mechanics), plant and machine operators and assemblers, elementary occupations (e.g. cleaners, kitchen helpers, and messengers)].

The original Finnish questionnaire was translated into the other Nordic languages and back from the respective language into Finnish but different languages are talked in all the Nordic countries. Two independent translators undertook this task in each country.

### Collecting Data Procedure

The questionnaire was mailed to all the participants but it differed how often it was allowed to send a reminder. In Finland it was allowed to send two reminders. In Denmark they sent two reminders and after that they phoned the non-responders once. In Iceland it was allowed to send one reminder both to the survivors and the referents. In Norway only one reminder was allowed to be sent to the survivors and non to the referents.

### Statistics

The completed questionnaires were saved into an electronic database for statistical analyses. Ordinary least squares multiple regression was used for continuous dependent variables (Gujarati, 2003). Binary logistic regression was used for dichotomous dependent variables (Long, 1997). The calculations were performed in SPSS 12.0.

### Permissions

The study was approved by all the Scientific Ethics Committees in all the respective countries and by the Data Protection Commissions as needed. In Denmark by the the Danish Data Protection Agency (j.nr. 2003-41-3331). In Finland by the Ethics Committee for Research in Occupational Health and Safety. In Iceland by the National Bioethics Committee (VSN 03-159-V1-S1) and the Data Protection Commission. In Norway by the Regional Committee for Medical Research Ethics of South Norway and approved by the Norwegian Data Inspectorate (NDI).

## RESULTS

The Nordic study population included 2247 female cancer survivors and 4710 female referents. Returned valid questionnaires from the survivors were 1580 (70.3%) whereas 2516 (53.4%) of the referents answered (Fig 1). A questionnaire was assessed valid if at least some questions had been answered.

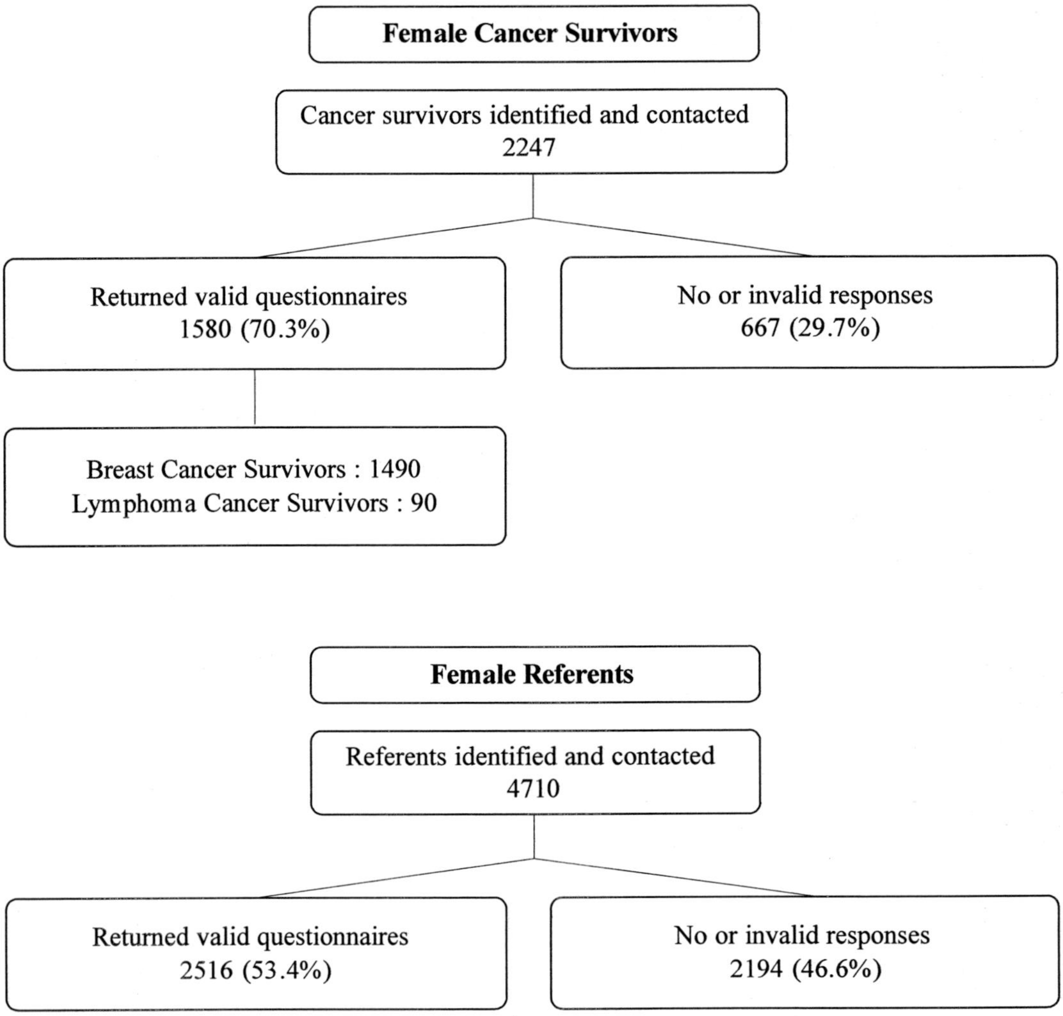


Figure 1. Cancer survivors and referents.

**Table 1. Descriptive statistics of the variables. Means and standard deviation (SD)**

| | Breast Cancer (N = 1490) | | Lymphoma (N = 90) | | Referents (N = 2516) | | Total (N = 4096) | |
|---|---|---|---|---|---|---|---|---|
| | Mean | SD | Mean | SD | Mean | SD | Mean | SD |
| Age in Years | 54.10 | 6.61 | 48.47 | 10.71 | 52.79 | 7.85 | 53.20 | 7.60 |
| Marital status | | | | | | | | |
| Single/divorced/widowed (coded zero) | ----- | ----- | ----- | ----- | ----- | ----- | ----- | ----- |
| Married/cohabiting | .74 | .44 | ..70 | .46 | .74 | .44 | | |
| Education | | | | | | | | |
| Compulsory school (1–9 years) (coded zero) | ----- | ----- | ----- | ----- | ----- | ----- | ----- | ----- |
| Secondary/vocational school/college (10–16 years) | .59 | .49 | .49 | .50 | .58 | .49 | .58 | .49 |
| Higher university degree (> 16 years) | .15 | .36 | .32 | .47 | .16 | .37 | .16 | .37 |
| Employment status | | | | | | | | |
| Not employed (coded zero) | ----- | ----- | ----- | ----- | ----- | ----- | ----- | ----- |
| Employed | .73 | .45 | .70 | .46 | .75 | .43 | .74 | .44 |
| Occupational status | | | | | | | | |
| Low (coded zero) | ----- | ----- | ----- | ----- | ----- | ----- | ----- | ----- |
| Medium | .46 | .50 | .45 | .50 | .42 | .49 | .44 | .50 |
| High | .41 | .49 | .44 | .50 | .44 | .50 | .43 | .50 |
| Dependent Variables (Indexes) | | | | | | | | |
| Organizational culture (range 1-5)* | 3.81 | .81 | 3.58 | .90 | 3.85 | .80 | 3.83 | .80 |
| Discrimination at work (range 1-5)* | 1.25 | .42 | 1.43 | .57 | 1.30 | .46 | 1.29 | .45 |
| Organizational commitment (range 1-5)* | 3.85 | .96 | 3.74 | .94 | 3.95 | .96 | 3.91 | .96 |
| Social support at work (range 1-5)* | 4.14 | .81 | 3.81 | .94 | 4.24 | .83 | 4.19 | .83 |
| Work motives (range 1-6)* | 3.86 | .53 | 3.94 | .46 | 3.95 | .53 | 3.92 | .53 |

* Only employed individuals included (N = 2950).

Table 1 shows that the lymphoma survivors were on average younger than the referents whereas the breast cancer survivors were on average older. The lymphoma survivors were more likely to be single, divorced or widowed than the other groups. A higher proportion of the lymphoma survivors had higher university degree than both the breast cancer survivors and the referents. The majority of all groups was employed when they answered the questionnaire.

**Table 2. Logistic regression of working status (working = 1, not working = 0) on survivors' diagnoses and control variables. Odds ratio (OR) and 95% confidence intervals (95% CI) are reported**

| Independent variables | OR | 95% CI |
|---|---|---|
| Referents | ----- | ----- |
| Breast cancer survivors | .95 | .81, 1.11 |
| Lymphoma survivors | .50* | .30, .85 |
| Single/divorced/widowed | ----- | ----- |
| Married/cohabiting | 1.18 | 1.00, 1.40 |
| Low education | ----- | ----- |
| Medium education | 2.12*** | 1.79, 2.50 |
| High education | 3.04*** | 2.35, 3.94 |
| Age in years | .91*** | .89, .92 |
| Chi-Square | 465.4 | |
| Nagelkerke $R^2$ | .16 | |

* $p < .05$; ** $p < .01$; *** $p < .001$ (two-tailed tests). Survivor diagnosis significantly improves model fit (Chi-square change 6.31; df = 2; p = .043).

We conducted logistic regression of employment status to examine whether the odds of working differed among the two cancer survivor groups and the reference group, controlling for marital status, educational attainment, and age. Results in table 2 indicate that lymphoma survivors were less likely to work than the referents and than the breast cancer survivors (OR =.53; CI: .31, .91; p = .020). Results show that the odds of working increase with educational attainment but decrease with age.

When we asked the cancer survivors if they had changed occupation during the 6/7 years 13.9% of the responding breast cancer survivors, 17.3% of the lymphoma survivors and 17.3% of the referents said they had done that. In all 33% of the responding breast cancer survivors and 16.7% of the lymphoma survivors said that the cancer partly or mainly was the cause of the change. Asked about the cause of the change of occupation only physical demands of the former occupation among the survivors emerged as statistically significant (not shown in a table).

**Table 3. Logistic regression of change of workplace or employer during the last 6/7 years (change = 1, no change = 0) on survivors' diagnoses and control variables. Odds ratio (OR) and 95% confidence intervals (95% CI) are reported**

| | Odds Ratio | 95% CI |
|---|---|---|
| Independent variables | | |
| Referents | ----- | ----- |
| Breast cancer survivors | .78** | .67, .92 |
| Lymphoma survivors | .87 | .52, 1.5 |
| Single/divorced/widowed | ----- | ----- |
| Married/cohabiting | .82* | .69, .97 |
| Low education | ----- | ----- |
| Medium education | 1.2 | .95, 1.40 |
| High education | 1.3* | 1.01, 1.63 |
| Age in years | .93*** | .92, .94 |
| Chi-Square | 247.1 | |
| Nagelkerke $R^2$ | .10 | |

* p < .05; ** p < .01; *** p < .001 (Two-Tailed Tests). Patient status significantly improves model fit (Chi-square change 9.45; df = 2; p = .009).

When we asked the cancer survivors if they had changed workplace/employer during the last 6/7 years 25.9% of the breast cancer survivors, 40.5% of the lymphoma survivors and 33.1% of the referents had done that. As shown in table 3, the difference between the breast cancer survivors and the referents was statistically significant. Also, women who were married/cohabiting were less likely than other women to have made such a change. High educational attainment increased the likelihood of change relative to women with low education. The odds of work change decreased with age.

**Table 4. Organizational culture (*What is the climate like in your work unit?*) regressed on survivors' diagnoses and control variables**

| | Regression Coefficient | Standard Error | 95% CI |
|---|---|---|---|
| Independent variables | | | |
| Referents | ----- | ----- | ----- |
| Breast cancer survivors | -.040 | .033 | -.104, .025 |
| Lymphoma Survivors | -.218* | .107 | -.427, -.009 |
| Single/divorced/widowed | ----- | ----- | ----- |
| Married/cohabiting | .136*** | .036 | .065, .206 |
| Low occupational status | ----- | ----- | ----- |
| Medium occupational status | .069 | .060 | -.048, .186 |
| High occupational status | .161* | .063 | .037, .285 |
| Low education | ----- | ----- | ----- |
| Medium education | -.008 | .045 | -.096, .081 |
| High education | -.070 | .060 | -.187, .048 |
| Age in years | .001 | .002 | -.004, .005 |
| Adjusted $R^2$ | .008 | | |

* p < .05; ** p < .01; *** p < .001 (two-tailed tests). Survivors' diagnosis significantly improved model fit (F-change = 3.95; $df_1$=2; $df_2$=2738; p = .019).

When asked about the organizational culture (*What is the climate like in your work unit?*) the lymphoma survivors were more negative than the referents but the outcome for the breast cancer survivors was not significantly different. Those who were married/cohabiting were on average more positive than those who were single, divorced or widowed, and the high occupational status group was more positive than the low occupational status group (table 4).

**Table 5. Discrimination at work regressed on survivors' diagnoses and control variables**

| | Regression Coefficient | Standard Error | 95% CI |
|---|---|---|---|
| Independent variables | | | |
| Referents | ----- | ----- | ----- |
| Breast cancer survivors | -.050** | .019 | -.086, -.014 |
| Lymphoma survivors | .091 | .060 | -.027, .208 |
| | | | |
| Single/divorced/widowed | ----- | ----- | ----- |
| Married/cohabiting | -.061** | .020 | -.101, -.022 |
| | | | |
| Low occupational status | ----- | ----- | ----- |
| Medium occupational status | -.062 | .034 | -.129, .004 |
| High occupational status | -.089* | .036 | -.159, -.019 |
| | | | |
| Low education | ----- | ----- | ----- |
| Medium education | -.010 | .025 | -.060, .039 |
| High education | -.001 | .034 | -.067, .065 |
| | | | |
| Age in years | .001 | .001 | -.001, .004 |
| Adjusted $R^2$ | .008 | | |

* $p < .05$; ** $p < .01$; *** $p < .001$ (two-tailed tests). Survivors' diagnosis significantly improves model fit (F-change = 3.64; $df_1$=2; $df_2$=2736; p = .026).

In table 5 we regressed questions on discrimination at work on survivors' diagnoses and a set of control variables. Breast cancer survivors experienced less discrimination than the referents. The lymphoma survivors did not score significantly different from the referents. However, compared to the breast cancer survivors the difference between lymphoma survivors and breast cancer survivors was statistically significant ($p < .05$). Those who were married/cohabiting experienced less discrimination than those who were single divorced or widowed. Those in the high occupational status group experienced less discrimination compared to the low occupational status group.

In table 6 we regressed commitment to the organization on survivors' diagnoses and a set of control variables. Breast cancer survivors experienced less commitment to the organization than the referents. Those who were married/cohabiting were more committed than those who were single, divorced or widowed. Those in the high occupational status group were more committed than those in the low occupational status group. Those who were older were more committed to the organization than the younger ones.

**Table 6. Commitment to the organization regressed on survivors' diagnoses and control variables**

| | Regression Coefficient | Standard Error | 95% CI |
|---|---|---|---|
| Independent Variables | | | |
| Referents | ----- | ----- | ----- |
| Breast cancer survivors | -.105** | .040 | -.182, -.027 |
| Lymphoma survivors | -.121 | .128 | -.372, .129 |
| Single/divorced/widowed | ----- | ----- | ----- |
| Married/cohabiting | .173*** | .043 | .089, .257 |
| Low occupational status | ----- | ----- | ----- |
| Medium occupational status | .007 | .072 | -.134, .149 |
| High occupational status | .191* | .076 | .042, .341 |
| Low education | ----- | ----- | ----- |
| Medium education | -.011 | .054 | -.117, .094 |
| High education | -.037 | .072 | -.178, .103 |
| Age in years | .013*** | .003 | .008, .018 |

*p < .05; ** p < .01; *** p < .001 (Two-Tailed Tests). Survivors' diagnosis significantly improves model fit (F-change = 4.65; $df_1$=2; $df_2$=2724; p = .010).

**Table 7. Social interactions at work regressed on survivors' diagnoses and control variables**

| | Regression Coefficient | Standard Error | 95% CI |
|---|---|---|---|
| Independent variables | | | |
| Referents | ----- | ----- | ----- |
| Breast cancer survivors | -.090** | .034 | -.157, -.023 |
| Lymphoma survivors | -.349** | .110 | -.565, -.133 |
| Single/divorced/widowed | ----- | ----- | ----- |
| Married/cohabiting | .073* | .037 | .000, .146 |
| Low occupational status | ----- | ----- | ----- |
| Medium occupational status | .249*** | .062 | .128, .370 |
| High occupational status | .340*** | .066 | .211, .469 |
| Low education | ----- | ----- | ----- |
| Medium education | -.056 | .046 | -.147, .035 |
| High education | -.132* | .062 | -.253, -.011 |
| Age in years | .000 | .002 | -.004, .005 |
| Adjusted $R^2$ | .015 | | |

* p < .05; ** p < .01; *** p < .001 (Two-Tailed Tests). Survivor status significantly improves model fit (F-change = 10.85; $df_1$=2; $df_2$=2732; p = .000).

In table 7. we regressed social interactions at work on survivors' diagnoses and a set of variables. Both the breast cancer survivors and the lymphoma survivors experienced less social support than the referents and the lymphoma survivors experienced less support than the breast cancer survivors (p < .05). Those married/cohabiting experienced more support than those who were single, divorced or widowed. Both medium and high occupational status groups experienced more support than those in the low occupational status group but those with high education experienced less support than those with low education.

**Table 8. Work motives regressed on survivors' diagnoses and control variables**

| | Regression Coefficient | Standard Error | 95% CI |
|---|---|---|---|
| Independent variables | | | |
| Referent group | ----- | ----- | ----- |
| Breast cancer survivors | -.093*** | .021 | -.135, -.051 |
| Lymphoma survivors | .001 | .070 | -.136, .137 |
| Single/divorced/widowed | ----- | ----- | ----- |
| Married/cohabiting | -.020 | .023 | -.065, .026 |
| Low occupational status | ----- | ----- | ----- |
| Medium occupational status | .054 | .038 | -.021, .128 |
| High occupational status | .077 | .040 | -.002, .156 |
| Low education | ----- | ----- | ----- |
| Medium education | -.037 | .029 | -.094, .020 |
| High education | -.062 | .038 | -.137, .014 |
| Age in years | .000 | .001 | -.003, .003 |
| Adjusted $R^2$ | .006 | | |

* $p < .05$; ** $p < .01$; *** $p < .001$ (Two-tailed tests). Survivors' diagnosis significantly improves model fit (F-change = 9.22; $df_1=2$; $df_2=2909$; $p = .010$).

In Table 8 we regressed work motives on survivors' diagnoses and a set of variables. Breast cancer survivors had less intrinsic and extrinsic motivation to work than the referents.

## CONCLUSION

The employment participation of breast cancer survivors in our study was not less than that of the referents whereas the lymphoma survivors were less likely to be working. Breast cancer survivors were on average less committed to the organization, perceived less social support at work and scored lower on work motives but experienced less discrimination than the referents. The lymphoma survivors were less content with the working climate in their unit/department than the referents and like the breast cancer survivors, perceived less social support at work than the referents. Marital status, educational attainment, occupational status and age had an effect on the outcomes in many instances. Those married or cohabiting and those with high occupational status and high education had on average more positive outcomes than others, however, those with high education perceived less support at the workplace than those with low education. Employment participation increased with educational attainment but decreased with age.

The high employment rate among the breast cancer survivors is consistent with results from other studies (Bouknight et al., 2006; Bradley et al., 2002; Ganz et al., 1996; Gudbergsson et al., 2006; Satariano, and DeLorenze, 1996; Taskila-Åbrandt et al., 2004; Taskila-Åbrandt et al., 2005).

Women who obtain health insurance from their employer may not exit the labour market and be unwilling to reduce the number of hours worked, especially if they have a serious health condition (Bradley et al., 2002). These authors therefore excluded women who were insured by either Medicaid or Medicare from their study on breast cancer and women's labour supply as they assumed that this type of insurance might constrain the women's participation in the labour market. In another study, the authors point out that the potential for a change/loss of health insurance may be an important consideration in the decision to leave one's job, given that cancer treatment is expensive and the potential for future medical expenses is great (Bradley, and Bednarek, 2002).

All the Nordic countries have public health insurance and a public social security system. In some of the Nordic countries, the social security system even enables people to retire due to a serious illness, especially in the case of persons approaching the statutory retirement age (Taskila-Åbrandt et al., 2005). The welfare systems in all the Nordic countries provide equal right for all to health care, regardless of employment status. The welfare systems of the Nordic countries and that of e.g. USA are in this way different (Ólafsson, 1999). This could be expected to hamper return to work of Nordic survivors, but our results do not indicate that this is the case. However, comparison of return to work after cancer diagnosis faces difficulties due to considerable differences in the organization of health care systems, benefits and insurance, climate, culture, and social networks (Gudbergsson et al., 2006).

A study of work absence after breast cancer diagnosis from Canada showed that self-employed women or those not belonging to a union were much less likely to take time off from work for initial treatments, even though their treatments resembled those of women who did take time off (Drolet et al., 2005). This shows that not only differences in health insurances and social security systems but also union participation can have an effect on the employment pattern of cancer survivors. In the Nordic countries, the right to paid sick-leave differs between trade unions, which could have an impact on return to work among cancer survivors. We did not have information on whether the participants in our study belonged to a union or not but this could certainly be of importance regarding return to work.

Our findings that those with medium or high education are more likely to be working than others could depend on the fact that they often have occupations that are not physically demanding. Cancer survivors with advanced education have been shown to have higher return to work rates than those with less education (Short et al., 2005; Taskila-Åbrandt et al., 2004). Those with low education and low occupational status are more likely to be manual workers with physically strenous work, which has been shown to be negatively associated with return to work (Bouknight et al., 2006; Satariano, and DeLorenze, 1996; Short et al., 2005).

Our results regarding the lymphoma survivors are in accordance with some prior studies (Abrahamsen et al., 1998; Razavi et al., 1993). The lower rates of return to work may be due to some functioning impairments that limit their activities (Joly et al., 1996). Men and women with Non-Hodgkin's lymphoma in Finland were only slightly less likely to work than their referents but the results for those with Hodgkin's disease were not significant (Taskila-Åbrandt et al., 2005). In comparison with prior studies, it should be noted that our study only included women and that we did not distinguish between Hodgkin's and Non-Hodgkin's survivors.

Reduced employment participation of cancer survivors may not entirely be attributed to cancer diagnosis. Only 33.3% of the breast cancer survivors and 16.7% of the lymphoma survivors in our study said that the cancer diagnosis was partly or the main cause for the change of occupation. Cancer survivors might have re-evaluated career and life priorities, the meaning of life, motivation and relevance of work relative to other aspects of their lives (Clark, and Landis, 1989; Gudbergsson et al., 2006; Joly et al., 1996; Main et al., 2005; Maunsell et al., 2004; Peteet, 2000). In our study the answers to the questions on commitment to the organization and on motives for work suggest that the survivors might have revaluated career and life priorities and that after the diagnosis, they value other things in their lives more than work.

In our study, physical demands stood out as the most important factor that caused change of occupation among the cancer survivors. This is in accordance with other studies that have shown that physical demands of the job are one of the factors that hinder return to work after cancer diagnosis (Satariano, and DeLorenze, 1996; Spelten et al., 2002).

The breast cancer survivors perceived less discrimination at work than the referents, whereas no such effect was seen for the lymphoma survivors. The results regarding breast cancer survivors are in accordance with the results of other recent studies (Maunsell et al, 2004) and may support the statement that times are changing and cancer survivors now seldom face blatant employment discrimination (Hoffman, 2005).

Many studies have reported that support at work, when needed, enhances workers' physical health, psychological well-being and job satisfaction. In addition there is evidence that work support can buffer the negative impact of workplace stress on health outcomes, particularly when there is a match between the nature of stressors and supports (Bond, Punnett, Pyle, Cazeca, and Cooperman, 2004; Karasek, and Theorell, 1990). Social support both from co-workers and employers is important for return to work and quality of life of cancer survivors (Bouknight et al., 2006; Ganz et al., 2002; Spelten et al., 2002; Steiner et al., 2004) and depends on factors like type of cancer, treatment, gender, age and education (Taskila et al., 2005). In our study the breast cancer survivors and the lymphoma survivors perceived less social support at work than their referents. In addition the lymphoma survivors perceived less support than the breast cancer survivors. Educational attainment and occupational status seem to play a role for the perceived support as those with medium or high occupational status perceived more support than those with low occupational status. However, those with high education perceived less support than those with lower education. This is difficult to interpret but is an important issue to study further.

As mentioned before, the balance between work and home has to be taken into account when measuring the well-being of the employees (Kivimäki, et al., 1998; Lorber, and Moore, 2002). The family can be an important source for support, which in many cases affects the well-being at work. Hence it is interesting to see that the married/cohabiting women experienced more social support at work, less discrimination, and they were more positive towards the organizational culture than those who were single, widowed or divorced.

In their reviews, Steiner et al. (2004) and Spelten et al. (2002) discuss many problems that should be addressed in studies on labour market participation of cancer survivors. Among other things they stress that a population-based sample of cancer survivors, ideally using a cancer registry or similar course to identify patients, is preferred to using patients who receive treatment at a single site, such as an academic cancer referral centre. In our study both these sources were used as in Denmark and Iceland the data source was the respective cancer registries but in Finland and Norway, it was academic cancer referral centres.

It has also been pointed out that samples have to be of sufficient size for both genders (Spelten et al., 2003). The Nordic study (NOCWO) was conducted both among men and women whereas only the results concerning the women are reported in this chapter. One of the strengths of our study was the size of the sample of breast cancer survivors. However, the sample of lymphoma survivors was small.

Our study is a cross-sectional one with the limitations of such studies (Spelten et al., 2002). However, the questions were mostly on the present situation and less retrospective so that recall problems should not be vexatious. On the other hand, there might be a potential effect of response bias as the response rate was clearly lower among the referents than the survivors. This may affect our findings. In addition it varied between countries how often it was allowed to send reminders and that must have had an effect on the response rate in the respective countries.

Another possible limitation is that we studied a long-term survivor population rather than the total cancer population. The survivors were contacted years after their diagnosis. These survivors are thus more likely to have been diagnosed in early stages and are expected to be less sick than patients diagnosed in later stages. The results are thus not applicable to all cancer patients. In this context the wording *survivor* refers to those who have not only survived their cancer diagnosis and treatment but survived years longer.

The questionnaire was based on validated sources, and the translation procedure was meticulous. On the other hand there are some differences in the Nordic countries that could not be captured by the questionnaire, e.g. the differences in the educational systems. For this reason we divided educational attainment into three groups, low, medium, and high to avoid misclassification.

Our study is not confined to one area only but includes cancer survivors in four countries. This can be seen as a strength as it provided us with a big sample of breast cancer survivors. On the other hand all countries did not succeed in fulfilling all the criteria of the study as neither Denmark nor Iceland could confirm the stage of the cancers, and in Iceland all women diagnosed either with breast cancer or Hodgkin's or Non-Hodgkin's lymphoma in the years 1998-2002 were included. As the number of Icelandic survivors was low and the respondents had survived at least 3 years, this fact is not likely to have had a serious impact on the outcome.

Our study provides important information on differences between cancer survivors and a non-cancer reference group regarding factors connected with return to and well-being at work. It also shows that the cancer type is important and thus all cancer survivors can not be grouped together. Hitherto studies in this field have been few (Bouknight et al., 2006; Bradley et al., 2002). With the increasing number of cancer survivors in the labour market, the work experience of this group is an urgent matter to study.

## ACKNOWLEDGEMENTS

We thank the Nordic Cancer Union (NCU) that supported the Nordic Study of Cancer and Work (NOCWO) and the following sponsors in the respective Nordic countries: Denmark: The National Labour Market Authority, the Danish municipal VAT foundation and the Danish Graduate School in Public Health Science, University of Copenhagen. Iceland: The Commersial Workers′ Union of Reykjavik, The Icelandic Nurses Association Science Fund, the Memorial Fund of Ingibjorg Gudjonsdottir under the auspice of the Cancer Union in Iceland, and the Icelandic Social Workers′ Association Science Fund. Finland: The Finnish Work Environment Fund and the Finnish Cancer Organizations. Norway: The Norwegian Foundation for Health and Rehabilitation (grant no. HO-54010/002).

Principal investigators of the Nordic Study of Cancer and Work (NOWCO) were as follows: Denmark: Kathrine Carlsen and Christopher Johansen. Finland: Marja-Liisa Lindbohm, Taina Taskila, Rami Martikainen, Päivi Hietanen, and Jari Hakanen. Iceland: Holmfridur K. Gunnarsdottir, Gudbjorg Linda Rafnsdottir, Nanna Sigurdardottir, Thora Jonsdottir, and Helgi Sigurdsson. Norway: Saevar B. Gudbergsson, Alv A. Dahl, and Sophie D. Fosså.

We want to thank our colleagues: Kathrine Carlsen, Nanna Sigurdardottir, Taina Taskila, and Thora Jonsdottir, especially for helping with information for this paper and for giving us useful comments after reading the manuscript.

## REFERENCES

Abrahamsen, A. F., Loge, J. H., Hannisdal, E., Holte, H., and Kvaløy, S. (1998). Socio-medical situation for long-term survivors of Hodgkin's disease: a survey of 459 patients treated at one institution. *Eur. J. Cancer, 34,* 1865–1870.

American Cancer Society. (2003). *Cancer facts and figures.* Retrieved November 22, 2006 from *http://www.cancer.org/downloads/STT/CAFF2003PWSecured.pdf*

Bond, M. A., Punnett, L., Pyle, J. L., Cazeca, D., and Cooperman, M. (2004). Gendered work conditions, health, and work outcomes. *J. Occup. Health Psychol, 9,* 28–45.

Bouknight, R. R., Bradley, C. J., and Luo, Z. (2006). Correlates of return to work for breast cancer survivors. *J. Clin. Oncol, 24,* 345–353.

Bradley, C. J., and Bednarek, H. L. (2002). Employment patterns of long-term cancer survivors. *Psycho-oncology, 11,* 188–198.

Bradley, C. J., Bednarek, H. L., and Neumark, D. (2002). Breast cancer and women's labor supply. *Health Serv. Res, 37,* 1309–1328.

Bradley, C. J., Neumark, D., Oberst, K., Luo, Z., Brennan, S., and Schenk, M. (2005). Combining registry, primary, and secondary data sources to identify the impact of cancer on labor market outcomes. *Med. Decis. Making, 25,* 534–547.

Charles, M., Grusky, D. B. (2004). *Occupational ghettos. The worldwide segregation of women and men.* Stanford: Stanford University Press.

Chirikos, T. N., Russell-Jakobs, A., and Jacobsen, P. B. (2002). Functional impairment and the economic consequences of female breast cancer. *Women and Health, 36*(1), 1–20.

Clark, J. C., and Landis, L. L. (1989). Reintegration and maintenance of employees with breast cancer in the workplace. *AAOHN, 37,* 186–193.

Doyal, L. (1995). *What makes women sick? Gender and the political economy of health.* London: MacMillan Press, Ltd.

Drolet, M., Maunsell, E., Mondor, M., Brisson, C., Brisson, J., Mâsse, B., et al. (2005). Work absence after breast cancer diagnosis: a population-based study. *CMAJ, 173,* 765–769.

Engeland, A., Haldorsen, T., Dickman, P. W., Hakulinen, T., Möller, T. R., Storm, H. H., et al. (1998). Relative survival of cancer patients: a comparison between Denmark and the other Nordic countries. *Acta Oncol, 37,* 49–59.

Eurostat. (2005). *Employment rate: females. Retrieved December 21, 2006 from http://epp.eurostat.ec.europa.eu/portal/page?_pageid=1996,39140985and_dad=portaland_schema=PORTALandscreen=detailrefandlanguage=enandproduct=STRIND_EMPLOIandroot=STRIND_EMPLOI/emploi/em012*

Fife, B. L., and Wright, E. R. (2000). The dimensionality of stigma: a comparison of its impact on the self of persons with HIV/AIDS and cancer. *J. Health Soc. Behav, 41,* 50–67.

Ganz, P. A., Desmond, K. A., Leedham, B., Rowland, J. H., Meyerowitz, B. E., and Belin, T. R. (2002). Quality of life in long-term, disease-free survivors of breast cancer: a follow-up study. *J. Natl. Cancer Inst, 94,* 39–49.

Gudbergsson, S. B., Fosså, S. D., Borgeraas, E., and Dahl, A. A. (2006). A comparative study of living conditions in cancer patients who have returned to work after curative treatment. *Support Care Cancer, 14,* 1020–1029.

Gujarati, D. N. (2003). *Basic Econometrics* (4th ed.). New York: McCraw-Hill, Inc.

Hoffman, B. (1991). Employment discrimination: Another hurdle for cancer survivors. *Cancer Invest, 9,* 589–595.

Hoffman, B. (2005). Cancer survivors at work: a generation of progress. *CA Cancer J. Clin, 55,* 271–280.

International Labour Office. (1990). *ISCO-88. International standard classification of occupations.* Geneva: International Labour Office.

Joly, F., Henry-Amar, M., Arveux, P., Reman, O., Tanguy, A., Peny, A-M., et al. (1996). Late psychosocial sequelae in Hodgkin's disease survivors: a French population-based case-control study. *J. Clin. Oncol, 14,* 2444–2453.

Karasek, R. A., and Theorell, T. (1990). *Healthy work: stress, Productivity and the reconstruction of working life.* New York: Basic Books.

Kauppinen, K. (1998). Gender and working conditions in the European Union. In S. Lehtinen, H. Taskinen, and J. Rantanen (Eds.), *Women at work* (pp. 204–209):

*Proceedings of an international expert meeting on Women at work.* People and Work. Research Reports 20. Espoo: Finnish Institute of Occupational Health.

Kivimäki, M., Vahtera J., and Pentti J. (1998). Psychosocial factors predicting medically certified sickness absence in men and women. In S. Lehtinen, H. Taskinen, and J. Rantanen (Eds.), *Women at work* (pp. 185–190): *Proceedings of an international expert meeting on Women at work.* People and Work. Research Reports 20. Espoo: Finnish Institute of Occupational Health.

Kornblith, A. B. (1998). Psychosocial adaptation of cancer survivors. In J. C. Holland (ed.), *Psycho-oncology* (pp. 223-254). New York: Oxford University Press.

Lindström, K., Elo A-L., Skogstad, A., Dallner, M., Gamberale, F., Hottinen, V., et al. (2000). *User's guide for the QPSNordic: General Nordic questionnaire for psychological and social factors at work.* (Tema Nord 603). Copenhagen: Nordic Council of Ministers.

Long. J. S. (1997). *Regression Models for categorical and limited dependent variables.* Thousand Oaks: Sage Publications.

Lorber, J., and Moore L. J. (2002). *Gender and the social construction of illness* (2nd ed.). Walnut Creek, CA: AltaMira Press.

Main, D. S., Nowels, C. T., Cavender, T. A., Etschmaier, M., and Steiner, J. F. (2005). A qualitative study of work and work return in cancer survivors. *Psycho-oncology, 14,* 992–1004.

Maunsell, E., Brisson, C., Dubois, L., Lauzier, S., and Fraser, A. (1999). Work problems after breast cancer: an exploratory qualitative study. *Psycho-oncology, 8,* 467–473.

Maunsell, E., Drolet, M., Brisson, J., Brisson, C., Mâsse, B., Deschênes, L. (2004). Work situation after breast cancer: results from a population-based study. *J. Natl. Cancer Inst, 96,* 1813-1822.

Ólafsson, S. (1999). *Íslenska leiðin: Almannatryggingar og velferð í fjölþjóðlegum samanburði* [The Icelandic way: Social security system and welfare, an international comparision]. [In Icelandic]. Reykjavík: Tryggingarstofnun ríkisins/Háskólaútgáfan.

Ólafsson, S. (2005). Normative foundations of the Icelandic welfare state. In N. Kildal and S. Kuhnle (Eds.), *Normative foundations of the welfare state: Scandinavian experiences* (pp. 214–236). London: Routledge, 2005.

Peteet, J. R. (2000). Cancer and the meaning of work. *Gen. Hosp. Psychiatry, 22,* 2000-2005.

Razavi, D., Delvaux, N., Brédart, A., Autier, P., Bron, D., Debusscher, L., et al. (1993). Professional rehabilitation of lymphoma patients: a study of psychosocial factors associated with return to work. *Support Care Cancer, 1,* 276–278.

Saarinen, K., Kurppa, K., Klaukka T., Karjalainen, A., Martikainen, R., Uitti, J., et al. (2001). Työperäisen astmaoireilun yleisyys ja merkitys: kartoittava tutkimus Tampereen seudulla. [The prevalence of work-related asthma symtoms: an explorative study in the region of Tampere]. [Report in Finnish]. Loppuraportti Työsuojelurahastolle. Helsinki: Työterveyslaitos [Finnish Institute of Occupational Health].

Satariano, W. A., and DeLorenze, G. N. (1996) The likelihood of returning to work after breast cancer. *Publ. Health Reports, III,* 236–241.

Short, P. F., Vasey, J. J., and Tunceli, K. (2005). Employment pathways in a large cohort of adult cancer survivors. *Cancer, 103,* 1292–1301.

Spelten, E. R., Sprangers, M. A. G., and Verbeek, J. H. A. M. (2002). Factors reported to influence the return to work of cancer survivors: a literature review. *Psycho-oncology, 11,* 124–131.

Spelten, E. R., Verbeek, J. H. A. M., Uitterhoeve, A. L. J., Ansink, A. C., van der Lelie, J., de Reijke, T. M., et al. (2003). Cancer, fatigue and the return of patients to work—a prospective cohort study. *Eur. J. Cancer, 39,* 1562–1567.

Steiner, J. F., Cavender, T. A., Main, D. S., and Bradley, C. J. (2004). Assessing the impact of cancer on work outcomes. What are the research needs? *Cancer, 101,* 1703–1711.

Taskila, T., Lindbohm, M-L., Martikainen, R., Lehto, U-S., Hakanen, J., and Hietanen, P. (2006). Cancer survivors' received and needed social support from their work place and the occupational health services. *Support Care Cancer, 14,* 427–435.

Taskila-Åbrandt, T., Martikainen, R., Virtanen, S. V., Pukkala, E., Hietanen, P., and Lindbohm, M-L. (2004). The impact of education and occupation on the employment status of cancer survivors. *Eur. J. Cancer, 40,* 2488–2493.

Taskila-Åbrandt, T., Pukkala, E, Martikainen, R., Karjalainen, A., and Hietanen, P. (2005). Employment status of Finnish cancer patients in 1997. *Psycho-oncology, 14,* 221–226.

van der Wouden, J. C., Greaves-Otte, J. G. W., Greaves, J., Kruyt, Ph. M., van Leeuwen, O., and van der Does, E. (1992). Occupational reintegration of long term cancer survivors. *J. Occup. Med, 34,* 1084–1089.

# INDEX

## A

## B

## C

## D

## E

## F



## G

## H

## I

## J



## K



## L

## M

## N



## O

## P

## Q

## R

## S

## T

## U

## V



## W



## X



## Y



## Z